BSAVA Manual of Small Animal Fracture Repair and Management

Edited by

Andrew R. Coughlan
BVSc PhD CertVA CertSAO FRCVS
Animal Medical Centre
511 Wilbraham Road, Chorlton
Manchester M21 1UF, UK

and

Andrew Miller
BVMS DSAO MRCVS
Veterinary Centre, 78 Tanworth Lane
Shirley, Solihull B90 4DF, UK

Publ

Brit
King
Shu
GL5

A C
Reg
Reg

Cop

All
stor
elec
pric

All the colour illustrations in this book have been designed and created by
Vicki Martin Design, Cambridge, UK and are printed with their permission.

A catalogue record for this book is available from the British Library

ISBN 0 905214 37 4

The publishers and contributors cannot take responsibility for information
provided on dosages and methods of application of drugs mentioned in this
publication. Details of this kind must be verified by individual users from the
appropriate literature.

Typeset and printed by: Fusion Design, Fordingbridge, Hampshire, UK

Other Manuals

Other titles in the BSAVA Manuals series:

Contents

Contributors

Ralph H. Abercromby BVMS CertSAO MRCVS
Ridgeway Veterinary Centre, 47 The Ridgeway, Flitwick, Beds MK45 1DJ, UK

Angus A. Anderson BVetMed PhD DSAS (Orthopaedics) MRCVS
Royal (Dick) School of Veterinary Studies, Edinburgh University, Summerhall, Edinburgh EH9 1QH, UK

David Bennett BVetMed BSc PhD DSAO MRCVS
Department of Veterinary Clinical Studies, University of Glasgow Veterinary School, Bearsden Road, Bearsden, Glasgow G61 1QH, UK

Warrick J. Bruce BVSc MVM CertSAO MRCVS
Institute of Veterinary, Animal and Biomedical Sciences, Massey University, Palmerston North, New Zealand

Steven J. Butterworth MA VetMB CertVR DSAO MRCVS
Weighbridge Referrals, Kemys Way, Swansea Enterprise Park, Swansea SA6 8QF, UK

Stuart Carmichael BVMS MVM DSAO MRCVS
Department of Surgery, University of Glasgow Veterinary School, Bearsden Road, Bearsden, Glasgow G61 1QH, UK

D. Gary Clayton Jones BVetMed DVR DSAO MRCVS
Pilgrims, Beech House, Salehurst, East Sussex TN32 5PN, UK

Hamish R. Denny MA VetMB PhD DSAO FRCVS
Cedar House, High Street, Wrington, Bristol BS18 7QD, UK

Jonathan Dyce MA VetMB PhD DSAO MRCVS
College of Veterinary Medicine, 601 Vernon L. Tharp Street, Columbus, OH 43210-1089, USA

John E.F. Houlton MA VetMB DVR DSAO DipECVS MRCVS
Department of Clinical Veterinary Medicine, University of Cambridge, Madingley Road, Cambridge CB3 0ES, UK

John P. Lapish BVetMed BSc MRCVS
c/o Veterinary Instrumentation, 62 Cemetery Road, Sheffield S11 8FP, UK

Christopher May MA VetMB PhD CertSAO MRCVS
Grove Veterinary Hospital, 2 Hibbert Street, New Mills, Stockport, Cheshire SK12 3JJ, UK

W. Malcolm McKee BVMS MVS DSAO MACVSc MRCVS
Willows Veterinary Centre, 78 Tanworth Lane, Shirley, Solihull B90 4DF, UK

Andrew Miller BVMS DSAO MRCVS
Willows Veterinary Centre, 78 Tanworth Lane, Shirley, Solihull B90 4DF, UK

Malcolm Ness BVetMed CertSAO DipECVS FRCVS
Croft Veterinary Surgeons, 36 Croft Road, Blyth, Northumberland NE24 2EL, UK

Marvin C. Olmstead DVM MS DipACVS
College of Veterinary Medicine, 601 Vernon L. Tharp Street, Columbus, OH 43210-1089, USA

Simon Roe BVSc PhD MS DipACVS
School of Veterinary Medicine, Veterinary Teaching Hospital, North Carolina State University, Raleigh, NC 27606, USA

Harry W. Scott BVSc CertSAD CertSAO FRCVS
Godiva Referrals, 207 Daventry Road, Cheylesmore, Coventry CV1 2LJ, UK

Tim M. Skerry BVetMed PhD CertSAO MRCVS
Department of Biology, University of York, York YO1 5YW, UK

A. Colin Stead BVMS DVR DSAO FRCVS
Royal (Dick) School of Veterinary Studies, University of Edinburgh, Summerhall, Edinburgh EH9 1QH, UK

Andy M. Torrington BVMS CertSAO MRCVS
Animal Medical Centre, 511 Wilbraham Road, Chorlton, Manchester M21 1UF, UK

Leslie C. Vaughan DSc DVR FRCVS
Burywick, Beeson End, Harpenden, Herts AL5 2AH, UK

Foreword

This new manual is a very welcome addition to the now world-renowned series of BSAVA publications. It complements the existing Arthrology and Diagnostic Imaging manuals and will be an invaluable help to practitioners at all stages of their careers. The full use of colour in both the line drawings and photographs adds to the clarity of the text. Practical tips and warnings are printed in coloured boxes to assist the veterinary surgeon checking on a clinical case.

The manual describes the background to fracture repair, radiographic assessment and the management of specific fractures. The operative techniques are described in a novel and most easily assimilated form, with every detail listed, including the instruments required and the need for assistance during the operation.

The editors are to be congratulated on their choice of contributing authors, who have a truly international standing and a background of academic and orthopaedic referral practice. This has resulted in a work which, I am sure, will rank as one of the main components of the practice bookshelf for years to come.

David F. Wadsworth
BSAVA President 1997-98

Preface

Our major objective in producing this manual was to create an orthopaedic text dedicated to the practical management of fractures in the dog and cat. Where surgical treatment is indicated, we did not wish to merely illustrate an idealised repair, but also to guide the surgeon through the procedure, emphasising both the potential pitfalls and practical tips already known to more experienced surgeons.

Parts 1 and 2 provide a comprehensive background to fracture management covering basic sciences and the principles to be applied later in the book, as well as a sobering review of the history of fracture treatment. Part 3 describes the management of specific fractures by region. In the first part of each chapter, types of fracture are described and the most appropriate treatment is indicated. The reader is then referred to the relevant Operative Technique at the end of the chapter. These may describe a particular technique as applied to that region, e.g. bone plating, or may describe the management of specific fractures, e.g. humeral condylar fracture, applying principles detailed in the first two parts of the manual. The surgical approaches illustrated are not comprehensive and it is intended that the Operative Techniques are read and used in conjunction with standard texts on surgical anatomy.

Our thanks are due to all the contributing authors who have produced comprehensive texts and we are grateful for their patience throughout the massive task of reformatting text into the current layout which we hope will add to the ease of use of the manual. We also wish to express our appreciation to Fusion Design who have played a major role in defining the layout, to Vicki Martin BSc BVSc who has produced figures of outstanding clarity, and to Marion Jowett, Publishing Manager for BSAVA, who has coordinated it all. Thank you to Simon Petersen-Jones who initially proposed the idea of a fracture manual and guided the development phase.

Finally, although we have endeavoured to produce a very practically orientated support text, we do encourage clinicians to recognize particularly challenging fractures and to seek advice from more experienced colleagues or to refer the case. We trust you will find this book both interesting to read and an invaluable companion in the day to day management of your fracture patients.

Andrew Coughlan
Andrew Miller
March 1998

PART ONE

Background to Fracture Management

CHAPTER ONE

Fracture Classification and Description

D. Gary Clayton Jones

INTRODUCTION

A method for classifying fractures is needed to be able to describe fractures for a variety of reasons. An accurate description of a fracture enables surgeons to discuss methods of diagnosis, treatment and prognosis and to compare results, thus providing easier verbal and written communication. The use of a similar fracture classification system for small animals and for humans could provide a basis for comparative studies between species. An accurate classification could assist in planning for patient requirements or ordering implants in quantity, which may be essential in a large hospital.

Many of the terms in current usage are many centuries old and relate to outmoded or superceded practices and problems. Initially fractures had to be described verbally, as the only alternative would have been to draw diagrams. The difficulty with verbal descriptions is that there is no internationally agreed definition for the terms that are commonly employed. For example, how angulated may a fracture plane be for the fracture still to be described as 'transverse'? The problem increases with the lack of a common language, as similar terms may have different meanings and therefore transmission of data between countries is made even more difficult. The value of exchange of data is obvious, as some fracture types are rare and individual experience may be very limited, apart from the important needs of educational exchange.

Prior to the advent of X-ray examination, photography, fax transmission and scanning, the use of prepared diagrams would have been very laborious and inefficient. Currently it is becoming more possible to scan fracture images and transmit the information electronically to some central point for pictorial analysis and recording by computer, or possibly for rapid advice from a specialist. An alternative is to classify fractures into groups identified from a series of definitions that can be identified by various alphanumeric symbols. The problem is to decide at the outset how much information is required from the data and thence the complexity of any coding system. The more complex the system, the more difficult it becomes for the user to classify each fracture in the same way as other workers and therefore the greater is the opportunity for variation and subsequently reduction in value of the data.

For this reason no single system of fracture classification or description has yet been adopted internationally for small animals. A system of fracture classification (Muller, 1990; AO/ASIF, 1996) has been developed for use in human patients by the AO/ASIF (Arbeitsgemeinschaft für Osteosynthesefragen/Association for the Study of Internal Fixation) Group using alphanumeric classifications combined with electronically stored X-ray images. The central store can be remotely accessed but requires considerable computer power at the recording centre, although a PC, scanner and modem are the only requirements at the hospital. Both recording of data and the requesting of data and information can be made from a hospital office. A computer-based CD-ROM or diskette system is now available for equine fractures (Fackelman, 1993).

METHODS OF DESCRIPTION

Early methods of describing fractures were based on various anatomical features or on using eponymous fracture descriptions, often named after the first observer (or sufferer). The most commonly recognized of such names are probably Colles, Potts and Monteggia. These human medical terms are occasionally used in veterinary practice but are of little value unless the explanation is already known. Such eponymous descriptions should therefore probably not be used in veterinary practice. The discovery of X-rays in the latter part of the nineteenth century allowed a more accurate form of description based on the radiological appearance of the fracture.

The earliest description of a fracture was whether or not the fracture was 'simple' (closed) or 'compound' (open). This stems from the period prior to antibiotic therapy when an open fracture carried a high risk of infection and potential loss of the limb or often of the patient. Today the words closed and open are more commonly used to refer to the same clinical features.

The expression 'simple' was used to imply ease or difficulty of treatment, but this was related to the aspect of fracture infection. Some simple fractures may be very difficult to reconstruct, while some open fractures can be straightforward two-piece fractures that are mechanically easy to mend. **Closed** is now also used to describe a single circumferential disruption of the diaphysis. (Small cortical fragments of less than 10% of the circumference are ignored as they probably have little significance for treatment or prognosis.)

Open (compound) fractures are now generally classified into various types which have a more modern clinical significance from the point of view of treatment and prognosis. 'Compound' does not indicate the number or type of fragmentation, though the word is commonly misused to imply a difficult or fragmented fracture.

Complex implies the difficulty or severity of the fracture, and can be defined as describing a multifragmented fracture of the diaphysis in which there is no contact between the proximal and distal segments after reduction.

Pathological (or secondary) fractures are a particular form, not related to trauma in every case, in which the fractures result from failure of bone strength from an underlying cause such as bone tumour, infection or osteodystrophy. The initiating defect may not always be readily identified by X-ray.

Complicated fractures are those in which there is major blood vessel, nerve or joint involvement. The description is not so commonly used in veterinary orthopaedics. These are often more serious in human patients, where loss of major arterial supply may cause permanent loss of function of a vital organ e.g. the hand, or even result in an amputation.

Closed (simple) fractures

There are various criteria that can be used to define different types of closed fracture:

Anatomical location

The bone shaft (diaphysis) has been conventionally divided into thirds: proximal (upper), middle and distal (lower).

Anatomical feature

General

- Capital
- Subcapital
- Metaphyseal
- Diaphyseal (shaft)
- Sub trochanteric
- Physeal
- Condylar
- Articular.

Specific

- Greater trochanter
- Tibial tuberosity
- Lateral condyle, etc.

Displacement of the fragments

- Greenstick (juvenile)
- Folded
- Fissure — undisplaced fragments which may displace at operation or under stress
- Depressed — fragments invade an underlying cavity, especially parts of the skull
- Compression — of cancellous bone, often vertebral body
- Impacted — cortical into cancellous bone.

Nature of the fracture line

- Complete — all of the cortices are broken with the separation of the fragments
- Incomplete — part of the bone remains intact.

Complete fractures may also be described in terms of:

Direction of fracture line

- Transverse — the angle of the fracture line to a perpendicular to the long axis of the bone is less than 30°
- Oblique — the angle is equal or greater than 30°.
- Spiral — the result of torsion
- Longitudinal, Y or T fracture, saucer.

Number or type of fragments

- Two-fragment, three-fragment, comminuted (many fragments, i.e. more than two); sometimes multifragment is preferred.
- Wedge fragments — the main fragments have some contact after reduction
- Segmental — large one or more complete or almost complete fragments of shaft
- Butterfly (intermediate) fragment
- Irregular — a diaphyseal fracture with a number of intermediate fragments with no specific pattern, usually accompanied by severe soft tissue lesions
- Multiple — more than one fracture in same or different bones.

Stability following reduction

This has been termed the Charnley classification and was used to determine which fractures would respond to closed reduction and fixation.

- Stable after reduction — tends to remain in place without force
- Unstable after reduction — fracture collapses as soon as reducing force is removed.

Nature of fracture origin

- Avulsion/apophyseal — pulled by tendon or ligament
- Chip — small fragments at articular margin following hyperextension injury
- Slab — larger fragment with a vertical or very oblique fracture of a small cancellous bone which may extend into both articular surfaces.

Articular fractures

- Extra-articular — not involving the joint surface but may be intracapsular
- Partial articular — involving only a part of the articular surface, with the remaining articular cartilage surface being attached to the diaphysis
- Complete articular — disrupting the articular surface and separating it completely from the diaphysis (e.g. Y or T fracture).

Special classifications

Growth plate or epiphyseal fractures (separations)

The most commonly used is the Salter–Harris system (Salter and Harris, 1963) in which six types of injury are recognized (see Chapter 11):

- Type I — complete, through the hypertrophied cartilage cell zone
- Type II — partially includes the metaphysis
- Type III — intra-articular fracture to the hypertrophied zone and then along the epiphyseal plate to the edge
- Type IV — intra-articular fracture that traverses the epiphysis, epiphyseal plate and metaphysis
- Type V — crushing injury that causes destruction of growing cells
- Type VI — new bone bridges the growth plate.

Classifications of special joint fractures

Certain specific fractures (mainly because of their importance in the racing Greyhound) have been classified to aid prognosis and treatment.

Accessory carpal bone (Johnson, 1987)

- Type I — intra-articular avulsion of the distal margin
- Type II — intra-articular fracture of the proximal margin
- Type III — extra-articular avulsion of the distal margin
- Type IV — extra-articular avulsion of the insertion of flexor carpi ulnaris at proximal palmar surface
- Type V — comminuted fracture of the body which may involve the articular surface.

Central tarsal bone (Dee et al., 1976)

- Type I — small dorsal slab fracture with minimal displacement
- Type II — dorsal slab fracture with displacement
- Type III — one-third to half of the bone fractured in the median plane and displaced medially or dorsally
- Type IV — combination of Types II and III
- Type V — severe comminution.

Various combinations of fractures of the tarsus (see Chapter 20) are regularly seen concurrently in the Greyhound, but are not classified, although they have been described as **triads** (Newton and Nunamaker, 1985).

Metacarpal/metatarsal fractures (Newton and Nunamaker, 1985)

- Type I — painful on palpation at the junction of the proximal fourth/third and distal two-thirds/three-quarters of the bone; endosteal and cortical thickening of the bone on X-ray
- Type II — hairline undisplaced fissure type fracture
- Type III — complete fracture with palmar/plantar displacement of distal fragment.

Open fractures

Open fractures possess a wound which communicates between the fracture bed and the outside environment. Usually this is via a visible surface wound but could describe a fracture of a skull bone which has penetrated the nose or a sinus cavity. Classification of open fractures is often helpful in determining optimal methods of treatment.

- Type 1 — a fracture produced from inside to outside by the penetration of a sharp fracture fragment end through the overlaying soft tissues. Such a fracture may become open some time following the initiating incident as a result of uncontrolled or unsupported movement. There is usually limited soft tissue injury and the bone fragments are all present, often without comminution.

- Type 2 — a fracture caused from outside to inside by penetration of a foreign object. There is usually more soft tissue damage with contusion around the skin wound and some mainly reversible muscle damage. Fractures may be more fragmented but there is little if any loss of bone or soft tissue.

- Type 3 — the most severe form of open fracture in which loss of tissue following penetration by an outside object has resulted. Loss of skin, soft tissue and bone material may have occurred and may be very severe. Some workers recognize a subdivision in which loss of the main arterial supply to the limb has occurred, as this indicates mandatory amputation.

Although not officially recognized, an estimate of the time elapsed since the injury may be helpful in classifying an open fracture. This acknowledges the dangers of bacterial invasion of a wound where, after an initial lag phase in which the bacteria become established, the organisms may begin to multiply, turning a contaminated wound into an infected one. This is the concept of a 'golden period' which should be taken into account but not relied upon implicitly.

A system for classification of the soft tissue injury has been developed for use in humans (Muller *et al.*, 1992) (Table 1.1). Certain evaluations in human patients are not made in veterinary patients and so the system may be too complicated for animals, although it could probably be used with a little variation.

Fracture classification suitable for computer analysis

The ability to classify fractures for computer analysis is clearly the best method: it would readily allow analysis and comparison of data as well as easily allowing worldwide cooperation. A number of methods have been attempted but currently no single method has gained acceptance.

A method of classification of femur fractures was developed at the University of Michigan (Braden, 1995) following a general analysis of fractures by Brinker (Brinker *et al.*, 1990). This system is only applicable to fractures of the femur and has a limited ability for fracture description. It is based on a paper

Integument Closed (IC)	
IC1	No injury
IC2	No laceration but contusion
IC3	Circumscribed degloving
IC4	Extensive closed degloving
IC5	Necrosis from contusion
Integument Open (IO)	
IO1	Skin breakage from inside out
IO2	Skin breakage from outside in > 5 cm, contused edges
IO3	Skin breakage from outside in < 5cm, devitalized edges, circumscribed degloving
IO4	Full thickness contusion, abrasion, skin loss
IO5	Extensive degloving
Muscle/Tendon (MT)	
MT1	No injury
MT2	Circumscribed injury, one muscle group only
MT3	Extensive injury, two or more muscle groups
MT4	Avulsion or loss of entire muscle groups, tendon lacerations
MT5	Compartment syndrome / crush syndrome
Neurovascular (NV)	
NV1	No injury
NV2	Isolated nerve injury
NV3	Localized vascular injury
NV4	Combined neurovascular injury
NV5	Subtotal / total amputation

Table 1.1: A system for classification of soft tissue injuries (designed for use in humans).

form which can be analysed by computer; thus no computer equipment is required at the hospital.

General classification of fractures was developed by Muller and others of the AO/ASIF group for human fractures (Muller, 1990; CCF, 1996). This has been modified by various workers to create similar methods for small animals and the horse. Two systems for small animals, the Prieur (Prieur *et al.*, 1990) and the Unger (Unger *et al.*, 1990), have been described in the literature although neither has yet been accepted universally.

These classifications describe the bone, the location and the type of fracture. Each of the proposed systems creates a four-digit record in a similar way to the human AO system.

The Prieur and Unger fracture classification systems can only be used for fractures of the long bones and are not used for fractures involving the skull, vertebral column, pelvis or small limb bones. Neither system discusses the soft tissue problems, which may well be of the greatest importance in determining treatment and outcome.

The Prieur system

This is the simpler system but it records slightly less information. Digits are allocated under each of four fields (bone; location; fracture area; fragment number) (Table 1.2), so that each fracture is described by four numbers (examples in Figure 1.1). The location zones of each bone are determined by drawing a square around the ends, of length and width equal to the widest dimension of the bone end (Figure 1.2).

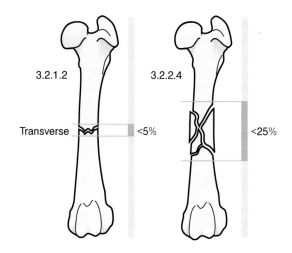

Figure 1.1: Examples of femoral fractures and their numerical identification using the Prieur classification system.

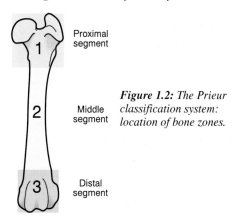

Figure 1.2: The Prieur classification system: location of bone zones.

Field	Number
Bone	
Humerus	1
Radius/ulna	2
Femur	3
Tibia	4
Location	
Proximal segment	1
Middle segment	2
Distal segment	3
Fracture area (percentage of bone length)	
< 5% (and/or not involving articular cartilage)	1
5—25% (specific fractures of femur neck)	2
> 25% (and/or involving articular surface)	3
Number of fragments	
Two	2
Three	3
Four or more	4

Table 1.2: The Prieur system.

The Unger system
This identifies fractures in a similar manner to the above but records somewhat more data by attempting to identify reducible or non-reducible wedges or the direction of the fracture line. Charts of both letters and numbers for each bone and the codes allocated for various fractures are required with this system, which attempts to record the fractures in a clinically related manner.

REFERENCES AND FURTHER READING

AO/ASIF (1996) *Comprehensive Classification of Fractures*. Pamphlets I and II, Maurice E Muller Foundation, AO/ASIF Documentation Centre, Davos, CH-7270 Switzerland.

Braden TD, Eicker SW, Abdinoor D and Prieur WD (1995) Characteristics of 1000 femur fractures in the dog and cat. *Veterinary and Comparative Orthopaedics and Traumatology* **8**, 203–209.

Brinker WO, Hohn RB and Prieur WD (1984) In: *Manual of Internal Fixation in Small Animals*, pp. 85–86. Springer Verlag, Berlin, Heidelberg and New York.

Brinker W, Piermattei D and Flo G (1990) *Handbook of Small Animal Orthopaedics and Fracture Treatment*, 2nd edn. WB Saunders, Philadelphia.

Dee JF, Dee J and Piermattei DL (1976) Classification, management and repair of central tarsal fractures in the racing Greyhound. *Journal of the American Animal Hospitals Association* **12**, 398–405.

Fackelman GE, Peutz IP, Norris JC *et al.* (1993) The development of an equine fracture documentation system. *Veterinary and Comparative Orthopaedics and Traumatology* **6**, 47–52

Johnson KA (1987) Accessory carpal bone fractures in the racing Greyhound classification and pathology. *Veterinary Surgery* **16**, 60.

Muller ME, Allgower M, Schneider R and Willenegger H (1992). In: *Manual of Internal Fixation, abridged 3rd edn,* pp. 118–158. Springer Verlag, Berlin.

Muller ME, Nazarian S, Koch P and Schatzker J (1990) *The AO Classification of Fractures of Long Bones.* Springer Verlag, Berlin, Heidelberg and New York.

Newton CD and Nunamaker DM (1985) Fractures associated with the racing Greyhound. In: *Textbook of Small Animal Orthopaedics.* Lippincott, Philadelphia.

Prieur WD, Braden TD and von Rechenberg B (1990) A suggested fracture classification of adult small animal fractures. *Veterinary and Comparative Orthopaedics and Traumatology* **3**, 111–116.

Salter RB and Harris WR (1963) Injuries involving the epiphyseal plate. *Journal of Bone and Joint Surgery* **45**, 587–622.

Steadman's Medical Dictionary, 25th edn. Williams and Wilkins, Baltimore.

Unger M, Montavon PM and Heim UFA (1990) Classification of fractures of long bones in the dog and cat, introduction and clinical application. *Veterinary and Comparative Orthopaedics and Traumatology* **3**, 41–50.

CHAPTER TWO

History of Fracture Treatment

Leslie C. Vaughan

INTRODUCTION

Evidence that survives about life in ancient civilizations shows that their people were aware of the effects of trauma. Fractures caused by accidents or combative violence were treated using principles which remain valid today. The bone setters appreciated that fracture healing depended on the broken bone being kept immobile for a long enough period, and splints were used to achieve this. Elliot Smith (1908) examined two sets of splints from Egyptian graves which had been applied to a fractured femur and forearm, respectively, about 5000 years ago. They were made of rough wood wrapped in linen and, together with pieces of bark, completely invested the limb, the whole held in place with linen bandages. Elliot Smith studied healed femoral fractures, many of which were shortened due to fragment displacement, and 100 forearm fractures, of which only one had not united while one had suppurated.

Egyptian papyri from about 1500 BC, found in Thebes in 1862, illustrate the treatment given to the injured and deformed (Guthrie, 1958). The Ebers papyrus deals with surgery, anatomy and pharmacy while the Edwin Smith papyrus describes fracture treatment with splints.

Other civilizations of similar lineage also practised fracture management. In India the Hindus employed bamboo for splints.

From writings and relics more is known about the physicians of many centuries later. Hippocrates (460–375 BC) wrote books on fractures and dislocations, using terms which are still familiar, and distinguished between open and closed fractures. Rigid support was provided with bandages impregnated with wheat glue, wax or resin, which set hard.

Celsus, remembered for describing the cardinal signs of inflammation, wrote a book in AD 30 detailing fracture treatment with splints fastened to limbs with bandages stiffened by starch.

After such early enterprise, fracture treatment might have been expected to progress at a greater pace in the following centuries than was the case. As Guthrie (1958) explained when tracing the development of human medicine, the decline of culture in Greece and Rome incurred a loss of original medical thought; and then, during the thousand or so years of the Dark Ages, learning was positively discouraged. It was not until the Renaissance in the fifteenth and sixteenth centuries that scientific enlightenment was revived in Europe. Interest in anatomy and surgery was rekindled but the real renaissance in surgery had to wait until the nineteenth century. This is not to say that the intervening years were devoid of originality in fracture management. Guthrie cites Guy de Chauliac (1300–1367) as possibly the first to employ extension and shows an extension device from Gersdoff (1517) that works on modern principles (Figure 2.1).

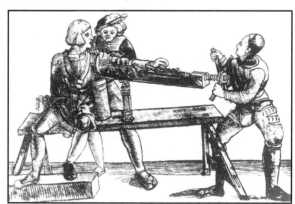

Figure 2.1: Gersdoff's (1517) application of extension apparatus to a fractured arm. (Reproduced from Guthrie, 1958 with permission.)

As ever, war was a teacher of surgery, and military surgeons became skilled in fracture care. Amputation was routine for open fractures but the mortality was high.

In the eighteenth century, among many distinguished surgeons, John Hunter (1728–1793) had a great impact. His work on fracture healing and bone growth, much of it learned from animal studies, established him as a pioneer of orthopaedics. About this time the term 'orthopaedic' was coined by Nicholas Andry, from the Greek *orthos* (straight) and *pais* (child), to describe the teaching of methods of treating and preventing deformities in children. It was not appropriated for use in a veterinary context until two centuries later.

The nineteenth century is particularly notable for

the many innovations that were introduced to avoid the untoward sequelae of closed reduction methods, such as joint stiffness and limb deformity. Attention began to be paid to the soft tissues and the development of means of fixation that enabled the limb to bear weight.

By the close of that century, three discoveries had been made which profoundly influenced surgery and fracture treatment. Morton (1846) demonstrated anaesthesia with ether, and Liston (1846) performed the first operation using ether: an amputation through the thigh. In 1865 Lister demonstrated an antiseptic system, employing carbolic acid, in a case of open fracture of the leg and 2 years later he recorded 11 such cases, with 9 complete recoveries.

The discovery of X-rays by Röntgen (1895) enabled fractures to be characterized and the efficacy of manual reduction and external fixation to be evaluated. Poor results could now be explained, and improved means of external and internal fixation were sought.

ANIMAL FRACTURES

For lack of evidence, it is not possible to determine what was known about animal fractures before the eighteenth century. Through the ages, the horse was depended on for labour, travel, sport and war and consequently its health and welfare received more attention than that of the other domesticated species. The need for hoof care was evident from the time when horses in the armies of Alexander (356–323 BC) were abandoned because of hoof wear. Ways of protecting the hoof were attempted with woven grass shoes, and later with leather or metal plates. The Romans used a 'hipposandal', a metal device strapped to the hoof, and by the fifth century in Europe metal shoes were fixed with nails.

The term 'farrier' was introduced in about 1562 and farriers, apart from shoeing, also dealt with general ailments of horses and other animals. Blundeville (1609) wrote the first English text of note on shoeing, under the influence of Italian and French works. Much of the early literature lacked a scientific basis but, even so, many of the terms used are still common.

Concern about farriery training standards led to the formation of the London Company of Blacksmiths in 1356 and this was the forerunner of the Worshipful Company of Farriers, which received its Charter in 1674.

The position of the treatment of fractures may be judged from the opinion in *Bartlet's Farriery* (1756) that there was 'no purpose in keeping horses who have any fracture except in the foot'. Nevertheless, Gibson (1729) treated fractures with splints while supporting the horse in slings.

The building of the first veterinary schools in Europe late in the eighteenth century marks the origin of veterinary science. Veterinary surgeons emerged who soon transformed the study of horse lameness and described the pathology and treatment of most common limb disorders, including fractures. In dogs, Blaine (1824) treated femoral fractures with a pitch plaster, spread on leather, and a wooden splint. Pliable wood was used to support the forearm. For open fractures the bone ends were sawn off, loose pieces were removed, the wound was closed and a splint was applied. Blaine blamed non-union on 'neglect of proper attention in the first place' and removed the soft bone ends with a fine saw.

Limb operations were performed on horses and dogs before anaesthesia and antisepsis were known, but with these aids this field expanded. The potential of radiography was immediately recognized and Hobday (1896) published probably the first veterinary skiagraph, of a cat's leg. The skiagraphs of canine fractures published by Hobday (1906) showed their value in diagnosis and for assessment of healing.

The trend of human surgery towards specialisms was evident in the late nineteenth century, and the recognition of orthopaedic surgery provided an impetus to promote the subject. Early in the twentieth century the work of Hey Groves, Lane and Sherman indicated the direction that advances in fracture treatment might take, but progress was slow. For example, in World War I the prompt application of a Thomas splint instead of a crude splint reduced mortality from femoral fractures to 20% from 80%, an indication that old methods needed to be changed. Even so, repair results were often unsatisfactory, as Robert Jones (1925) complained in a lecture, 'Crippling due to fractures'. Failure to achieve anatomical alignment, or to avoid injury to soft parts, was too common. The remedy, he believed, was to have special units run by surgeons skilled in this work.

In the veterinary field a similar *cri de coeur* in the 1950s changed attitudes to specialization and resulted in veterinary orthopaedics developing along similar lines to those in human medicine.

Such has been the revolution in the theory and practice of fracture treatment in modern times that the main categories under which this has occurred demand separate consideration. In animals, for practical reasons, it is the dog and cat that have benefited most from these advances.

EXTERNAL FIXATION

Rigid external limb support has been provided with many different materials. For humans, splints have been made of wood and metal, and casts of bandages impregnated with substances that harden, such as resin, starch, sodium silicate and plaster of Paris. Munro (1935) traced the early use of plaster of Paris to Arabia, and showed how cast application changed over many years, eventually to allow weightbearing and to avoid confinement to bed.

In animals, wood, metal, gutta percha, leather, cardboard and poroplastic felt have been used for splints, and casts were moulded with bandages soaked in starch or pitch. Williams (1893) and Hobday (1900) advocated plaster of Paris for dogs. Lacroix and Cozart (1924) preferred soaked wood because of its lightness and Ehmer (1925) employed yucca board attached with bandages soaked in sodium silicate. Barrett (1936) and Wright (1937) conformed unpadded strips of plaster of Paris to the shape of the limb (Figure 2.2).

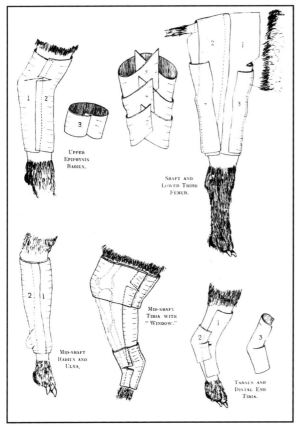

Figure 2.2: Method of applying plaster slabs. (Reproduced from Wright, 1937, with permission of The Veterinary Record.*)*

In dogs, adequate results could be achieved with external supports for fractures which were readily reduced, especially those distal to the elbow and stifle joints. The method proved less satisfactory for the humerus and femur, where muscle mass and limb shape made reduction and support difficult. In humans, reduction could be achieved with mechanical traction but, due to lack of patient cooperation, it was not practical in animals. Steiner (1928) treated 40 dogs with femoral fractures by suspending them by their hindlegs and found the results satisfactory but the humanity of this is doubtful. Dibbell (1930) provided traction with a wire splint devised for humans by Thomas (1875), and he checked the reduction by fluoroscopy before incorporating tongs attached to the bone end in an external support (Dibbell, 1931). Schroeder (1933a,b, 1934) employed skin and skeletal traction and developed the Thomas splint for dogs.

McCunn (1933) and Wright (1937) also made use of the Schroeder-type splint. Gunn (1936) achieved continued traction with an apparatus involving the insertion of pins into both bone ends (Figure 2.3).

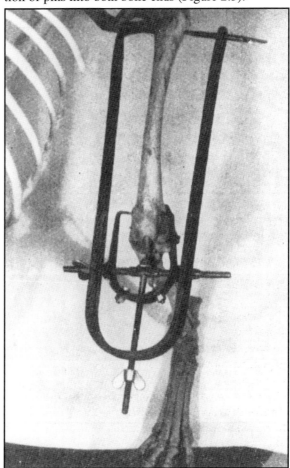

Figure 2.3: Mechanical fracture traction apparatus for overriding fractures in dogs. (Reproduced from Gunn, 1936, Australian Veterinary Journal, *12, 139.)*

Coaptation splinting and casting remained the main option for fracture treatment until superseded by internal fixation. While the Thomas splint has become outmoded except as a first aid measure, casts still have an important role in the treatment of minor injuries and in supplementing surgical repairs. Plaster of Paris has been replaced with synthetic materials such as fibreglass and resin, which have the advantages of being light, waterproof and resistant to self-mutilation.

EXTERNAL SKELETAL FIXATION

The advantages of stabilizing a fracture without exposing the site or burying foreign material have long been recognized. In 1849 Malgaigne (Venable and Stuck, 1947) devised adjustable metal hooks that pierced fracture fragments close to the skin surface (Figure 2.4). Parkhill (1897) inserted four pins at right angles into the bone and secured them externally with bolts and clamps (Figure 2.5). Lambotte (1907) used a half-pin apparatus.

Hey Groves (1916) employed a double transfixation device to treat open and comminuted fractures, which allowed ambulation and avoided confinement to bed (Figure 2.6). In the 1920s various attempts were made to control reduction and fixation externally.

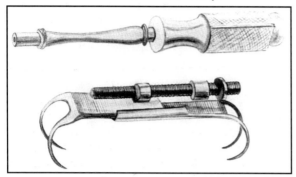

Figure 2.4: Malgaigne's clamp (1849) used for fractures of the patella and olecranon. The prongs projected through the skin. (Reproduced from Venable and Stuck, 1947, with permission of Blackwell Science. Originally printed in Stimson, Fractures and Dislocations, *1910.)*

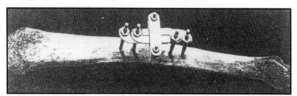

Figure 2.5: A new apparatus for the fixation of bones after resection and in fractures with a tendency to displacement. (Reproduced from Parkhill, 1897, American Surgery Association Transactions, *15, 251.)*

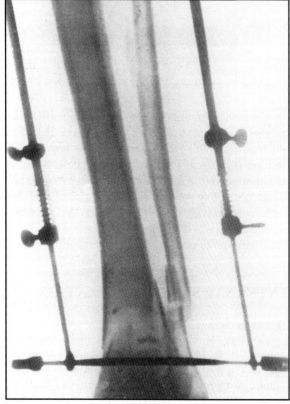

Figure 2.6: Double transfixion apparatus. (Reproduced from Hey Groves, 1916, On Modern Methods of Treating Fractures, *published by John Wright and Sons.)*

Anderson (1934) inserted half-pins under local anaesthesia for radius/ulna fractures and embedded their ends in a plaster cast after mechanical reduction. Later he modified this method to include clamps and connecting rods in various configurations.

For dogs, Stader (1934) described a full-pin transfixation splint, with K-wires embedded externally in a wooden strip, while Self (1934) used steel wires and fastened them to a metal splint. Stader (1937) next introduced a half-pin device to provide reduction and fixation. By 1939 the Stader Reduction Splint was available in three sizes (and was also used in US servicemen in World War II). Ehmer (1947) developed a half-pin splint (Kirschner—Ehmer) which allowed flexibility of pin angles and which, after attachment of a reduction gear, allowed the fragments to be manoeuvred — a design that is still manufactured.

Such apparatus gained popularity in North America but not in the UK. The risk of tracking infection and pin loosening were common fears. Knight (1949) found that results were not consistent but Turnbull (1951), Weipers (1951) and Kirk (1952) reported favourably on them. At this time internal fixation was being perfected; antibiotics had overcome the fear of surgical infection and it was inevitable that intramedullary fixation and plating would become the chosen methods.

In the 1970s interest in external skeletal fixation was revived, particularly for open and comminuted fractures, shearing injuries and mandibular fractures. The results achieved were better than previously, due to the upgrading of methods of application and aftercare. There is now a burgeoning literature on this subject which reflects a worldwide acceptance of these techniques. Sophisticated systems may be purchased or home-made devices constructed to suit the individual case (Carmichael, 1991; Harari, 1992).

INTERNAL FIXATION

The advantages of maintaining fracture components in apposition by mechanical means were appreciated long before this became possible practically. The introduction of aseptic surgery and of radiography enabled such techniques to advance, though the concept was not immediately accepted. The early implants were similar to those in present use but experience has brought about changes in their design, the materials of which they are made and the manner of their insertion.

Wire

The apposition of bone ends with wire is probably the oldest of the internal fixation methods (Figure 2.7). In humans, silver was used first but in 1883 Lister repaired a fractured patella with iron wire and Lambotte employed annealed iron wire. Hey Groves

(1916) preferred iron to silver and believed that the wire should perforate rather than encircle the bone, though he thought wiring was unsatisfactory. Despite the relative weakness of wire and its inability to overcome angulation forces, it found favour over the next 20 years because it meant introducing less metal into the wound than did a plate. This is an indication of the fear of complications that plating had engendered, which did not abate until the introduction of biologically inert metals.

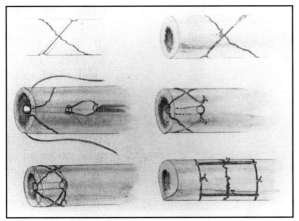

Figure 2.7: Types of wire 'bone sutures' devised to provide more rigid internal fixation. (Reproduced from Venable and Stuck, 1947, with the permission of Blackwell Science. Redrawn from Seer's Practical Surgery, *1901.)*

Metal bands were stronger than wire loops and various designs were made, the most notable being by Parham and Martin in 1916. Erosion tended to occur beneath bands and this could so weaken the bone that it fractured; such changes were attributed to pressure necrosis before the destructive effects of electrolysis were realized.

In dogs, Hobday (1906) mentioned the union of fractures with silver wire inserted in hemi-cerclage fashion, while French (1906) treated pseudarthroses with silver wire sutures. Ehmer (1925) plated and wired dog fractures but found after-care with external supports was unsatisfactory. Perrin (1923) repaired a dog's femur with wire but it became infected. A fractured calcaneum was wired by McCunn (1933), and Weipers (1951) had used silver and phosphorbronze wire in the 1930s. Larsen (1927) and Moltzen-Nielsen (1949) used Parham bands and Knight (1949) employed silver wire for some years.

Cerclage wiring gained popularity for small animals largely as an adjunct to intramedullary pinning, to secure long oblique bone ends and to hold fragments in place (Turnbull, 1951). Repair failures were not uncommon, due to wires loosening or breaking, which sometimes led to non-union or osteomyelitis, and this provoked a controversy about the hazards of cerclage (Newton and Hohn 1974). Interference with blood supply was thought to be responsible for some of these failures, though a narrow loop was less likely to reduce vascularity than a band. Bands were discarded and more satisfactory results were achieved when cerclage application improved (Hinko and Rhinelander, 1975).

A more recent innovation using wire is the tension-band technique, which converts a distracting or tension force into a compressive one. It has special advantages for treating avulsions and allows an early return to weightbearing, which is beneficial for animals.

Intramedullary devices

Short pegs that crossed the fracture line and impacted in the medullary cavity were used in the late nineteenth century, especially for delayed unions. Hey Groves (1912, 1916) tried pegs of ivory, bone and nickel-plated steel, 1.5—2.0 inches (38—51 cm) long, for recent fractures. They were difficult to insert, they were limited to simple transverse fractures and they failed to provide rigid alignment. When he introduced full-length pinning for femoral fractures, his critics believed this would cause marrow destruction, fat embolism and sepsis. According to Hobday (1906) pegs were used to treat non-union fractures in dogs.

The concept of intramedullary fixation was revived when Kuntscher (1940) successfully repaired experimental fractures in dogs with V- or trefoil-shaped nails. By 1950 nailing was routine in humans (Watson-Jones, 1950) and it proved satisfactory in dogs (Jenny *et al.*, 1946; Marcenac *et al.*, 1947; Griesmann, 1948; Moltzen-Nielsen, 1949; Schebitz, 1949; Jenny, 1950). It was, however, the round section Steinman pin rather than the nail that found favour for long bone fractures in dogs and cats, possibly because it was easier to insert and cost less. Its early advocates were Bernard (1948), Brinker (1948), Frick *et al.* (1948), Knight (1949), Knowles (1949), Lauder (1949), Moltzen-Nielsen (1949), Turnbull (1949), Henderson (1950), Leighton (1950) and Weipers (1951). The canine femur proved not to be ideally suited for pinning because its medullary cavity varies in width along its length, making it difficult to achieve adequate bone/pin contact. Consequently fragment rotation or even non-union might occur unless the repair were supplemented. Obel (1951) impacted the medulla with two or more pins. Pins with a threaded end were thought to give a better grip. The addition of cerclage wires or an external skeletal fixator could also resist rotation.

An intramedullary extension splint was devised by Jonas and Jonas (1953) which included a spring-loaded device intended to make insertion easier. Enthusiasm for the splint waned when it was associated with untoward reactions and proved difficult to remove.

A round-section pin which has a sledge-runner tip at one end and a hook at the other relies on its spring-like action to contact the inner wall of the cortex. Although initially developed for humans (Rush and Rush, 1949), it was adapted for small animals (Carney, 1952) and remains popular, especially for condylar fractures in miniature breeds of dog.

Plates and screws

The first metal bone plates and screws were devised by Hansmann (1886). Made of nickel-plate, they were inserted in such a way that the screws and one end of the plate protruded through the skin to make removal easy (Figure 2.8). Trials with plates in the late nineteenth century led Lane (1907) to design a pattern of steel plate that remained standard for many years. Lane's belief that success depended on strict antisepsis caused him to recommend a 'non-touch' technique. Lambotte (1907) preferred plates of soft steel plated with gold or nickel, having tried aluminium, silver and brass. As experience with plating grew, it was reported that Lane plates tended to break at the junction of the bar and first screw hole (Figures 2.9 and 2.10). The plates were 1/16—3/16 of an inch (1.6—4.8 mm) thick and 1/4 of an inch (6.3 mm) wide. Since the screws penetrated only one cortex, the repair was weak. Sherman (1912), advised by engineers, introduced a substantially stronger plate that was slightly curved and had fewer screw holes. It was made of vanadium steel, which was twice as tough as the tool steel in Lane's plates; the screws were machine type with self-cutting threads, which provided greater holding power than wood-type screws.

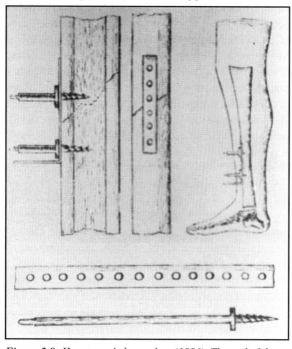

Figure 2.8: Hansmann's bone plate (1886). The end of the plate and the screws protruded from the wound. (Reproduced from Venable and Stuck, 1947, with the permission of Blackwell Science. Originally printed in A. Hansmann's A new method of fixation of fragments in complicated fractures, Verh. d. Deutsch Gesellsch. f. Chir, *1886.)*

Hey Groves (1912, 1916) experimentally tested the efficacy of plating in cats and rabbits and found that short plates attached with screws through one cortex were unable to retain the bones in position. He advocated longer, thicker plates fixed with screws or cotter pins through the full width of the bone. For some fractures a plate was applied to each cortex, both held

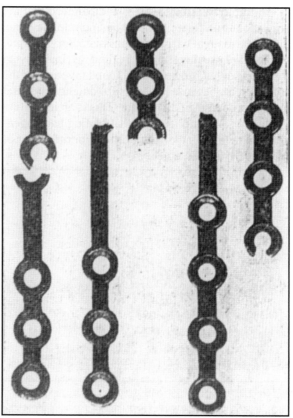

Figure 2.9: Lane bone plates broken at their weakest point. (Reproduced from Sherman, 1912, Surgery, Gynecology and Obstetrics, **14,** *629.)*

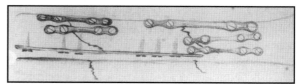

Figure 2.10: Lane bone plates applied to a fractured femur. (Reproduced from Venable and Stuck, 1947, with the permission of Blackwell Science. Originally printed in Lane, Operative Treatment of Fractures.*)*

together with bolts. He was ahead of his time in stressing the importance of fracture planning and the value of motor-driven drills.

Over the next two decades, plating became associated with an unacceptable level of complications such as plate loosening, wound breakdown and failure of union. The severe bone reactions ('rarefying osteitis') that developed were attributed to infection or faulty technique until Venable *et al.* (1937) showed that the problem was due to the metals used. Metals could disintegrate in tissues through electrolysis, but this could be avoided by using metals that are biologically inert. The inert alloy, vitallium, was introduced to bone surgery (Venable and Stuck, 1941) and stainless steel was modified to improve its inertness. The qualities of 18-8 S Mo steel in this respect led to its universal acceptance in implant manufacture. The lesson regarding metal corrosion was learned slowly and it was some years before old stocks of inferior implants were discarded from hospitals (Cater and Hicks, 1956).

In dogs, Larsen (1927) reported the repair of fractures with Lane plates, the first being in 1910 (Figure 2.11). Chambers (1932) and Stainton (1932) referred to plating but gave no clinical details. Moltzen-Nielsen (1949) described 30 repairs with Lane plates between 1928 and 1939. Bateman (1948) repaired calcaneal fractures in Greyhounds with a slotted plate fixed to the tibia and tuber calcis. Sherman plates of vitallium were used by Knight (1949), Chappel and Archibald (1951) and Kirk (1952). Two steel plates were used in tandem to repair a fractured calcaneum in a bull (Kirk and Fennell, 1951). The plating of long bone fractures became increasingly common in the 1960s, tending to replace intramedullary pinning in large dogs. The type of plate depended on the size and shape of the bones, which vary greatly in the different breeds, unlike the standard morphology of bones in humans. Sherman plates were inherently weak at the screw holes and so the straight-edged Venable plate was indicated for large and heavy dogs. The Burns plate combined features of the latter two, while the Eggers Contact plate had long slots instead of screw holes and was claimed to provide compression of the fracture during weightbearing. The finger plates designed for human phalanges were suitable for long bones in the miniature breeds.

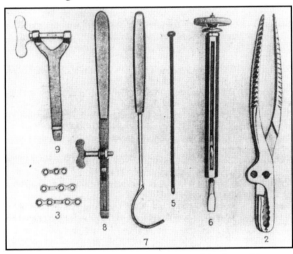

Figure 2.11: *Bone plating equipment used in dogs. (From Larsen, 1927,* Maanedsskrift für Dyrlaeger, *39, 337.)*

In 1958 a group of Swiss surgeons formed an association for the study of the problems of internal fixation with a view to evaluating the operative treatment of fractures in humans. The research undertaken in their laboratories at Davos had far-reaching effects on fracture repair in humans and animals. Attention was focused on achieving a mechanically stable unit with lag screws, compression plates and intramedullary nails, in order to allow early, pain-free limb use and thus avoid some of the serious joint and soft tissue complications. Primary bone healing was said to follow such a fixation although more probably the improved healing was promoted by rigid immobilization of the bone fragments.

Implant development has been an important aspect of this vigorous reappraisal. At first compression was achieved with a plate attached to the bone using a compression device, but in 1969 Perren *et al.* tested in animals a new style of "dynamic compression plate' (DCP), which relies on the geometry of the holes and eccentric placement of the screws to produce compression. It was successfully used in humans by Allgower *et al.* (1969) and is arguably the outstanding innovation in bone plating in the last half-century.

The various systems now commercially available provide implants of high quality but also require practical skills of equal quality for their correct insertion. In 1970 an international veterinary association for the study of internal fixation was formed, with similar aims to those of the original organization. Implicit in the ethos is the acquisition of skills to the benefit of fracture treatment and many veterinary surgeons worldwide take advantage of the courses that are available where practical knowhow may be learned.

The fact that rigid fixation tends to overprotect bone union has led to the introduction of plates made of materials that allow some flexibility, such as carbon fibre. Biodegradable materials might answer some of the problems created by metals, and plates with low contact interfere less with vascularity. These and many other developments are being tested in response to clinical challenges and are part of a never ending process which began when the first attempts were made to assist nature in the healing of fractures many centuries ago.

REFERENCES

Allgower M, Ehrsam R, Ganz R *et al.* (1969) Clinical experience with a new compression plate 'DCP'. *Acta Orthopaedica Scandinavica* (Supplement) **125**, 45.

Anderson R (1934) Fractures of the radius and ulna. A new anatomical method of treatment. *Journal of Bone and Joint Surgery* **16**, 379.

Barrett EP (1936) The treatment of fractures in small animals by means of the unpadded cast. *Veterinary Record* **48**, 1086.

Bartlet (1756) *A Gentleman's Farriery or, a Practical Treatise on the Diseases of Horses*, 3rd edn. Nourse, London.

Bateman JK (1948) A fresh approach to the repair of the os calcis in the Greyhound. *Veterinary Record* **60**, 674.

Bernard BW (1948) Method of repair of femoral and humeral fractures. *Journal of the American Veterinary Medical Association* **113**, 134.

Blaine D (1824) *Canine Pathology*, 2nd edn. Boosey and Sons, London.

Brinker WO (1948) The use of intramedullary pins in small animal fractures. *North American Veterinarian* **29**, 292.

Carmichael S (1991) The external fixator in small animal orthopaedics. *Journal of Small Animal Practice* **32**, 486.

Carney JP (1952) Rush intramedullary fixation of long bones as applied to veterinary surgery. *Veterinary Medicine* **47**, 43.

Cater WH and Hicks JH (1956) The recent history of corrosion in metal used for internal fixation. *Lancet* **2**, 871.

Chambers F (1932) Fracture of the femur in the dog. *Veterinary Record* **12**, 91.

Chappel CI and Archibald J (1951) Vitallium bone plating in dogs. Description of a practical technique and clinical observations. *Veterinary Medicine* **46**, 291.

Dibbell EB (1930) Splints for fixation of fractures and dislocations in small animals. *North American Veterinarian* **11**, 29.

Dibbell EB (1931) Lower third femoral fractures in dogs. *North American Veterinarian* **12**, 37.

Ehmer EA (1925) Our method of handling fractures. *North American Veterinarian* **6**, 47.

Ehmer EA (1947) Bone pinning of fractures of small animals. *Journal of the American Veterinary Medical Association* **110**, 14.

Elliot Smith G (1908) The most ancient splints. *British Medical Journal* **1**, 732.

French C (1906) *Surgical Diseases and Surgery of the Dog*. French, Washington, DC.

Frick EJ, Witter RE and Mosier JE (1948) Treatment of fractures by intramedullary pinning. *North American Veterinarian* **29**, 95.

Gibson W (1729) *The Farrier's New Guide*, 6th edn. Osborn and Longman, London.

Griesmann H (1948) Marknagelung eines Oberschenkelbruches beim Hund. *Deutsch tierarztliche Wochenschrift* **55**, 275.

Gunn RMC (1936) The treatment of limb bone fractures in animals. *Australian Veterinary Journal* **12**, 139.

Guthrie D (1958) *A History of Medicine (with supplements)*. Thomas Nelson and Sons, London.

Harari J (1992) *The Veterinary Clinics of North America* **22**, 1.

Henderson W (1950) Intramedullary repair of femoral fractures in the dog and cat. *Veterinary Record* **62**, 168.

Hey Groves EW (1912) Some clinical and experimental observations on the operative treatment of fractures. *British Medical Journal* **5**, *1102*.

Hey Groves EW (1916) *On Modern Methods of Treating Fractures*. John Wright and Sons, Bristol.

Hinko PJ and Rhinelander FW (1975) Effective use of cerclage in the treatment of long bone fractures in dogs. *Journal of the American Veterinary Medical Association* **166**, 520.

Hobday FTG (1896) The new photography in veterinary practice. *The Journal of Comparative Pathology and Therapeutics* **9**, 58.

Hobday FTG (1900) *Canine and Feline Surgery*. W and AK Johnston, Edinburgh and London.

Hobday FTG (1906) *Surgical Diseases of the Dog and Cat*, 2nd edn. Bailliere, Tindall and Cox, London.

Jenny J (1950) Kuntscher's medullary nailing in femur fractures of the dog. *Journal of the American Veterinary Medical Association* **117**, 381.

Jenny J, Kanter U and Knoll H (1946) Die Behandlung von Femurfrakturen des Hundes durch Marknagelung. *Schweizer Archiv für Tierheilkunde* **88**, 547.

Jonas S and Jonas AM (1953) Self-retaining medullary extension splint. *Journal of the American Veterinary Medical Association* **122**, 261.

Jones R (1925) Crippling due to fractures: its prevention and remedy. *British Medical Journal* **1**, 909.

Kirk H (1952) Modern methods of fracture repair in large and small animals. *Veterinary Record* **64**, 319.

Kirk H and Fennell C (1951) Treatment of fracture of os calcis of a bull by plating. *Veterinary Record* **63**, 363.

Knight GC (1949) A report on the use of stainless steel intramedullary pins and Sherman type vitallium plates in the treatment of small animal fractures. *British Veterinary Journal* **105**, 294.

Knowles JO (1949) Fracture repair by bone pinning. *Veterinary Record* **61**, 648.

Kuntscher G (1940) Die Behandlung von Knochenbruechen bei Tieren durch Marknagelung. *Archiv für wissenschaftliche praktische Tierheilkunde* **75**, 262.

Lacroix JV and Cozart JM (1924) Wood splints and the treatment of fractures of long bones. *North American Veterinarian* **5**, 408.

Lambotte A (1907) *L'Intervention Opératoire dans les Fracteurs*. Lamartins, Brussels.

Lane WA (1907) Clinical remarks on the operative treatment of fractures. *British Medical Journal* **1**, 1037.

Larsen S (1927) Operativ Frakturbehandling. *Maanedsskrift für Dyrlaeger* **39**, 337.

Lauder JSJ (1949) Fracture repair by bone pinning. *Veterinary Record* **61** 866.

Leighton RL (1950) A new method of permanent intramedullary pinning. *Journal of the American Veterinary Medical Association* **117**, 202.

Marcenac N, Bordet R and Jenny J (1947) Osteosynthèse fémoral par enclouage métallique centromédullaire. *Bulletin Académie Vétérinaire France* **20**, 61.

McCunn J (1933) Fractures and dislocations in small animals. *Veterinary Record* **13**, 1236.

Moltzen-Nielsen H (1949) Recent experiences in the treatment of fractures by surgical methods. *Veterinary Record* **61**, 791.

Munro JK (1935) The history of plaster-of-Paris in the treatment of fractures. *British Journal of Surgery* **23**, 257.

Newton CD and Hohn RB (1974) Fracture nonunion resulting from cerclage appliances. *Journal of the American Veterinary Medical Association* **164**, 503.

Obel N (1951) Intramedullar fixation med rostfria stavar vid fraktur pa femurdiafysen nos hund. *Nordisk Veterinarmedicin* **3**, 723.

Parkhill C (1897) A new apparatus for the fixation of bones after resection and in fractures with a tendency to displacement. *American Surgery Association Transactions* **15**, 251.

Perren SM, Russenberger M, Steinemann S *et al.* (1969) A dynamic compression plate. *Acta Orthopaedica Scandinavica* (Supplement) **125**, 31.

Perrin F (1923) The treatment of fractures. *North American Veterinarian* **4**, 490.

Rush LV and Rush HL (1949) Evolution of medullary fixation of fractures by longitudinal pin. *American Journal of Surgery* **78**, 324.

Schebitz H (1949) Die Marknagelung bei Haustieren. *Monatshefte für Veterinarmedizin* **4**, 27.

Schroeder EF (1933a) The traction principle in treating fractures and dislocations in the dog and cat. *North American Veterinarian* **14**, 32.

Schroeder EF (1933b) Fractures of the femoral shaft of dogs. *North American Veterinarian* **14**, 38.

Schroeder EF (1934) Fractures of the humerus in dogs. *North American Veterinarian* **15**, 31.

Self RA (1934) Open reduction and mechanical devices in treating fractures in small animals. *Veterinary Medicine* **29**, 120.

Sherman WO (1912) Vanadium steel bone plates and screws. *Surgery, Gynecology and Obstetrics* **14**, 629.

Stader O (1934) A method of treating femoral fractures in dogs. *North American Veterinarian* **15**, 25.

Stader O (1937) A preliminary announcement of a new method of treating fractures. *North American Veterinarian* **18**, 37.

Stader O (1939) Treating fractures of long bones with the reduction splint. *North American Veterinarian* **20**, 55.

Stainton H (1932) The fractured canine femur. *Veterinary Record* **12**, 187.

Steiner AJ (1928) Treating femur and pelvic fractures. *Journal of the American Veterinary Medical Association* **73**, 314.

Thomas HO (1875) *Diseases of the Hip, Knee and Ankle Joints*. T. Dobb and Co., Liverpool.

Turnbull NR (1949) Fractures of the humerus and femur repaired by intramedullary pins. *Veterinary Record* **61**, 476.

Turnbull NR (1951) The problems of the displaced epiphysis. *Veterinary Record* **63**, 678.

Venable CS and Stuck WG (1941) Three years experience with Vitallium in bone surgery. *Annals of Surgery* **114**, 390.

Venable CS and Stuck WG (1947) *The Internal Fixation of Fractures*. Blackwell Science, Oxford.

Venable CS, Stuck WG and Beach A (1937) The effects on bone of the presence of metals: based on electrolysis. *Annals of Surgery* **105**, 917.

Watson-Jones R (1950) Medullary nailing of fractures after fifty years. *Journal of Bone and Joint Surgery* **32B**, 694.

Weipers WL (1951) Matters canine. *Veterinary Record* **63**, 659.

Williams W (1893) *The Principles and Practice of Veterinary Surgery*. John Menzies and Co., Edinburgh.

Wright JG (1937) Some observations on the incidence, causes and treatment of bone fractures in the dog. *Veterinary Record* **49**, 2.

Note on Illustrations: The BSAVA has been unable to contact the original publishers for Figures 2.3, 2.5, 2.6, 2.9 and 2.11. We are pleased to acknowledge the source and apologize for any unintended discourtesy.

CHAPTER THREE

Biomechanical Basis of Bone Fracture and Fracture Repair

Simon Roe

INTRODUCTION

Every aspect of fracture management is influenced by extrinsic or intrinsic forces. It is therefore essential for successful orthopaedists to appreciate the mechanical nature of the art of fracture repair and to meld it with their understanding of the biological aspects of the tissue and its response to trauma. This chapter addresses the mechanics of bone as a material and a structure, of fractures and fracture healing, and of implants used to impart stability. Terms in bold type are defined further in the Glossary at the end of the chapter.

MECHANICS OF BONE

Bone as a material

It is often helpful to understand a material before considering the structure that it builds. An engineer must be familiar with how steel behaves before building a bridge. When he looks at the bridge, he considers the loads that are likely to be borne and then decides if the structure and the material it is made of are strong enough. In a similar way, a surgeon must assess a fracture and its repair. The loads that must be considered are discussed later in this chapter. This section considers the **stress** and **strain** that might be expected within the material with which the surgeon is working. Appreciating these internal forces and deformations is important in understanding the limits of bone as a mechanical material.

A common approach to understanding mechanical materials is to subject them to a load while measuring the resulting deformation. For simple materials (which includes most of those associated with fracture mechanics), the response is linear and the slope of the line represents the **stiffness** of the structure tested. This is often the most important parameter as it conveys how much movement will occur for a certain load. In fracture repair mechanics, it relates directly to the amount of movement that might be expected at the fracture site. If the specimen being tested is a pure material that has known dimensions, then the stress *versus* strain response can also be produced. The slope of this line is termed the **modulus** of the material. This

parameter is used to compare different materials, not different structures.

Bone is a complex material composed mostly of organized collagen fibrils and a hydroxyapatite mineral matrix. Although many other components are present, these two contribute most significantly to the mechanical behaviour of bone. At a very basic level, cortical and cancellous bone are quite similar.

When a material is not homogeneous, its mechanical behaviour is influenced by the direction of loading relative to its orientation and it is termed **anisotropic**. A graphic depiction of how bone properties are influenced by specimen orientation is presented in Figure 3.1. The response also varies with the type of load applied. Due to the organization of the mineral phase, bone is very resistant to compression in all directions. The interaction of the mineral crystals causes it to fail by **shear**, usually at 45° to the long axis. Because the mineral crystals are much more resistant to compression than the collagen fibres are to tension, peak compressive loads are much greater than failure loads measured in tensile evaluations.

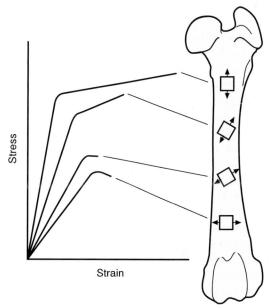

Figure 3.1: *The tensile strength of four specimens prepared from the same piece of cortical bone is recorded on the graph. Specimens oriented other than in line with the osteons were weaker in tension, demonstrating the anisotrophy of bone.*

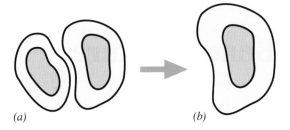

Figure 3.2: (a) Section through a radius and ulna to demonstrate the cross-sectional area that bears the load in the limb. (b) After removal of the ulna, the dimensions, cross-sectional area and area (AMI) and polar moments of inertia (PMI) increase. If a diaphysis responds to load by increasing its cortical thickness by 20%, the cross-sectional area increases by 90% and the AMI and the PMI increase by 250%, to produce a structure with greatly enhanced resistance to bending and rotation.

Bone as a structure

The structural arrangement of bone (as a material) has both microscopic and macroscopic components. The two primary types of bone when considering fracture management are cortical and cancellous.

Cortical

On a microscopic level, cortical bone is very dense and very regularly aligned, thus imparting considerable strength to diaphyses of long bones. The arrangement of bone in the diaphysis demonstrates a major mechanical concept, **area moment of inertia** (AMI), that applies to many aspects of fracture management and will be the basis of understanding many situations described in this chapter.

The cylindrical structure of the diaphysis provides resistance to bending and rotation forces while optimizing the mass of the bone. The dynamic nature of the response of bone to its mechanical environment is revealed by the way in which it responds to increases in load (Figure 3.2). If a portion of the ulna of young pigs is removed, the load borne through the radius increases. The radius responds by increasing in thickness and in outer diameter, greatly increasing its AMI.

The dimensions of the structure also determine the **polar moment of inertia** (PMI), which influences the resistance to torsional load. PMI reflects the distribution of the structure around the central axis of rotation. Material further from the axis will increase this parameter and produce a structure with superior resistance to rotation.

An important point to remember is that the bending and torsional strengths of a structure are determined by the strength of the material as well as AMI and PMI. Mineralized disorganized callus is not as strong as cortical bone and so, during healing, the amount and dimensions of callus tissue are increased to provide bending and torsional strengths that are able to withstand the loads applied.

Cancellous

The properties of cancellous bone are determined by its density and by its architecture. It also displays anisotropy. There are few conditions in animals in which the mechanics of cancellous bone need to be considered. The primary concern is its ability to hold implants when fractures occur in the metaphysis or epiphysis, particularly in the young and very old. Some specific conditions (beyond the scope of this chapter) that have stimulated considerable research into cancellous bone mechanics are osteoarthritis, osteoporosis and joint replacement.

Fracture of bone

Cortical

The majority of fractures involve primarily cortical bone. The way in which a cortical shaft breaks will be determined by the type of loading and the rate at which the load is applied. It is easiest to consider the specific patterns created by simple loads applied slowly (Figure 3.3):

- Compression results in fracture lines 45° to the axis
- Tension produces a straight separation of the material
- Rotation results in a spiral fracture line
- Bending is more complex as it produces tension on one side of the cylinder and compression on the other. A simple transverse fracture begins on the tension side (because bone is weaker in tension). As the forces become compressive, the weakest plane is at 45° and often two fracture lines diverge and a 'butterfly' fragment develops.

In clinical situations, loading is usually very complex. Weight bearing and muscle contraction in anticipation of a trauma often create large compressive forces within a bone that may be subject to rotation, bending or a combination of both.

Another factor of the fracture process that influences the final degree of damage is the rate of loading. The process of development and propagation of fracture lines is very complex and the following discussion is a simplification to highlight the major principles involved. When a load is applied relatively slowly, a fracture begins in the material at the weakest point. As more energy is applied to the bone, the fracture line follows the weakest path through the material. A single line of fracture occurs and its configuration is influenced by the type of load applied and any inherent weaknesses in the structure. However, if load is applied rapidly to bone, the energy stored in the structure can cause multiple sites of disruption of the material. As these develop into fracture lines, the large amount of energy being rapidly applied to the structure may be dissipated in multiple directions, and not necessarily along the weakest plane. In the clinical situation, high energy trauma is associated with a high degree of

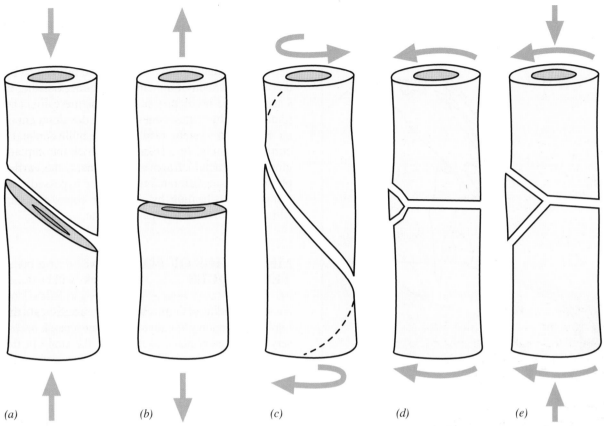

Figure 3.3: *The fracture configuration is a function of the forces acting on the bone. (a) Compression: the mineral structure shears at 45° to the long axis, producing oblique fracture lines. (b) Tension: bone is weaker in tension because the mineral crystals contribute little, failure occurs by separation in a straight line. (c) Rotation: shear forces create a spiral fracture pattern. (d) Bending: tension develops on the convex surface and compression on the concave surface as the bone bends. Because the bone is weaker in tension, the fracture begins transversely. As it travels across the bone, the forces change to compression and the fracture often progresses in both 45° directions to create a 'butterfly' fragment. (e) Combined bending and compression: an increase in the compressive stress results in shear failure earlier and a larger 'butterfly' fragment results.*

comminution. The highly comminuted femur fracture in Figure 3.4 occurred when the dog leapt from a truck travelling at 35 mph. When the dog's foot contacted the ground and stopped moving forward, his body continued, creating a massive torsional load in the limb. This was combined with a massive compressive load from the landing body and the contraction of the thigh muscles in an attempt to prevent falling.

Cancellous

Fracture of cancellous structures follows some of the patterns seen for cortical bone. In compression, however, collapse and compaction occur. It is important that this type of change be noted when evaluating a fracture as it will influence the ability to reconstruct the bone and to apply an implant to it. This type of fracture is most commonly seen in vertebrae.

MECHANICAL ASPECTS OF FRACTURE HEALING

The various stages of callus maturation are influenced by local humoral and physical factors. The

stress and strain experienced by the tissues within the fracture influence their development and differentiation. The types of tissue present in various regions of the callus are often dictated by their tolerance of the local deformations.

Early in the healing process, the fracture gap fills with granulation tissue. The loose, fibrous nature of this tissue allows it to tolerate strains in the region of 40%. Because strain is calculated from the original length of the tissue being loaded, one way that nature is able to reduce tissue strain is by increasing the width of the fracture gap. Resorption of fracture ends occurs when large motions are present (Figure 3.5).

As the biological processes drive callus differentiation, regions with less strain become more fibrous and cartilaginous matrix is deposited. This tissue is stiffer – less movement of the fracture fragments will occur with the same load. However, it is also less tolerant of strain. If it is distorted by more than 5%, tissue injury will occur, differentiation will be retarded, and more granulation tissue will be laid down. If the stiffening of the callus does control movement, mineralization and woven bone formation begin. Again, this commences first in regions of the callus with the least motion. The tissue is stiff but more

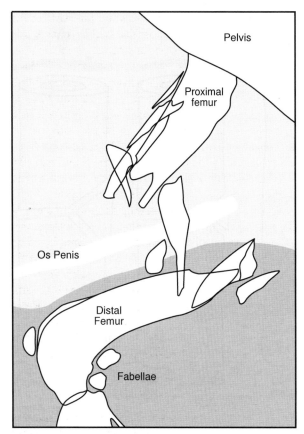

Figure 3.4: *Line drawing of a radiograph of a highly comminuted femur fracture that occurred when the dog leapt from the back of a truck moving at 35 mph. When the foot landed and stopped and the body continued moving, massive torsional forces were applied. These combined with the compressive forces of body weight and of the thigh muscles. The fracture developed many comminutions because of the large amount of energy and the rapid rate of loading.*

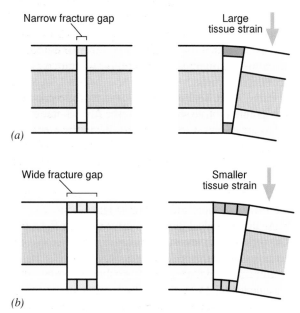

Figure 3.5: *(a) When the fracture gap is small, the tissues within the gap experience a large amount of strain because a small amount of movement is distributed over a short length of tissue. (b) When the fracture gap is wider, the strain is reduced as the same amount of deformation is distributed over a longer length.*

susceptible to injury – more than 0.2% strain will damage the mineralized matrix. If tissue strain is minimal during the bridging period, the newly formed bone can provide sufficient strength to join the fracture ends.

The final maturation process is also influenced by the mechanical environment of the bone. Loading is sensed by the osteocytes of the immature callus and remodelling by 'cutter cones' and the development of an Haversian system result in re-establishment of cortical structure. In a fracture in which the implant eliminates fracture fragment movement, the earlier phases of tissue differentiation may be bypassed, and primary bone healing by the cutter cones and gap filling will combine to repair the bone.

MECHANICS OF FIXATION TECHNIQUES

An understanding of the mechanical characteristics of the implants commonly employed in fracture repair is necessary if a surgeon plans to minimize the strain in the fracture callus so that healing can occur. This section will begin by presenting a method used by the author to assess implants in general and individual fracture repairs. This method simplifies the likely forces acting on an implant and provides a basis for evaluating stability of a repair.

Forces acting on an implant

During a gait cycle, weight bearing and muscle contraction result in a complex array of forces within a bone or bone-implant construct. Studies of these forces are difficult and have provided limited data, but for improving clinical judgement in orthopaedics it is usually sufficient to take a much more simplistic approach. The forces acting on a bone or implant are a combination of axial compression, bending and rotation (Figure 3.6). In some specific instances, fragments associated with the origin or insertion of major muscle groups may experience mostly tension. This scenario will be addressed in a separate subsection.

Axial compression is the component of the forces aligned down the shaft of the bone. When acting on a fracture, it causes collapse and shortening. Weight bearing and muscle contraction will contribute to this component. When evaluating an implant for its ability to counter this force, the purchase obtained in the major proximal and distal fragments must be considered. The ability of a fracture repair to resist compression will also be influenced by the completeness of reconstruction.

Bending is present whenever a bone is bearing load and it is not perpendicular to the ground. Eccentric muscle contractions can also apply bending forces in any direction. An implant's resistance to bending is determined by the elastic modulus of the material it is made of and its area moment of inertia (AMI). Implants made from 316L stainless steel can be generally

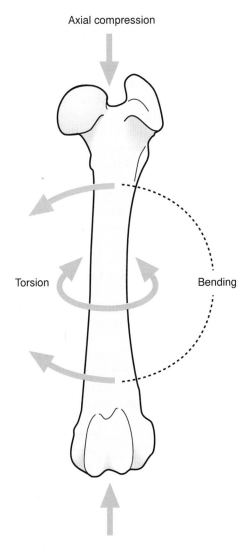

Axial compression

Torsion

Bending

Figure 3.6: *Diagrammatic representation of the three force categories considered when evaluating a fracture, a fixation method, or a repaired fracture. Weight bearing and muscle contractions contribute to compressive forces down the long axis. When the bone is at an angle to the ground or when the muscles pull more on one side than on the other, bending will be induced. This may be in any direction. Torsion will occur when the mass of the body changes direction while the limb is bearing weight.*

compared based on their AMIs. Titanium has a lower modulus and implants of similar AMI will be less stiff. However, titanium resists fatigue damage under repeated loading better than stainless steel. Since most implants fail by fatigue rather than from a single excessive loading event, this property must also be allowed for when assessing an implant's suitability to maintain fracture stability until healing has occurred.

Because calculation of the AMI of a structure is based on the direction of bending, it is necessary to estimate this for a repair. In most bones, a primary direction is not evident and the smallest AMI, which determines the weakest direction, is used to characterize the weakest point in bending. In the femur, the eccentric location of loading through the femoral head dictates a lateral to medial bending direction.

It is also necessary to determine the AMI at the weakest point of the structure that will be loaded. It is easy to calculate the AMI for circular or rectangular structures but, if a hole in a bone plate or interlocking nail is bearing load, then this will be the weakest point. The AMI of the solid portion of a 3.5 mm plate is 29.9 mm^4 while through a hole it is 14.8 mm^4 – a 50% reduction. If a screw hole in an interlocking nail is located close to a fracture, it should also be considered a weak point in the construct. For the 8 mm nail, the AMI drops from an impressive 201 mm^4 for the solid section to 64.7 mm^4 in the weakest direction.

Torsion is induced by changes in the direction of the body while the limb is bearing weight. Assessment of rotational stability is often more complex than compression or bending. The polar moment of inertia (PMI) of the implant is not usually a weak point in the construct. Stability is estimated by how well the implant engages the primary fracture fragments. Rotational stability may also be imparted by interaction of the fracture fragments. The way in which different systems are assessed will be discussed in the specific sections below.

External coaptation

Splints and casts provide immobilization of fracture ends by encasing the limb. They do not directly contact bone and so must act through the skin and muscles of the limb. The cast or splint material is the most rigid portion and it must be built with sufficient strength to withstand the forces that will be applied to it for the appropriate duration. Bending forces are the most significant forces because casts span joints and there is a great propensity for the limb to want to bend at the level of the joint. There are a number of ways of improving cast design and construction to counteract the bending forces. Thickness of the wall of the cast is the most obvious approach but the disadvantage is that the cast becomes heavier. If the primary bending direction is known, the cast may be reinforced in that specific plane. This will increase the AMI (because the added dimension is in the plane of bending) without adding too much weight. It is also beneficial to form a cast that is relatively straight but this tends to lengthen the limb and is more awkward for the patient.

The interface between the cast and the bone will also influence the ability of the cast to immobilize the fracture fragments. The greater the stiffness of this interface, the better will the rigid cast material support the fracture. High stiffness is produced by using little or no cast padding and by applying the cast wrap with pressure. Both these approaches increase the likelihood of pressure injury to the skin and soft tissues between the cast and the bone. The surgeon must therefore judge the correct amount of padding and cast wrap pressure that will avoid soft tissue injury but will still provide adequate immobilization of the fracture fragments.

External skeletal fixators

Pin factors

The strength of the purchase of the pins in the fracture fragments is an important factor in the success of external fixation (Figure 3.7). Individually, smooth pins rely on compression of the bone against the pin shaft to resist pull-out. In most frames, multiple pins are placed and they are purposefully angled to each other so that they brace each other. Threaded pins are more securely anchored in bone. Negative thread profiles were used initially because they are easier to manufacture; however, they are weak at the point where the shaft and threads meet and pin breakage was frequently seen. The Ellis pin was designed with a short negatively threaded portion so that only the far cortex was engaged with thread and the thread–shaft junction was protected by being inside the bone. Breakage was seen occasionally following resorption of the bone of the near cortex.

Positive profile threaded pins are now available. The threads are created by a lathing or rolling process. The shaft diameter is not significantly reduced and therefore the bending strength of the pin is not compromised. Because the thread diameter is greater, the purchase of the pin is also greater than for negative profile pins. This larger diameter does make these pins a little more awkward to place as the threaded portion does not fit through the hole in the external fixator clamp.

The surgeon must select the appropriate diameter pin for each situation. The larger the diameter, the stronger the pin will be in bending and the stiffer the frame will be, overall. This must be countered by the size of the bone into which the pin must be placed. As a general rule, the diameter of the pin should not exceed 30% of the diameter of the bone so as not to weaken the bone. This may be difficult to comply with when placing pins in the mediolateral plane of the radius or in the metacarpals or metatarsals.

The rigidity of a fixator is increased by increasing the number of pins in each fragment. Two is a minimum and four is considered the maximum in most small animal applications. Obviously, pin diameter and fragment size will dictate what can actually be achieved. Pins should be spaced evenly over each fragment, as this increases torsional rigidity of a frame. They should be placed as close to the fracture as is considered safe. This is determined by the possible presence of fissures and the size of the bone. If there are no fissures, an estimate of this safe distance is three times the diameter of the pin being used. Because stiffness of a structure is influenced by its length, the pins closest to the fracture should be angled towards each other so that the span of the connecting bar that bridges the fracture is minimized.

A final factor that influences the stiffness of a fixator is the length of the pin. Clamps are oriented so that the clamping bolt is closest to the skin. Sufficient distance must be left between the clamp and the skin to allow for some swelling. The surgeon can reduce the length of the pin by selecting a location with the least soft tissue. This also reduces the tissue irritation caused by the pin and appears to reduce the incidence of pin track drainage and infection.

In the beginning of this section, the advantages of threaded pins in increasing the immediate strength of the pin–bone interface was described. It is of equal importance for the surgeon to consider the long-term stability of the pin–bone interface. Loosening of pins is the most common complication of external fixation. It causes discomfort for the patient and may affect the healing process. The mechanical aspects of pin placement feature heavily in the maintenance of a stable interface. Threaded pins loosen less frequently, because they mechanically lock into the bone. The more pins that are present in a fragment, the less is the load at each interface and, therefore, the less likely is loosening.

The amount of bone injury that occurs during pin placement is also a major determinant of how the bone around the pin will change during healing. Significant thermal injury causes bone necrosis.

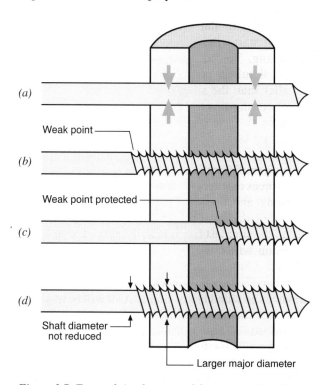

Figure 3.7: *Types of pins for external fixators. (a) Smooth pins rely on friction with the bone or bracing against other pins in the frame. (b) Negative-profile threaded pins engage the bone more securely but are susceptible to failure at the shaft–thread junction. (c) Ellis pins have a small length of negative-profile thread, designed to engage only one cortex. The weak point of the pin is protected from bending forces. (d) Positive-profile threaded pins have a larger major diameter, so holding strength is increased. Because the shaft diameter is not reduced, they are better able to resist the cyclic bending forces associated with weight bearing.*

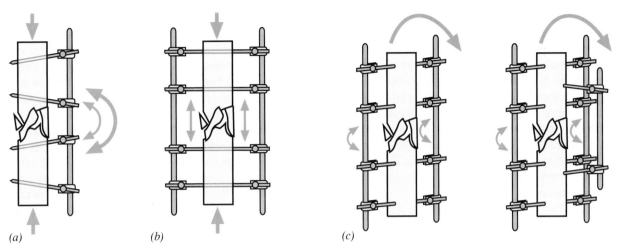

Figure 3.8: *(a) Axial compression down the shaft of a fractured bone supported by a unilateral external fixator results in bending of the pins and the connecting bar. (b) Axial compression of a bilateral frame results in bending of the exposed lengths of the pins. (c) Bending forces directed out of the plane of a bilateral frame result in bending of the connecting bars. By adding a third bar in another plane, the frame is better able to resist these forces.*

Microcracking reduces the strength of the supporting bone and stimulates a repair response. Resorption to remove the dead and damaged bone may reduce the strength of the interaction between the bone and pin. Movement at the interface will prevent new bone formation and a fibrous interface will develop. Movement will also injure these tissues, causing pain and stimulating an inflammatory response. Once it starts, the process often becomes self-perpetuating. To reduce thermal injury to bone, pin tracks should be pre-drilled with a drill only slightly smaller than the shaft diameter, or pins with efficient cutting tips should be used. Pre-drilling also reduces the amount of microcracking in the surrounding bone.

Frame configuration

The forces that act on a fracture – axial compression, bending and torsion – must be considered when assessing the suitability of a fixator frame configuration. The simplest frame is a unilateral design. Compression will cause bending of the connecting bar (Figure 3.8a). The diameter of the bar and the size and number of pins will influence the performance of the frame. The inherent stability of the fracture must also be considered. If the fracture is transverse, it will not be able to collapse and the bone will reduce the load placed on the fixator. If the fracture fragments do not interact, the frame must bear all of the load through the limb. Bending forces will be resisted similarly by a unilateral frame. To increase the resistance of a unilateral frame to bending, a second connecting bar will increase the AMI. Torsional forces are resisted by friction between the clamp and connecting bar in a unilateral frame. The clamp bolt must be very firmly tightened to ensure that it is secure.

If the surgeon feels that a unilateral frame will not be able to provide sufficient resistance to the bending forces in a particular patient, then a more complex frame should be applied. A bilateral frame employs connecting bars on each side of the bone. Axial compressive forces will now be resisted by the pins (Figure 3.8b): their diameter, number and exposed length will determine the stiffness. Bending in the plane of the fixator is also well resisted because the connecting bars protect each other. Bending in the plane perpendicular to the fixator is resisted by the connecting bars only: their exposed length and diameter are determining factors of rigidity. Torsional forces also are better resisted by bilateral frames as the connecting bars are distributed around the axis of rotation.

Triangular configurations are selected to improve the bending stiffness of a frame (Figure 3.8c). The connecting bar in the second plane imparts resistance to bending perpendicular to the plane of the bilateral portion of the fixator. A multi-planar fixator may also be indicated when the primary fragments are small. When only two pins are possible in one plane, a third pin may be placed in a different plane to improve fragment purchase.

Complex, multi-planar fixators have been criticized as potentially being too rigid. They may significantly reduce the load being borne by the callus and thus reduce the stimulus for callus development and maturation. To counter this effect, destabilization of the frame should be considered once callus development has begun. The optimal time at which to increase the load borne by the callus has not been determined. In a large gap fracture model, six weeks of healing seems most advantageous. The extent of the bone and soft tissue injury should be taken into account for each case. Destabilization is preferably achieved by removing connecting bars from a frame but can also be achieved by removing pins.

Fixator frames can be constructed with acrylic or epoxy materials. They have the advantage that pins can be positioned in any plane; soft tissue interference can be minimized and wounds can be avoided. This is particularly helpful for shearing injuries and for fractures of the jaw. Acrylic connections can also be used when the small metal system is too large, such as in toy breeds and birds. Polymethylmethacrylate is the most common material used. One commercial system supplies tubing and prepackaged methacrylate for connecting bars similar in strength to the small and medium metal systems. The acrylic can also be mixed to its dough state and applied without tubing. Epoxy putty is of similar strength to the acrylics and is easier to use for small fixators.

Points to remember

- Maximize pin diameter
- Maximize pin number per fragment
- Reduce pin length
- Add more connecting bars
- Reduce connecting bar span
- Use full pins and bilateral frames when possible.

Intramedullary pins and interlocking nails

Pins

Intramedullary pins provide little resistance to axial compression. If the fracture configuration is not inherently stable (i.e. simple, transverse), collapse will occur. Intramedullary pins are able to resist bending forces because of their large AMI. They are not able to resist torsional forces and, again, must rely on interdigitation of fracture fragments to be stable as a single device. Stacked pinning increases the rotational stability only very slightly and should not be relied upon if the fracture is not inherently stable. Because of these deficiencies, intramedullary pinning as the only fixation method is only indicated in simple fractures in which there is good interdigitation of fragments. If this is not the case, adjunct fixation must be added or another fixation method chosen.

Pins can often be used for metaphyseal and epiphyseal fractures, particularly if they are placed dynamically. These fractures are often quite transverse and so they have inherent resistance to collapse. Two small pins placed on either side of a fragment will impart rotational stability if they engage well proximally. Dynamic placement entails directing the pins into the medullary cavity and having them deflect off the inner wall of the cortex and continue up the medullary canal into the far metaphysis. The interaction of the pin with the cortical wall provides a stable anchorage against rotational forces. The crossed pin technique can also be used: these pins begin on one side of the bone and penetrate the cortex on the other side. For optimal rotational stability, the pins should be directed so that the point at which they cross is above the fracture line.

Interlocking nails

Interlocking nails resist all three of the forces acting on a fracture. The screws that lock the proximal and distal fragments to the nail prevent collapse under compressive forces and prevent rotation when torsional forces are applied (Figure 3.9). The central location of the nail and its large AMI provide good resistance to bending. Interlocking nails are weakened at the screw holes and this weakening is not reduced by placing a screw in the hole. It is therefore important to position the nail so that screw holes are not close to the fracture. In some situations, this may mean selecting a nail with only one locking screw. New nail systems are being developed for veterinary use. The influence of factors such as screw size, number of holes and nail diameter will need to be determined to guide the surgeon in the selection of the appropriate nail for each case.

Orthopaedic wire and cerclage

Orthopaedic wire is malleable stainless steel that is formed into cerclage, hemi-cerclage, interfragmentary or tension-band wires. The wire is often stressed during placement and tying, and is susceptible to fatigue failure. Small nicks and notches in the wire also weaken its resistance to repetitive loading.

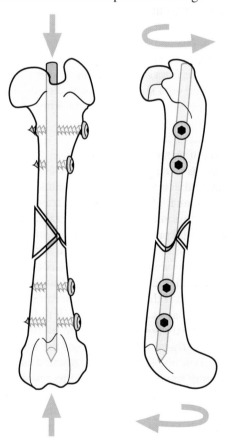

Figure 3.9: *Interlocking nails provide good stability because the primary fracture fragments are 'locked' to the device. Compressive and rotational forces are resisted by the screws. Because the nail has a large area moment of inertia, it resists bending forces well.*

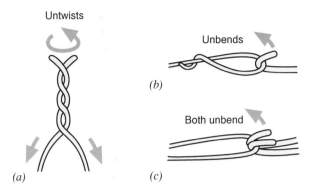

Figure 3.10: The three common cerclage knots. (a) Twist knot. When loaded past its yield point, the knot untwists. (b) Single loop. Greater tension is generated than for a twist knot. The loop yields at a similar load to twist knots by the free arm unbending. (c) Double loop. A greater tension is generated and it resists a much greater load before yield. Both arms unbend during this process.

Full cerclage acts to compress fragments of the diaphysis together. The complete circumference must be rebuilt and fragments accurately reduced because the wire will no longer be tight if there is any reduction of the circumference around which they are tied. Cerclage comparisons are based on the tension that is generated when they are formed and the resistance of the knot to loosening.

- Twist knots must be formed by evenly wrapping both wire strands around one another (Figure 3.10). This knot is used commonly because it can be formed with inexpensive equipment. When loaded past their yield point, the wires untwist
- The single loop knot is formed using a wire with a loop made in one end: the free end passes around the bone and through the loop. The wire is tensioned in a wire tightener with a rotating crank. Once tight, the free end is bent over, cut and flattened. The single loop cerclage generates greater tension than the twist cerclage but has similar yield properties – the free arm unbends as the wire yields
- The double loop cerclage is formed from a piece of wire bent double in the middle: both ends are passed around the bone and back through the bend. Both arms are tightened using a wire tightener with two cranks and bent, cut and flattened in a similar fashion to the single loop cerclage. This cerclage generates three times the tension of the single loop cerclage and resists twice the distracting load.

A minimum of two cerclages should always be used; otherwise bending forces are not countered. Long oblique fractures of two or three segments are the most suited to their use but they are not considered strong enough to be the only means of fixation of a fracture. They can be used in some shorter oblique fractures,

especially in conjunction with one or two skewer pins so that their line of action is directed more perpendicular to the fracture line.

Hemi-cerclage is chosen when the cylindrical nature of the diaphysis can not be rebuilt. When used in conjunction with an intramedullary pin, the wires should also encircle the pin. Interfragmentary wires are used to appose fragments in flat bone fractures, particularly those of the mandible. Twist knots are the most common.

Tension-band wires are employed to counter bending forces on pins or screws used to attach avulsed bone fragments. They should be positioned opposite the direction of pull on the fragment. Although they are passive structures, the cyclic stresses are reduced if they are tightened firmly. The wires are frequently placed in a figure-of-eight configuration and tied with one or two twist knots (Figure 3.11).

Bone screws and plates

Screws
Screws convert the torque of insertion into compression along their shaft. They are used individually to compress or hold fragments, or in conjunction with a bone plate. In most instances of individual use, they are applied in lag fashion so that fragments are compressed together. The near fragment is drilled to the diameter of the threads while the far fragment is drilled to the core diameter and, for most screws, threads are cut with a tap. As the screw is tightened, the head of the screw compresses the near fragment on to the far fragment. The amount of compression that can be achieved is dictated

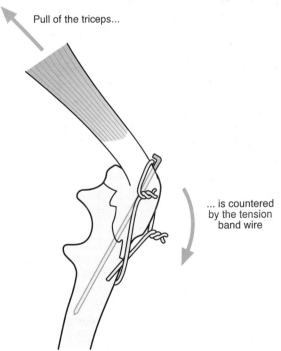

Figure 3.11: A tension band wire is a passive structure that resists the pull of a distracting muscle that is acting on the end of a pin or screw.

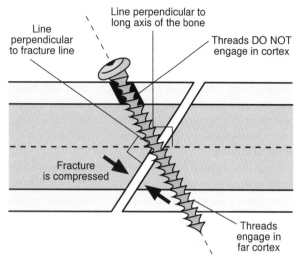

Figure 3.12: *A screw placed in lag fashion is used to compress two fragments together. Screw threads engage the far cortex but not the near cortex. As the screw is tightened, compression is achieved. The optimal orientation for the screw in shorter oblique fractures is half way between a line drawn perpendicular to the fracture line and a line drawn perpendicular to the long axis of the bone.*

by the strength of the bone threads in the far cortex. For optimal compression, the screw is ideally placed perpendicular to the fracture line. When the fracture is short and oblique, this is not feasible and will often result in sliding of the fracture fragments. The optimal angle is then half-way between perpendicular to the fracture and perpendicular to the axis of the bone (Figure 3.12). (The same principle holds if skewer pins and cerclage wires are used for a similar purpose.)

In a number of instances the screw must resist bending and the surgeon must select the appropriate sized implant. The bending strength of a screw is determined by the AMI of its core diameter. This relationship involves raising the radius to the fourth power. A 4.5 mm cortical screw is 2.5 times as strong as a 3.5 mm screw.

Plates

Bone plates are effective in resisting all three of the forces that must be countered – compression, bending and torsion. They are most susceptible to bending forces because of their eccentric position relative to the axis of the bone. Their mode of placement dictates the level of risk associated with a repair. If a fracture is anatomically reduced and the fragments are compressed by the plate, the bone and plate share the load, their combined AMI is large, and the construct is strong (Figure 3.13a). If the bone is not reconstructed, particularly the cortex away from the plate, the plate alone must resist bending forces. The solid section of a plate is usually strong enough but if a screw hole is located within the fracture the screw hole is the weakest point. The AMI is greatly reduced and there is a concentration of stress (Figure 3.13c).

To reduce the stress concentration effect, the limited contact plate (LCP) was designed with a scalloped profile to the surface that is in contact with the bone. Because the AMI is similar over the length of the plate, there is little concentrating effect of the stress. The solid section of the LCP is significantly weaker than the solid section of the regular dynamic compression

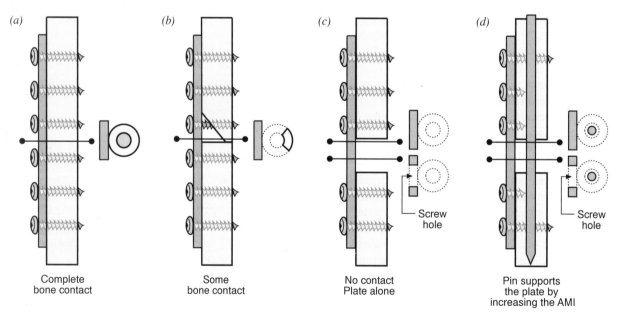

Figure 3.13: *The bending strength of a fractured bone repaired with a bone plate is affected by the integrity of the bone after the repair. (a) If the bone is fully rebuilt, its dimensions can be included in the estimation of the AMI at the weakest point of the repair. The bone protects the plate from bending loads. (b) If the far cortex makes contact, this will also contribute to the AMI at the weakest point. Because the bone contact is some distance from the plate, this provides some mechanical advantage. (c) If there is no contact between the bone fragments, the plate must resist all the bending forces. The AMI of the weakest point must be considered when assessing the stability of the repair. (d) By combining a plate with an intramedullary pin, the AMI of the comminuted area is greatly enhanced.*

plate (DCP). LCPs rely on the presumption that, when the solid section is bearing the load alone, the bone will usually also contribute to the strength of the repair. If a hole does need to be left unfilled, the plate is only as strong as its weakest point and the reduced strength of the solid section will have little effect on outcome. Also, the original LCPs were made of pure titanium, which, though weaker and less stiff, has superior fatigue resistance. The scalloped contour also reduces the amount of cortical bone that is devitalized by the plate's interference with periosteal blood supply.

Plates may still be used for repair in fractures in which it is not possible to reconstruct portions of the shaft or in which it is felt that the extensive dissection necessary to incorporate all fragments into a repair would compromise healing. Lengthening plates, which come with a range of lengths of the solid section, can be used in bones that are large enough to accommodate a 4.5 mm screw. Another approach that can be used in bones of all sizes combines a plate applied to the primary proximal and distal fragments with an intramedullary pin (Figure 3.13d). The plate effectively prevents fragment collapse and rotation but, without the pin, the central span that is unattached to the bone is subjected to bending. By adding the intramedullary pin to the repair, the AMI of the implants is greatly increased and the risk of plate failure greatly reduced.

GLOSSARY

This section gives more detail of terms highlighted in bold earlier in the chapter, in the order in which they first appeared.

Stress
When an external load is resisted by a structure, internal forces are generated. These internal forces are termed stress. In complex structures with complex forces (such as bones), the stress is also complex. Two approaches are used to simplify the understanding of stress. The forces can be simplified to a single important direction or the stresses can be considered only in certain important directions. One important point to remember is that stress is distributed over the cross-sectional area of a structure, and so the magnitude at any one point will be influenced by this dimension. The usual units for stress are Newtons/mm^2 (N/mm^2) or Pascals (Pa).

Strain
When an external load is resisted by a structure, the structure deforms. Often, the internal deformations that compound to produce the overall change in shape must be considered. These internal deformations are termed strain. Because they describe deformation within a material, they are expressed as a ratio of the change in length to the original length; the usual terminology is percentage. Strain, like stress, is complex within complex structures and similar techniques are used to simplify their understanding. For example, if a piece of cortical bone 10 mm long is compressed, it will shorten as the load increases. Because we know that the failure strain of bone in compression is approximately 2%, we know that if the load applied reduces the height of our piece of bone to 9.8 mm, it will probably break.

Stiffness
When a load is applied to a structure and it deforms, the relationship between the load and deformation represents the stiffness of the structure. In most simple cases, stiffness is assumed to be linear and is denoted by a single number with units of Newtons/mm. It is represented graphically by the slope of the load *versus* deformation curve. In fracture mechanics this is often an important parameter to consider: the stiffer the structure, the less motion will be present at the fracture site.

Modulus
If the stress and strain are calculated for a structure that had a load *versus* deformation test, the slope of that curve is termed the modulus. It denotes the stiffness of the material, in contrast to the stiffness of a structure. Its units are the same as stress - Newtons/mm^2 or Pascals. Modulus is useful for comparing materials and making assumptions about how structures might behave based on their material. An example would be the comparison of a bone plate made of stainless steel *versus* one made of titanium. The modulus of steel is greater than that of titanium; so, for a similar load and given that the plates have the same dimensions, there would be less movement with a steel plate.

Isotropic and anisotropic
If a material is homogeneous, the expected response will be the same, no matter what is the direction of the applied load. This material is isotropic. The steel of implants is isotropic.

When a material or a structure has a direction in how it is put together, its response to a load will depend on the direction from which the load is applied. This material is anisotropic. Most biological materials are anisotropic and to appreciate the properties of the material fully it is important to denote its orientation relative to the forces impacting it.

Shear
Shear is generated when an applied force causes two parts of the structure to want to slide past one another. This is most easily demonstrated at interfaces between two objects when one goes one way and the other another, but is also present within a structure when the base is held firm and the top is pushed. Shear can refer to a way in which a force is applied and to the types of stress that are present within a material. Shear stress is created when torsional forces are applied to bone.

Area moment of inertia

Area moment of inertia (AMI) is a structural parameter important in assessing resistance to bending. It quantitates not only the cross-sectional area, but also how the material is distributed. In pure compression or tension, cross-sectional area alone provides an estimate of a structure's strength. In bending, one side of a structure experiences tension and the other compression. There is a plane along the structural centre that experiences no force; this is termed the neutral plane. Material further from the neutral plane is better able to resist the forces in the structure, and so the formulae for calculation of this parameter emphasize this distance. For a circular structure, the formula is $(\pi.r^4)/4$, where r is the radius. The influence of increasing the diameter on a structure's ability to resist bending is easily appreciated. For a rectangular structure, the equation is $(b.h^3)/12$, where b is the width and h is the height. Because the terms width and height relate to the orientation of the rectangle relative to the bending force, it is important first to determine in which direction bending will occur before computing this parameter. For example, a 3.5 mm bone plate (10 x 3 mm) on the lateral aspect of the femur would be expected to fail in mediolateral bending before craniocaudal bending, because the AMI in the mediolateral direction is 29.9 mm^4 and in the craniocaudal direction is 250 mm^4. It is also important to realize that AMI is influenced by the plane chosen in measuring the dimensions. When analysing an implant or fracture repair, consider the weakest portion. Using the 3.5 mm bone plate example, the AMI in the mediolateral direction through a hole is only 14.8 mm^4.

Polar moment of inertia

Polar moment of inertia is a similar concept to area moment of inertia except that it defines the dimension of a structure at a certain plane relative to its ability to resist torsional forces. This parameter quantitates the way in which the structure is distributed around the centre of the torsional effect. This is obviously easy for circular structures but becomes more complex with complex shapes. For a hollow cylinder (like a bone) being twisted around its longitudinal axis, the equation is $^1/_2.\pi.(r^4 - r'^4)$, where r is the outer radius and r' is the inner radius.

CHAPTER FOUR

Fracture Healing

Tim M. Skerry

INTRODUCTION

Fracture healing is a specialized form of wound repair in which there is regeneration of the injured issue without scar formation. The mechanisms behind such a remarkable response involve bone growth, modelling and remodelling. The control of fracture repair therefore involves the same local and systemic influences capable of affecting bone in other circumstances.

The purpose of this chapter is to provide a brief introduction to the cellular processes that are activated when bone fractures, and to explain:

- The implications of concurrent injury, disease or treatment on the progress of a healing fracture
- The mechanisms behind the novel treatments for enhancement of healing which are beginning to appear in the clinics.

ACUTE EVENTS AFTER BONE FRACTURE

In addition to the local events that occur immediately after fracture, there is an acute inflammatory response to the injury. The major systemic effect of this inflammation is the acute phase response (APR), a process that appears to have a protective function for the organism (for reviews see Lewis, 1986; McGlave, 1990). Local inflammation associated with injury causes changes in the circulating concentrations of the acute phase proteins. These include proteins with coagulation and complement system functions, their inhibitors, transport proteins and C-reactive protein. The APR is also associated with changes in hormones (insulin, glucocorticoids and catecholamines), vitamins and minerals — primarily iron and zinc. There is also activation of proteolytic enzyme cascades connected with clotting, complement, kinin and fibrinolytic pathways, and a change in amino acid metabolism, with breakdown of muscle protein.

Locally, the acute events after fracture follow the same initial sequence seen in other tissues, with bleed-

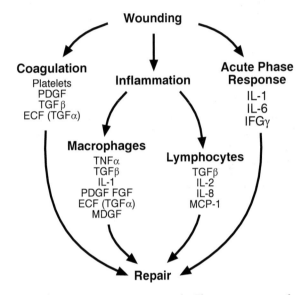

Figure 4.1 The inflammatory cascade. The consequences of injury include the different stages of the inflammatory process in which are expressed many of the same cytokines as those with effects on bone physiology.

ing, progressing through organization of the clot, angiogenesis and fibrosis. At this stage, events in bone begin to differ from other tissues, as the fibrous callus is replaced by cartilage which undergoes endochondral ossification and eventually remodelling.

It is important to consider the mechanisms of these acute changes, because the so-called inflammatory cytokines (Figure 4.1) are in many cases regulators of normal bone function (Table 4.1). This is entirely in accordance with the needs of an early inflammatory response to injury. However, persistent inflammation (as a sequel to infection, for example) may cause aberrant or inappropriate effects by direct actions on the cells that are attempting to repair the fracture.

TYPES OF FRACTURE HEALING

Indirect fracture healing

In normal circumstances after a fracture, there will be some degree of instability of the bone ends. The movement between the bones will not support imme-

Cytokine	Osteoclast formation/activity	Osteoblast growth/activity	Resorption *in vivo*	Formation *in vivo*
IL-1β	+ / +	+ / –	+	+
TNFα	+ / +	+ / –	+	
IFNγ	– /	– / ~	–	
IL-6	+ /	– / ~		
GM-CSF	~ /	+ /		
TGFβ	~ / ~	+ / +	~	+
FGF		~ / ~		
PDGF		~ / –		

Table 4.1: Cytokines implicated in bone formation and resorption. Most of the cytokines in this table are also implicated in the inflammatory response, showing the pleiotropic actions of these agents. The complex actions of cytokines are illustrated by the divergence between actions of individual agents on specific cells in vitro, *seen as ~ which denotes different results by different workers. In addition, the lack of correlation between* in vitro *and* in vivo *actions, or stimulation of both formation and resorption by a single agent, suggest that the picture presented by these data are far from complete. + = expression; – = no expression; space = no data.*

diate formation of new bone, and a tissue with the ability to deform more than bone must be made as an intermediate. Fibrous tissue is therefore produced by fibroblasts in the organizing clot around the fracture. In the organization process, capillary invasion and angiogenesis occur so that the clot becomes accessible to other precursor cells via the circulation. The fibrous tissue stabilizes the fracture enough to permit cartilage survival, and a wave of metaplasia passes from each side of the periosteal cuff of the callus across the fracture gap. The cartilage is then replaced by bone in endochondrial fashion.

Biologically, this indirect fracture healing is a sensible process. Since the clot forms a mass around the fracture site, the ensuing callus forms a large cuff around the bone ends so that, as the organization process occurs, the sequential stiffening of the tissues provides good mechanical stability. When the bones have united, the fracture is stronger than the surrounding normal bone, and remodelling (see below) reduces the superfluous mass so that eventually complete restoration of normal function and strength can occur.

Direct fracture healing

There are circumstances in which the presence of fracture callus is a serious obstacle to a return to function. This is rarely the case in midshaft fractures of long bones, but where a fracture includes part of an articular surface, rapid anatomical realignment of the fragments is the primary consideration. If this is performed and the fragments are held rigidly, direct fracture healing can occur with little or no callus formation. In this circumstance, Haversian systems can cross the fracture gap and repair the cortical bone directly without any endochondral processes. Where defects exist in cancellous bone, with sufficient stability, it is possible for trabeculae to regenerate directly. This can occur by axial growth of new elements along collagen and elastin fibres which form within the defect (Aaron and Skerry, 1994).

Direct fracture healing does not occur without surgical intervention. The ASIF developed the ideas that anatomical reduction, rigid fixation and rapid return to normal function were the ideal goals of treatment (see Chapter 9). In many fractures, perfect anatomical reduction is not necessary for good function, and rigid fixation can have adverse effects on the rate of healing. Fractures fixed with plates, which heal by direct union, are weaker than the surrounding bone and take much longer to unite than those that heal by indirect union. It is tempting to assemble the 'jigsaw' in order to obtain a satisfactory postoperative radiograph, but the reduction of use of plate fixation in human orthopaedics, and the increase of use of intramedullary nails and external fixators, implies that other considerations may be more important (see Chapter 10).

FRACTURE REPAIR, BONE GROWTH AND REMODELLING

When the processes involved in fracture repair are dissected into their component parts, there are many similarities with bone growth and remodelling (Table 4.2) . In both growth and fracture repair, endochondral ossification occurs to convert a mineralized cartilage template into new bone tissue, using the same regulated chondrocyte differentiation pathway. Because of these similarities, understanding of fracture healing is simplified if the controlling influences of the individual component processes are considered separately.

	Growth (endochondral)	Growth (apposition)	Remodelling	Fracture repair
Chondrocyte differentiation	+			+
Cartilage resorption	+			+
Bone formation	+	+	+	+
Bone resorption	+	+	+	+

Table 4.2: *Similar component cellular processes are combined differently to give rise to such diverse tissue actions as longitudinal bone growth and fracture healing.*

Endochondral ossification and appositional growth

During the normal endochondral ossification process, chondrocytes in the growth plate undergo an ordered developmental sequence. Chondrocytes in callus, probably originating from cells within the periosteum or from differentiating cells in the organizing haematoma, undergo the same sequence of events.

After mineralization of cartilage, there is capillary invasion and recruitment of cells resembling osteoclasts. Since they resorb cartilage, not bone, they are termed chondroclasts, but there is no evidence that they are a separate cell type. The cells resorb crescent-shaped pieces of calcified cartilage matrix, analogous to the Howships' lacunae resorbed from bone by osteoclasts. New bone is then formed in those defects.

New bone formation at this stage is similar to the appositional formation that occurs with periosteal expansion during growth. Mature osteoblasts line the surfaces, and secrete matrix in a highly polarized fashion, so that it is deposited on the side nearest to the bone. This highly regulated polarization is controlled by specific cytokines and moderators of their function at different levels in the periosteum. For example, transforming growth factor ß (TGFß) is expressed by osteoblasts on the bone surface and in a more peripheral zone two or three cell layers further away from the surface. Interestingly, the zone between these two layers does not contain TGFß, and in the more peripheral zone the actions of the peptide are moderated by expression of the latent TGFß-binding protein, which is absent on the bone surface.

The new bone matrix differs from cartilage in that the predominant collagen is type I (type II is the predominant fibrillar collagen in cartilage), although the same chondroitin sulphate and some keratan sulphate proteoglycans are also present. Mineralization of this osteoid proceeds with focal calcifications occurring around matrix vesicles. While most osteoblasts advance with the deposition of matrix, some remain and become incorporated in the new bone as osteocytes. It was thought that this was a passive process. However, during the development of fish bone, all the osteoblasts continue to advance with the periosteal surface, so that no osteocytes are formed. This suggests that mammalian osteocytes are osteoblasts that made a committed step to stop advancing by substituting polarized secretion with a generalized secretion of matrix proteins.

Bone formation during fracture healing, whether endochondral or appositional, results in replacement of the large mass of the soft periosteal and endosteal callus with bone. However, at this stage, although there is restoration of function in that the bone is able to withstand loading, the mass of the callus is excessive. In addition, the bulk of the callus may interfere with normal muscle and tendon movements. To convert the relatively disorganized bony callus into a restored cortical tube, the callus must be remodelled — a process entailing bone resorption.

Bone resorption and callus remodelling

Bone resorption is accomplished by osteoclasts, which must perform two roles: removal of the hydroxyapatite mineral phase of the bone with acid; and degradation of the collagenous and non-collagenous proteins with enzymes. Osteoclasts are highly polarized cells that initiate resorption after attaching to the bone surface at the periphery of their zone of contact. This sealing or clear zone contains contractile proteins including osteopontin, which are secreted by the osteoclast to facilitate attachment. Osteoclast attachment to bone matrix is also facilitated by integrins — a class of cell matrix attachment molecules found in many tissues. Interestingly osteoclast attachment is mediated by an $\alpha V \beta 3$ integrin, whose ß3 subunit appears to be exclusive to these cells and is different from the ß2 subunit expressed by closely related cells of the monocyte macrophage lineage. This specificity may have therapeutic implications, as neutralizing antibodies to the osteoclast integrins inhibit bone resorption (Horton *et al.*, 1991).

Tight attachment allows the osteoclast to maintain specific conditions in the resorption space where the pH may drop as low as 3 (Silver *et al.*, 1988). Acidification of the resorption space is the result of secretion of hydrogen ions, produced by the action of carbonic anhydrase and transported across the osteoclast's 'ruffled border' cell membrane by a specific proton pump. This appears to be uniquely expressed in osteoclasts and different from the classical vacuolar and potassium ATPase pumps found in other cells. A chloride/bicarbonate exchanger in the basal membrane of the cell maintains the osteoclast's intracellular pH, which would otherwise rise with acidification of the resorption space. Degradation of matrix proteins is accomplished by neutral protease enzymes such as cathepsins, which are secreted into the resorption space.

Bone resorption in remodelling is responsible for removal of the now superfluous mass of periosteal and endosteal callus. At the same time, Haversian remodelling occurs in the intracortical callus to restore normal compact bone structure.

Haversian remodelling

Haversian remodelling is an ordered process of bone resorption and formation within the cortex, which gives the classical histological appearance of concentric lamellae in adult bone. It is important to distinguish this from the primary osteonal bone seen in younger animals, which is a feature only of rapid growth and not previous resorption.

Primary osteons arise when a periosteal bone surface expands rapidly in young growing animals. The osteoblasts in periosteum form osteoid matrix, as described previously, but in an irregular way so that some areas of the advancing front proceed faster than others. The consequence of this is that gaps lined with osteoblasts are left in the new bone surface and these fill in concentrically. Primary osteons are therefore characterized by concentric lamellae of bone, which do not interrupt the more linear lamellae that represent the line of the advancing mineralizing front (Figure 4.2). In appearance they are not dissimilar from knots in wood.

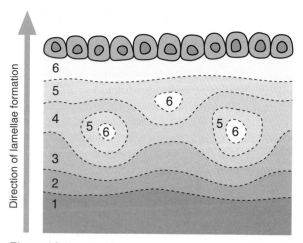

Figure 4.2: As osteoblasts appose new bone on a periosteal surface, primary osteons result from concentric infilling of spaces left as the developing front of formation advances unevenly. The lamellae between the primary osteons are continuous and are not interrupted by the osteons. Numbers show the order of deposition of lamellae.

Secondary osteons or Haversian systems are superficially similar to primary osteons, but arise when a group of osteoclasts tunnel into a surface and proceed along the length of the bone (Figure 4.3). At the same time as the tunnelling is proceeding, capillary growth occurs to maintain supplies to the cells, and to bring in osteoblast precursors. The osteoblasts fill in the tunnel concentrically as the osteoclasts continue to resorb bone, so that in cross-section a Haversian system, like a primary osteon, contains concentric lamellae. However, the concentric lamellae of the Haversian system cut through the pre-existing lamellae of the bone.

ENHANCEMENT OF FRACTURE HEALING

Increased understanding of the control of bone cells and the way that local interactions occur has led to some exciting new ideas with direct relevance to the clinician. The idea of using biological materials to enhance fracture healing or to stimulate filling of defects has progressed beyond bone grafting, and may explain some of the mechanisms by which that technique can be so effective. Experiments have shown the profound effects of demineralized bone matrix in stimulating bone formation *in vivo* (Syftestad *et al.*, 1984), and this appears to be due to stimulatory effects of some of the extracellular matrix components as well as mitogenic growth factors such as the insulin-like growth factors, transforming growth factor ß (TGFß) and the bone morphogenetic proteins (BMPs) which are present in large quantities in bone. Direct application of exogenous TGFß or BMPs have been shown to stimulate profound bone formation in healing fractures (Bolander, 1992). The actions of these agents may be related to their roles in development, where limb morphogenesis is linked to BMP expression (Jones *et al.*, 1991). Such therapies are not confined to the laboratory. Growth factor-loaded bone cements and bone substitutes are in development for clinical use, and may offer radical advances for treatment of inactive non-unions, where biological activity has ceased.

Finally, it is appropriate to consider mechanical loading as a method of effecting fracture healing. Bone cells are rapidly responsive to strain in the matrix (Skerry *et al.*, 1989), and interfragmentary movement has been shown to stimulate more rapid progression of indirect healing than totally rigid fixation (Goodship and Kenwright, 1985). It is of extreme importance to distinguish these micromovement regimes from the gross movements that occur at inadequately fixed fracture sites. The latter will not enhance healing! The use of controlled micromovement has become accepted to the degree that fixators are now dynamized to allow small movements at the fracture

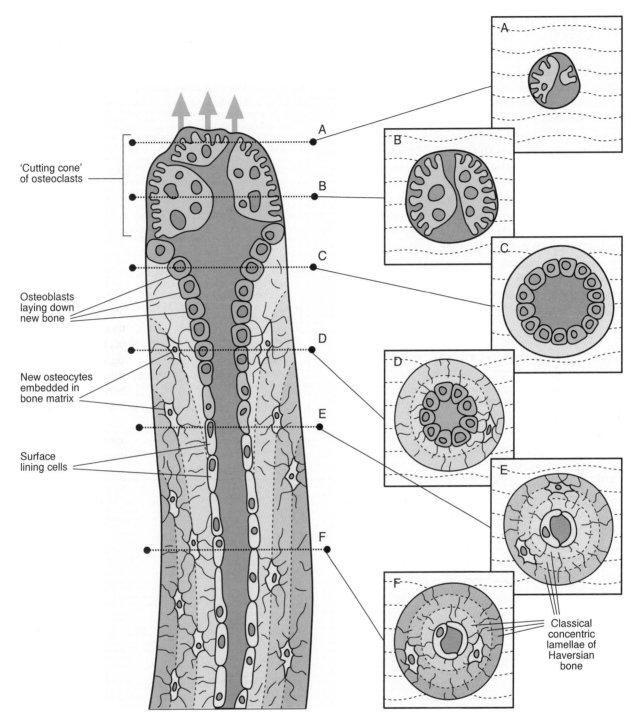

Figure 4.3: *Central figure: Haversian or secondary osteons are the result of tunnelling into the bone cortex by a 'cutting cone' composed of osteoclasts. Immediately behind the osteoclasts, populations of active osteoblasts lay down new bone and gradually become less active as lining cells which cover the surface. Some osteoblasts become incorporated into the new bone matrix as osteocytes. (A)–(C) Cross-sections show progressive expansion of the resorbing Haversian canal as the cutting cone of osteoclasts erode out of the plane of the diagram. (D)–(F) Osteoblasts fill in the defect, resulting in the classical concentric lamellae of secondarily remodelled Haversian bone. These lamellae interrupt the original lamellae of the primary bone.*

site, in order to stimulate the cells and enhance the healing. Recent research into the early consequences of loading on bone cell gene expression has already led to the identification of a number of possible pharmacological targets which could mimic the effects of loading in situations where the application of movement is impractical. The discovery that bone cells communicate via excitatory amino acids, previously thought to be involved only in intercellular communication within the CNS, is one example of a route by which the healing of fractures might be enhanced (Mason *et al.*, 1997).

CONCLUSIONS

Fracture healing is a remarkable process in that it is one of the most successful repair mechanisms in the body. When one considers the immense complexity of the cellular interactions that occur to restore the continuity of fractured bones, it is surprising that so few problems occur. Increased understanding of the fundamental physical and biochemical influences on bone is having a considerable impact on clinical treatments, and will continue to do so. The relative ease of production of recombinant osteotropic biochemicals and the development of novel methods of application and delivery mean that fracture treatments are likely to advance beyond recognition in a short time. Since technological advances invariably appear to exceed predictions, the only certainty about the future is that it will be even more exciting than anything which is currently perceived to be possible.

REFERENCES AND FURTHER READING

Aaron JE and Skerry TM (1994) Intramembranous trabecular generation in normal bone. *Bone and Mineral* **25**(3), 211.

Bolander ME (1992) Regulation of fracture repair by growth factors. *Proceedings of the Society for Experimental Biology and Medicine* **200**, 165.

Currey JD (1984) What should bones be designed to do? *Calcified Tissue International* **36**(S1), 7.

Goodship AE and Kenwright J (1985) The influence of induced micromovement upon the healing of experimental tibial fractures. *Journal of Bone and Joint Surgery* **67B**, 650.

Horton MA, Taylor ML, Arnett TR and Helfrich MH (1991) Arg-Gly-Asp (RGD) peptides and the anti-vitronectin receptor antibody 23C6 inhibit dentine resorption and cell spreading by osteoclasts. *Experimental Cell Research* **195**, 368.

Jones CM, Lyons KM and Hogan BLM (1991) Involvement of bone morphogenetic protein-4 (BMP-4) and Vgr-1 in morphogenesis and neurogenesis in the mouse. *Development* **111**, 531.

Lewis GP (1986) *Mediators of Inflammation*, Wright, Bristol.

Mason DJ, Suva LJ, Genever PG *et al.* (1997) Mechanically regulated expression of a neural glutamate transporter in bone. A role for excitatory amino acids as osteotropic agents. *Bone* **20**, 4–9.

McGlave P (1990) Bone marrow transplants in chronic myelogenous leukaemia: an overview of determinants of survival. *Seminars in Haematology* **27**, 23–30.

Nathan CF and Sporn MB (1991) Cytokines in context. *Journal of Cell Biology* **113**, 981.

Rosati R, Horan GSB, Pinero GJ *et al.* (1994) Normal long bone growth and development in type X collagen-null mice. *Nature Genetics* **8**, 129.

Silver IA, Murrills RJ and Etherington DJ (1988) Microelectrode studies on the acid microenvironment beneath adherent macrophages and osteoclasts. *Experimental Cell Research* **175**, 266.

Skerry TM and Fermor B (1993) Mechanical and hormonal influences *in vivo* cause regional differences in bone remodelling. In *Mechanical Interactions with Cells,* ed. F Lyall and AJ El Haj, p. 97. Cambridge University Press, Cambridge.

Skerry TM, Bitensky L, Chayen J and Lanyon LE (1989) Early strain-related changes in enzyme activity in osteocytes following bone loading *in vivo. Journal of Bone and Mineral Research* **4**, 783.

Syftestad GT, Triffitt JT, Urist MR and Caplan AI (1984) An osteo-inductive bone matrix extract stimulates the *in vitro* conversion of mesenchyme into chondrocytes. *Calcified Tissue International* **36**, 625.

Vaes G (1988) Cellular biology and biochemical mechanism of bone resorption. A review of recent developments on the formation, activation, and mode of action of osteoclasts. *Clinical Orthopaedics* **231**, 239.

CHAPTER FIVE

Imaging of Fracture Healing

D. Gary Clayton Jones

INTRODUCTION

The monitoring of the healing of fractures is based upon both the clinical progression of the patient and the evaluation of the process by ancillary examination. By far the most common method of examination is radiography and this is likely to be the situation for the foreseeable future in veterinary practice. The initial diagnosis of fractures and the planning of treatment methods is generally based on the X-ray examinations and therefore an initial base line of information is already available to enable comparison with the subsequent healing process.

Standard views should be made during any subsequent examination, generally using two views at right angles. Occasionally other views may be indicated to examine a particular feature of the fracture process, e.g. oblique or stressed views. If all exposure factors are recorded and kept constant along with the other radiographic parameters, then useful comparisons may also be made later in terms of bone density/calcification. When large metallic implants are present then they may obscure the fracture line in one view and this can make for more difficult interpretation as only one view may be possible. Similarly, allowances need to be made when radiographs are taken through a cast or splint, particularly if the cast or splint is only partially radiolucent.

It must be remembered that radiographic changes of bone will often appear to lag behind changes that may be perceived clinically and that the rate of radiographic change will depend on:

- Age of the patient
- Method of repair
- Type of fracture
- Associated soft tissue injury.

TIMING OF RADIOGRAPHS

Films may usefully be obtained at a number of time periods following a fracture. However, economics or the condition/nature of the patient may preclude some of these examinations.

Immediate post-operative
This study provides the base line for further examination and indicates the quality of the reduction and the position of any implants (Figures 5.1 and 5.2).

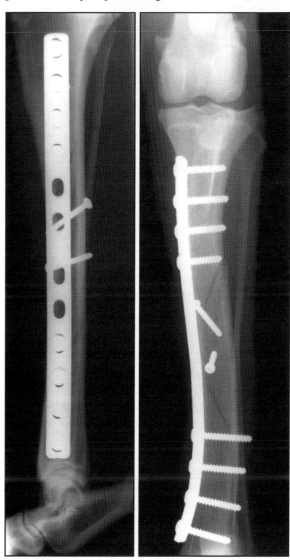

Figure 5.1: Immediate post-operative films of a Bernese Mountain Dog's tibial fracture, treated using lag screws and a plate and screws. These films allowed evaluation of overall reduction of the fracture fragments, size of the fracture gaps, effectiveness of contouring of the plate with respect to the bone surface and the length and position of the lag screws and the plate screws.

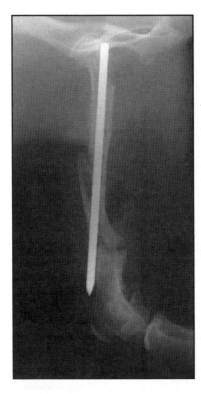

Figure 5.2: Immediate post-operative film of intramedullary pinning of a non-union, showing failure of the implant to engage in the distal femoral segment. The dog had to return to the theatre for repositioning of the pin.

Ten to 14 days
This will be at around the time of suture and soft dressing removal and would be the period when soft tissue changes should be resolving, or commencing if a post-operative infection is establishing.

Four to 6 weeks
Fracture healing is generally advancing significantly by this time. Where callus is expected or required it will normally be adequately calcified at this stage to be readily visible. There may be little to see sooner than this, especially in adult animals, even when fracture repair is progressing well. Implant failures due to cyclic loading will often be noted at about this time.

Towards the end of healing
This is the time at which a decision will be made as to whether the animal can be allowed more normal activity and whether implant removal is to be considered. The time taken to reach this point will vary.

Prior to implant retrieval
It is always better to make a radiographic assessment of healing rather than to rely on an elapsed calendar period to determine implant removal. This assessment is often complicated by poor visualization of the fracture because of overlay of the image of a plate. The nature of the region around the fracture is also examined as extensive covering of implants by new bone formation may complicate the retrieval operation.

After removal of implants
This is the examination that may now allow assessment of the fracture line on all views and sometimes it may be noted that an apparently healed fracture is less well repaired than expected, indicating that some secondary treatment may be required.

At secondary procedures
When a fracture has not healed by the first procedure and further treatments have to be made, or when fracture repair progresses more slowly than normal, then further radiographic examinations may be required, as indicated by the particular features of the individual case.

EXAMINATION OF THE FILM

All of the visible structures on the film should be examined systematically to obtain the maximum information. These include:

- Skin
- Soft tissues – muscle planes, ligaments, tendons, lymph nodes
- Joints – articular surfaces, joint space, regions of attachment of ligaments and joint capsule
- Bone – periosteum, cortex, endosteum, medullary cavity and fracture ends
- Implants – shape and position and the bone/implant interface.

The possible changes that can be seen in bone are quite limited and will involve loss of bone, production of bone or no change in the bone.

Bone loss (resorption or loss of density/fine structure)
Loss of bone is generally associated with hypervascularity and may be the result of motion, infection, dystrophy, allergy, metalosis or tumour.

- At the fracture line a small amount of resorption is probably normal, even when there is rigid internal fixation. However, when significant it indicates instability, infection or corrosion (Figures 5.3 and 5.10).
- At the bone implant junction it usually indicates motion, infection, corrosion or early stress protection (see Figure 5.8).
- Beneath the implant it indicates established infection/neoplasia or stress protection.
- All of the complicating conditions mentioned may ultimately involve the bone substance at some distance from the vicinity of the fracture.
- Disuse osteoporosis is usually noted distal to the fracture, often involving the smaller bones of the carpus or tarsus (Figures 5.4 and 5.5).
- Severe progressive resorption of fracture ends is seen in the uncommon atrophic non-union (see Chapter 26).

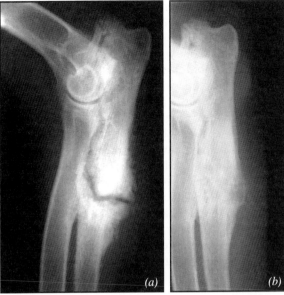

Figure 5.3: *Mastiff, 18 months old. (a) Widened osteotomy line, one month after osteotomy of the ulnar shaft for treatment of ununited anconeus. The osteotomy is only supported by the radial shaft and so there is movement at the fracture plane. Note the hypertrophic bone formation and the irregular periosteal reaction of active irritation callus extending proximally and distally on the ulnar shaft. (b) The same case 3 months later with bridging of the gap and infilling with woven bone, almost complete resolution of the periosteal reaction and remodelling of the callus.*

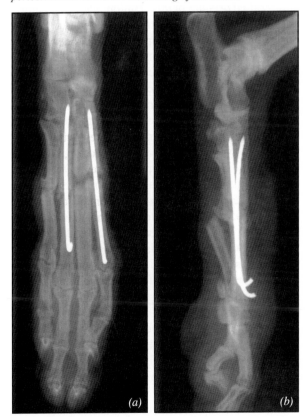

Figure 5.4: *Immediate post-operative film of long-standing non-union of metatarsal fractures treated with intramedullary pinning. The ends of the bones of digit III (the unsupported digit) show a long-standing resorption of the fracture ends but no evidence of any callus formation, in spite of previous external support treatment.*

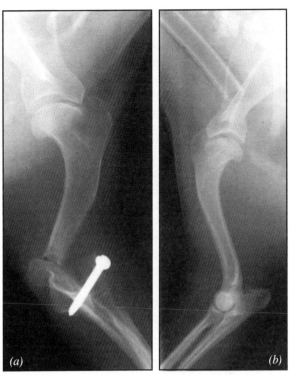

Figure 5.5a,b: *Yorkshire terrier with a distal humeral non-union. Note the loss of density of the humeral condylar fragments as well as the loss of density and coarse trabecular appearance in the bones of the forearm below the fracture. The opposite leg contrasts the loss of density and bone structure with an identical radiographic exposure.*

Bone production

At the *fracture line*, bone production may indicate primary union if the gap is filled evenly and at right angles to the fracture line. Gap healing is seen when the bone is formed parallel to the fracture line. When bone forms parallel to the fracture gap but fails to bridge the gap, this may progress so as to seal the medullary cavity and indicates there is motion in the fracture gap and a non-union is developing.

At the *bone/implant junction*, motion may result in formation of a sclerotic line at a slight distance from the surface of the implant. At the junction of the end of the implant and the bone a small mound of bone can be formed because of the sudden difference in rigidity between the bone/implant montage and the bone alone (stress riser).

At the *periosteum* level, bone production is either periostitis or the natural healing response at a fracture, termed periosteal callus. New bone may form below the periosteum or above the surface.

- *Periostitis* (irritation callus) (Figure 5.3)
  develops as the result of infection or instability,
  or following trauma due to surgery. It tends to be
  more obvious in younger patients, in which it
  may be difficult to avoid entirely. It is rapid in
  development and has an irregular, poorly defined
  surface. The density and the fine structure are

also irregular. It may be very large in hypertrophic non-unions. Periosteal reaction is also seen in pathological fractures associated with neoplasia as well as being a reaction to the neoplastic process itself.

- *Bridging callus* is the combination of periosteal reaction, endosteal reaction and callus induced within the fracture gap. It bridges the fracture ends and is noted most frequently in cases treated by unstable methods such as external coaptation using casts and splints. It is a less irregular reaction than periostitis. Once the gap has been bridged and the fracture is stable, the surface of the reaction becomes smooth and the density and fine structure are more even.
- *Involucrum* is a specific type of periosteal callus that endeavours to surround the dead bone of sequestra.
- *Endosteal callus* is formed in similar circumstances to periosteal reactions but at a slower rate.

No change in bone

Apparently inert bone is noted occasionally during fracture repair, and repeated radiographs over a period of weeks or months will usually show that there is in fact some very gradual change taking place (Figure 5.4). For bony change to occur there must be a viable blood supply or nearby cellular activity. Thus inert bone indicates loss of blood supply or absence of cellular activity in the neighbourhood.

Avascular fragments or bone ends will remain apparently inert until revascularization occurs.

Biologically inactive non-unions are occasionally noted that show inactivity that is marked by the absence of callus formation at the bone ends or of any change in cortical density or fine structure (see Chapter 26). Bone ends of a fracture supported by a large plate or pin may also be inert if no load bearing is passed through the bone substance (stress protection).

Sequestra are by definition dead bone fragments separated from a blood supply, usually in association with infection. Initially they are not always separated physically from the original bone. They remain as radiodense fragments (often appearing more dense than surrounding inflamed bone that loses density because of hypervascularity) and they only gradually become devoured by phagocytic activity (see Figure 5.10). They then become ragged in outline and have a moth-eaten appearance.

RADIOGRAPHIC APPEARANCE OF HEALING FRACTURES

It is difficult to provide hard and fast rules as to when a fracture is healing normally. The healing of a fracture may occur and be successful in spite of therapy or problems, so that the requirement of radiography is not just to monitor the state of union but to try to assist in determining whether or not any further intervention is required from the surgeon. The age of the patient will have considerable effect on the rate of normal union: fractures in juvenile animals may heal to radiographic union within as little as 3 weeks, whereas they may take two or three times as long in an old animal. The ability of bone to develop a profuse periosteal callus is frequently noted in juvenile patients but the development of a similar callus in an older animal would signify some major problem.

When internal fixation has been performed the 'quality' of the operation will have a direct bearing on the repair. The manner of soft tissue and bone handling will affect periosteal reaction, interference with blood supply may significantly delay healing and the method of repair will determine the type of healing process to be expected.

Healing of bone under stable conditions

This type of healing is noted in bone fragments that are in contact and usually supported by a plate and/or screw fixation so that there is no movement of the fracture ends in relation to one another – so-called *rigid* internal fixation. This type of repair is often promoted by compression of the fracture fragments and is sometimes called *primary* or *direct* union. The only requirement is for there to be good vascularity of the fragments. In the laboratory under experimental conditions this type of repair can be demonstrated reasonably easily. In practice it is rare that true accurate apposition of the fracture ends is achieved perfectly by the surgeon; by the time surgery is performed the fracture fragments will almost always be deformed by splintering, rubbing or the initiating trauma itself, so that there is almost always a combination of *gap healing* and *contact healing* along various parts of the fracture line.

Immediately post-operatively, fine lines or small pockets of air from the surgical procedure can be seen in the soft tissues. These often tend to follow the tissue planes and they should disappear within one or two days. Soft tissue swelling is variable: in cases where there was pre-operative oedema there will usually be a significant reduction in soft tissue swelling within a week as circulation is re-established.

The initial fine lines of the fracture gap and ends remain relatively unchanged for 1 to 2 weeks and may even appear clearer after this time. This is the result of loss of blood supply from the fracture line back to the nearest intact Haversian/Volkmann system, so the bone remains inert until revascularization. Once revascularization has developed, there is a progressive remodelling of the fracture ends by regrowth of Haversian systems by invasion of new osteones. As remodelling is a combination of osteoclastic and osteoblastic activity there may be removal of some bony cortex close to the fracture ends so that there may be a transient apparent slight widening of the fracture gap. The gap becomes more hazy due to new bone production so that by 8 to 12 weeks the fracture lines are filled. Remodelling of the repaired cortex results in virtual absence of the fracture lines after a few months (Figure 5.6).

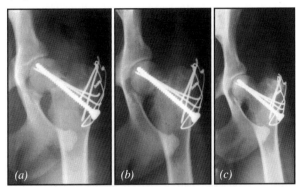

Figure 5.6: *Fracture of the femoral neck in an adult Weimaraner treated by a lag screw and anti-rotational wires via trochanteric osteotomy repaired with pins and tension-band wire. (a) Immediate post-operative film showing the fracture line with clearly defined margins. (b) After 6 weeks the fracture line is still evident but is now hazy, with less well defined margins, and no callus is seen. (c) Fifteen months later the whole region is repaired, with well organized bony bridging and no excess callus, indicating that the repair was stable during the healing period. Clinically the dog made good use of the limb at all times.*

Fracture callus is said not to develop in fractures successfully managed by this method. In practice this is largely true, although a small periosteal callus is sometimes seen. This may be more a reflection of the development of periosteal reaction secondary to the inevitable handling necessary for fracture reduction and the separation of periosteum from the cortex in the region of the fracture by the original trauma, rather than a requirement on the part of the body for a periosteal bridge to be created. Thus only minimal amounts of periosteal new bone should be expected and excessive amounts should be evaluated as indicating some form of fracture complication. Some callus new bone will be produced in those parts of the fracture line where there is a need for gap healing. This initially has an amorphous dense appearance; it fills the gap, and may even be seen to project a little way into the medullary region as endosteal new bone until it remodels to develop a more conventional cortical pattern in later months.

If a gap is present in the cortex opposite the plate then a small bridging callus will often be seen here which develops following micro-movement in this region. When greater than 1 mm, gaps may become filled by fibrous tissue or cartilage rather than bone and remain radiographically apparent until they finally fill with bone.

When a plate has been used for the fracture repair there will be some localized change beneath and near the ends of the plate. Some reduction of bone density

may be noted within a few weeks of the fracture repair. This may be as early as 3 to 4 weeks in younger patients. This is the result of vascular changes in the cortex beneath the plate and also a possible stress protection effect. The vascular changes can be minimized by the use of low contact dynamic compression (LCDC) plates, but the cost of such implants and the apparent unimportance of such changes clinically means that they are rarely used. A small mound of periosteal bone, forming next to the ends of the plate, is noted after a few weeks because of the stress change occurring in the bone at this level. This can be observed to consist of an elevated margin all around the plate when it is removed. However, the new bone on the lateral sides of the plate is difficult to display radiographically. The cortex beneath this periosteal reaction may also become slightly sclerosed (Figure 5.7).

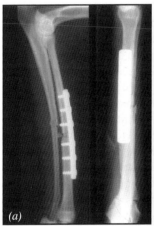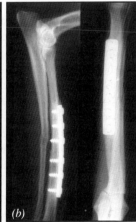

Figure 5.7: *DC plate repair of a radius and ulna fracture in a Poodle. (a) Immediate post-operative film shows a good reduction of the radius and slight displacement of the ulna. A small cortical fragment is visible between the radius and ulna. (b) At 4 months the fractures are healed: the cortices of the radius are continuous, with re-establishment of a normal medullary cavity. No callus formed in this bone but callus formation has united the ulna, which needs remodelling. The cortical fragment has been resorbed. Small mounds of periosteal bone are present at the ends of the plate and the cortex beneath the plate proximally appears slightly sclerotic because of the bone formation along the sides of the plate. Distally a fine lucent line is seen between the plate and the bone, indicating minor cortical resorption from mild stress protection or vascular inhibition. The trabeculae in the medullary cavity are more dense and hazy at the levels of the proximal and distal screws because of the extra stress being transmitted from plate and screws to unsupported bone.*

Healing after partial reduction with minor instability

This type of healing is to be expected with repairs using intramedullary (IM) pins and wires and the external fixator. In these circumstances there is little or no dynamic or static compression at the fracture surface and some minor movements of the fracture fragments may be expected. Reduction is often less well achieved than when compression plates and screws are used. The radiographic changes will then depend on the degree of stability of the fracture site and the size of any gaps or defects. Callus formation is therefore to be expected, and both periosteal and endosteal callus will be noted. IM pin placement may damage the endosteal blood supply so a preponderance of periosteal callus is more likely, especially in those animals where a large diameter pin which almost fills the cavity has been used. The amount of callus depends on the amount of fragment movement and the age of the animal. As IM pins are often used by inexperienced surgeons, the amount of iatrogenic periosteal trauma may also be quite large and this can contribute to the periosteal reaction that is seen. Similarly the placement of cerclage wires often results in circumferential stripping of soft tissue attachments with a resultant reaction.

When healing is progressing normally the callus production will be noted to be fairly limited to the fracture region, to bridge the gap and to have a smooth remodelling outline within a few weeks. A profuse callus, with extension some distance above and below the fracture level, that fails to bridge the fracture gap and has a rough exterior surface suggests an irritation callus secondary to infection or movement. Infection tends to cause a more widespread reactive appearance than movement, which is limited to the ends of the bone near the fracture gap. However, infection and movement are often present simultaneously in the same fracture so that the distinction may be blurred both radiographically and clinically (Figure 5.8).

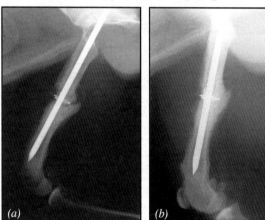

Figure 5.8: Femoral fracture in adult Boxer Dog treated by intramedullary pin and cerclage wires 8 weeks previously. (a) There is a delayed union, with the fracture gap still evident and mineralized callus formation that has not bridged the gap. The callus is large on the caudal cortex and further mineralization is present in the soft tissues. The wires lie in a lucent region, possibly indicating a low-grade infection. Periosteal reaction is evident along the shaft of the bone, almost reaching the metaphysis proximally and distally. (b) Six weeks later the fracture has progressed to union, with healing by callus formation. Much of the periosteal reaction is now smooth and well mineralized and will gradually resorb.

The callus will rapidly remodel once bridging has been achieved, leaving just a small bulge in the outline of the bone and a more dense sclerotic scar that can persist for months or years (Figure 5.8).

External fixators are often used for extensively comminuted or open fractures. In these cases soft tissue trauma may be extreme; reduction may be incomplete or impossible and this will influence the healing noted. Callus formation is usually essential for the repair of such fractures and will be a combination of periosteal, endosteal and induced callus. The callus is often irregular as infection comes under control and because of defects and periosteal damage. Where fragments are displaced from the fracture bed or are separated from their attachments, little change may be noted until the fragments are either revascularized or incorporated into a callus process. Fragments at a

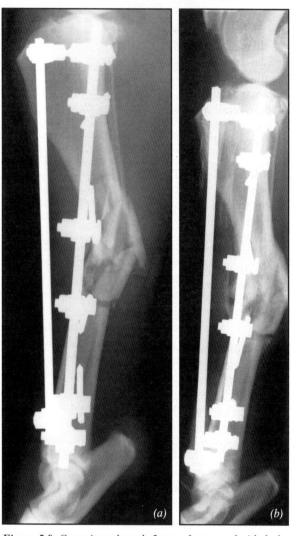

Figure 5.9: Comminuted grade 2 open fracture of mid-shaft tibia in Dobermann treated with type 2 external fixator. (a) Immediate post-reduction film shows soft tissue swelling and gas shadows close to the fracture. Small, separated, dense fragments are visible caudally, level with the distal fracture line. (b) Six weeks later there is extensive periosteal, endosteal and medullary callus engulfing and almost obscuring the comminuted fragments. The small dense fragments are now incorporated in the callus and some have been resorbed. Bridging of the fracture is almost complete. The circumscribed nature of the callus suggests that little motion is present in the fracture region. (Dense linear streaks parallel to the connecting bars are layers of dressing covering the clamps.)

significant distance from the fracture bed may not become incorporated into the healing process but may actually gradually become resorbed. This is a sterile process which is normal if the fragment is no longer required for weight bearing, and does not signify an infection (Figure 5.9).

At the implant/bone junction there is normally a small amount of periosteal and endosteal bone production around the pins, especially at the cortex closest to the connecting bar. A small halo of lysis is often noted next to the pin but this will usually extend to the full thickness of the cortex only if the pins are loosening due to movement. Ring sequestra are rarely noted at the implants but, if present, may also indicate loosening of the implants. There is usually some soft tissue swelling around the pin tracks which persists while the implants are in place. In cases treated by external fixator, soft tissue swelling of the limb is often extensive at the time of original surgery; a general reduction in the overall soft tissue swelling around the limb is a feature of successful repair and may be noted within two weeks of surgery.

Healing by spontaneous repair with moderate instability

Cases treated by conservative methods or by use of coaptation with splints or casts may be considered to be of this type. These will usually be closed fractures and are often only partially reduced. Healing is thus entirely as the result of callus formation without the presence of implants. In these cases there is a gradual formation of periosteal and endosteal callus and it is to be expected that the amount of callus will be greatest in these cases. The callus may often appear to obstruct the medullary canal partially or completely. The amount of callus depends on the amount of fracture movement and the effectiveness of the reduction. The callus is often radiographically visible by 1 to 2 weeks after reduction and bridging is usually complete by 2 to 4 weeks. Soft tissue swelling may be slower to reduce than may be noted in a fracture treated by open reduction, as movement of fracture ends (even within a cast) will continue to induce soft tissue inflammation. The large bridging callus often has a smooth outline and may be seen to be remodelling and reducing in volume at its limits while continuing to enlarge in the region of the fracture gap. Remodelling of the callus is relatively rapid once union has occurred but some change in bone outline may persist for the rest of the life of the animal, though re-establishment of the medullary cavity will often occur. Synostosis of paired bones (e.g. radius and ulna) is common with this method of repair and medullary canal re-establishment may not occur in these cases. This may be of no clinical significance.

Healing of bone graft

Cancellous bone graft is the type of graft most commonly employed in clinical practice, to stimulate healing in a delayed union or non-union or to replace a comminuted segment of bone. In either circumstance it is intended to promote callus. Initially it is relatively radiolucent and may be almost invisible or appear as poorly defined radio-dense fragments at the fracture site on the post-operative film. This may reduce in density over the first 2 weeks but then be replaced by a more widespread amorphous shadow within and around the defect which increases in density and size so as to become a bridging callus. This will consist of a combination of periosteal callus as well as new bone induced within the graft itself.

Cortical grafts are less commonly used and consist of fragments of cortical bone usually separated from their blood supply. In general they are radiographically inert for long periods of time, provided that they are not infected. Callus formation is usually seen at the bone ends of the host bone as they become incorporated. It has been shown that cortical grafts may not develop vascularity for a number of years so they function as a physical strut rather than being truly incorporated. Cancellous bone is often placed around the ends and it is probably this that largely contributes to any radiographic change.

DISTURBANCES OF UNION

These may be the result of delayed union or non-union, infection or implant failure. The radiographic identification of impending problems is important in fracture management and will often be pre-empted by clinical signs. Interpretation is often made because of a departure from what would be expected to be the normal process, which is determined by the mode of treatment that was originally selected (see Chapters 25 and 26).

Acute infection

Acute infection is very important but has few obvious radiographic signs. Soft tissue swelling and possible gas shadows in the soft tissues may be the only early signs during the first few days. This will usually become associated with a faint palisade periosteal reaction which may be quite extensive along the shaft of the bone within 2 to 3 weeks. In a young animal infection can track between the periosteum and the cortex so that the cortex remains smooth, with a lucent line between it and the periosteal shadow. Extension of the periosteal reaction, continuing soft tissue swelling and the development of sequestra are the sequelae as the infection becomes fully established.

Chronic infection

The changes described for acute infection become established and more radiographically apparent and either continue with an extending bony destruction and periosteal reaction or develop to a condition which no longer progresses but remains established with draining tracks, sequestra and involucral new bone around the fragments and draining tracks. There is usually a halo of lysis around any implants which become progressively loose and have a gradually diminishing function. An implant in effect becomes a metallic sequestrum (Figure 5.10).

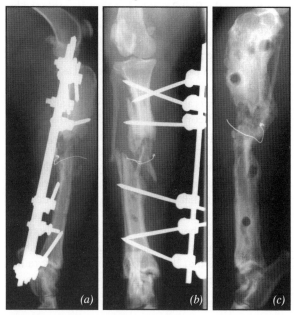

Figure 5.10: Mature Greyhound pet with infected non-union of tibia previously treated by an external fixator. (a,b) The fracture region is surrounded by soft tissue swelling which contains hazy mineralization of ectopic bone formation. The fracture line is poorly marginated, irregular and widened with woolly periosteal reaction. Sequestra are seen in the fracture gap with a broken fragment of cerclage wire. Some resorption of the cortices is evident in the region of the fracture and lucent tracks from previous external fixator pins are visible in the distal segment. (c) Six weeks later the fixator has been removed, leaving large lucent tracks. The original pin tracks have healed. Callus is now partially bridging the fracture caudally, and the bone ends and margins are more clearly defined. The sequestra have been removed. Soft tissue swelling is now much less evident. Further external support was provided and the fracture went on to heal.

Delayed union

A delayed union is one in which the anticipated changes of repair are not as rapid as expected and it has no specific radiographic signs. As most fractures occur in young immature animals there is a general expectation that all fractures heal rapidly, so that when an older animal is presented normal progress for a mature patient becomes diagnosed as delayed union. In a true delayed union the fracture will go on and repair without alteration of the treatment method.

Non-union

Non-union is a pathological process which requires treatment. The diagnostic features radiographically are that bridging of the fracture does not occur and the fragments remain separate. Various types of non-union occur with atrophy of the bone ends, minimal callus, or hypertrophic callus, as well as signs of infection in some cases. The medullary cavities become closed by new bone and develop well-defined sclerotic ends. In long-standing cases a pseudarthrosis develops, in which the ends of the bone remodel until they form a crude ball-and-socket type joint. In the distal limb the socket is distal and the ball is proximal. These features may be reversed in the upper limb.

Stress protection

This process is not well defined and is not often noted in small animals. It occurs when the implants are strong enough to unload the underlying bone so that most or all of the weight bearing is through the implant (usually a plate) and not through the bone. This results in atrophy of the unloaded part of the bone. It is sometimes noted in radius and ulna fractures after synostosis has occurred between the proximal fragments and the distal radial fragment, but in which the distal fragment of the ulna is not united and gradually resorbs. Fractures have generally united but the cortices beneath the plate undergo a progressive reduction in density as well as a reduction in thickness. A gap may develop beneath the implant and the bone. Careful removal of implants with temporary protection of the weakened bone until it regains its strength is indicated.

FURTHER READING

Brinker WO, Hohn RB and Prieur WD (1984) *Manual of Internal Fixation In Small Animals*. Springer Verlag, Berlin/ Heidelberg/ New York.
Morgan JP and Leighton RL (1995) *Radiology of Small Animal Fracture Management*. WB Saunders, Philadelphia.
Rittmann WW and Perren SM (1974) *Cortical Bone Healing after Internal Fixation and Infection. Biomechanics and Biology*. Springer Verlag, Berlin.

Principles of Fracture Management

PART TWO

Principles of Fracture Management

CHAPTER SIX

Evaluating the Fracture Patient

Ralph H. Abercromby

INTRODUCTION

To the biased observer, fracture management is one of the most exciting and rewarding disciplines of veterinary surgery. However, care must be taken not to become preoccupied with the obvious fracture, thereby neglecting the remainder of the patient.

Frequently tissues other than bone, and often unrelated to the musculoskeletal system, are injured. The entire patient must therefore be examined and assessed, and investigations and treatments prioritized. Definitive fracture management may have to be delayed should it prove of less critical concern.

Assessment of the patient is made in several phases:

- Telephone advice
- Initial examination of the patient
- Detailed examination of body systems.

Telephone advice
Fracture evaluation and management may begin at the time of the initial phone call from a distressed owner. First aid advice, such as clearing airways, stemming haemorrhage or temporary splinting, can be given by phone and may be life saving or may limit further damage to osseous or soft tissues. It must be judged whether it is in the interests of the patient for a veterinary surgeon to attend at the site of injury, with limited facilities, or whether the patient should be transferred urgently to a well equipped, prepared clinic having previously advised the owner with regard to covering open wounds, control of haemorrhage and temporary stabilization of lower limb fractures. Conclusions will have to be drawn from information provided by untrained and perhaps distressed personnel as to the presence of life-threatening injuries or whether irreparable damage may occur to vital structures if the patient is moved by such persons.

Initial examination of the patient
A rapid but careful initial assessment of the patient is made and a thorough history taken when the patient is first encountered. Priority is given to life-threatening injuries. An accurate patient assessment completed in the first few minutes after arrival is often pivotal to patient survival. Only once the ABC (airway, breathing, circulation) of emergency medicine has been dealt with can a full examination be performed. A patent airway must be confirmed or established (suction or an emergency tracheotomy may be required), haemostasis must be established (using either pressure or ligation/stapling) and the circulation may require support. Fluid therapy at this stage is usually given to reverse hypovolaemic shock, perhaps caused by obvious haemorrhage or less apparent loss of circulating blood volume into a potentially massive fracture haematoma.

Fluid therapy is indicated in the shocked patient. Blood volume expansion will increase cardiac output, systemic blood pressure and tissue perfusion. Isotonic crystalloid solutions such as 0.9% saline or Ringers are useful but high volumes are required to maintain circulating blood volume (CBV) because of fluid redistribution. Alternatives include hypertonic saline, which has a profound effect on CBV for a relatively small amount of i.v. fluid, or the use of colloid solutions, either plasma or synthetic plasma expanders. Whole blood should be administered when blood loss is great.

Cranial trauma or shock must be considered if the patient is unconscious.

Detailed examination of body systems
Once obvious life-threatening conditions have been dealt with, a more thorough examination must be given. Analgesics may be required on humane grounds and the calming effect of reduction of pain may facilitate a more efficient further examination.

A protocol should be established which is memorable and comprehensive, ensuring that all body systems are examined and assessed. This may be a system/organ-based examination (heart, lungs, intestines, eyes) or a regional one beginning, say, cranially and extending caudally and distally. The author considers a system-based examination less likely to result in omissions. For example, when examining the neurological system, the effects and responses of the brain, spinal cord and nerves are considered, which includes assessment of structures such as the eyes and muscles which, in turn, demand their own examination – so ensuring that tissues are assessed from at least one perspective, and probably two or more.

A full examination requires a variety of skills and equipment. Experience and well trained senses can be more valuable than expensive monitoring or diagnostic equipment. Observation and regular reassessments are paramount. Essential equipment includes stethoscope, torch, percussion hammer or similar, and sterile needles/catheters and syringes (for detection of free fluid or air within the thorax or abdomen).

Truly life-saving findings and decisions are likely to be made within the consulting room. Subsequent to stabilization and thorough clinical examination, further investigations may require techniques such as radiography, ultrasonography, endoscopy, electro-cardiography and laboratory facilities.

THORACIC EXAMINATION

The respiratory and cardiovascular systems should be assessed in their entirety, not just those parts contained within the limits of the thorax (Figure 6.1).

Although the major trauma may be apparently unconnected with the thorax, the patient should receive careful thoracic auscultation and radiography, ECG examination and perhaps ultrasonography. Needle thoracocentesis, in addition to being easily performed, can provide rapid confirmation of clinical suspicions of pneumo/haemothorax and allow early (perhaps life-saving) management before results of more involved tests are available.

Conditions of concern include pneumothorax, pneumomediastinum, haemothorax, pulmonary parenchymal haemorrhage, fractured ribs, diaphragmatic rupture, haemopericardium, traumatic myocarditis and neurogenic pulmonary oedema.

Surgeons are sufficiently aware of the majority of the above to establish their presence or absence. The possibility of traumatic myocarditis is, however, quite often overlooked and may explain otherwise unexpected sudden anaesthetic or post-surgical deaths. Blunt trauma to the heart results in areas of cardiac contusion +/– myocardial infarction which are conducive to the

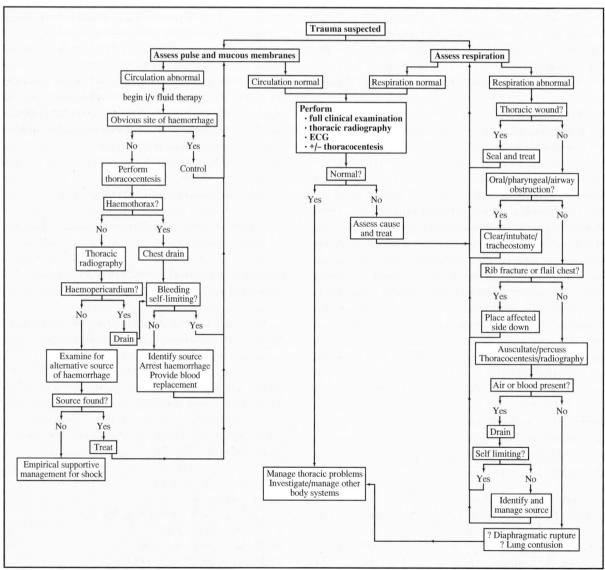

Figure 6.1: Algorithm for initial management of thoracic trauma.

development of cardiac arrhythmias. Most are evident within the first 48 hours but may not be apparent at the time of presentation or for some time thereafter. A wide variety of arrhythmias may present but the most common ones are relatively non-specific ST segment and T-wave changes. The majority of patients will be clinically unaffected but some may progress to conditions such as ventricular tachycardia or ventricular fibrillation, and death, if appropriate management is not instigated. For this reason it is probably advisable to arrange for a lead 2 ECG to be performed several times on the day of admission and occasionally thereafter and to delay surgery until the ECG reading is normal, unless there are very good reasons to do otherwise.

ABDOMINAL EXAMINATION

The organs or muscles of the abdomen are not uncommonly damaged in conjunction with musculoskeletal injuries. Plain radiography (indicated in virtually all cases of traumatic injury), ultrasonography and peritoneal lavage may be useful in identifying abdominal haemorrhage or rupture of viscera. More extensive investigations of organ integrity or function may require contrast studies.

The ability of an animal to pass urine or faeces does not eliminate the possibility of injuries to the relevant system. Animals with ruptured bladders, ureters or urethra will regularly pass relatively normal urine in an acceptable fashion. With the exception of urinary obstruction, ruptures of the gastrointestinal tract tend to be of more pressing importance than are injuries to the lower urinary tract.

As far as is practicable an animal's ability to pass urine or faeces under control should be assessed. The cause and implications of any problem must be considered.

Extensive abdominal or retroperitoneal haemorrhage may prove rapidly fatal. When treatment can be given, the patient may benefit more from supportive care and abdominal compression to limit further bleeding than from immediate and heroic surgical intervention. The latter may merely facilitate iatrogenic exsanguination of the patient unless large amounts of replacement blood are immediately available.

The integrity of the diaphragm must be established, especially if anaesthesia is being considered.

NEUROLOGICAL EXAMINATION

Critical assessment of the neurological system is vital and the reader should consult standard texts for details on examining this system. (The *BSAVA Manual of Small Animal Neurology* gives an excellent description of the requirements and the interpretation of a neurological examination.) The results of the exami-

nation are unlikely to identify a specific lesion: they are more likely to localize and grade the severity of any problem. Assessment of gait, mental status, posture, cranial nerve reflexes, proprioception and local spinal reflexes enables identification of the presence or absence of a neurological problem and typing of it as upper or lower motor neuron. The area affected may be localized to a general region, e.g. to the head or spine between T3 and L3, or to a more specific site, e.g. a fibular nerve injury.

Some injuries, such as those causing increased intracranial pressure, may require immediate investigation and management, whilst others may significantly affect the prognosis for a return to acceptable post-treatment quality of life. Injuries to the neurological system may present with signs suggestive of musculoskeletal injury, and vice versa. Careful assessment is required to prevent treatment of the wrong body system.

A critical neurological examination can be difficult to perform in the severely traumatized patient. Abnormal signs noted may be transient, reflecting swelling or contusion rather than anatomical disruption, or may be static or progressive. **Repeat examinations at regular intervals are therefore essential.**

Ophthalmic examination is likely to be performed in conjunction with the neural system.

Clinical findings may suggest that more extensive examination is required, e.g. myelography or MRI scan. Electrodiagnostics such as electromyography can be useful but valid conclusions may require a delay of 3–7 days.

ORTHOPAEDIC EXAMINATION

> **Examination and management of the fracture site, with the exception of early management of haemorrhage and covering open wounds, is likely to be of lower priority than that of most other systems.**

To limit further skeletal or associated soft tissue injury, however, examination of these should not be allowed to cause unnecessary movement of the patient. Temporary support (e.g. splints such as rolled-up newspapers, gutter splints or binding to the contralateral limb) may be applied to damaged areas (Figure 6.2). Early application of splints and support bandages, both before and after critical limb examination, has the following advantages:

· Fracture stabilization
· Reduces pain
· Reduces further soft tissue damage
· Prevents or reduces oedema
· Reduces periosteal strip
· Reduces self-inflicted trauma
· Helps to reduce overriding.

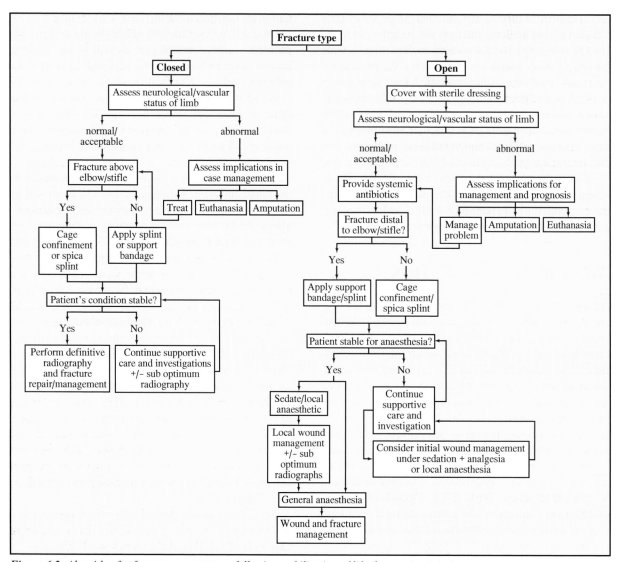

Figure 6.2: *Algorithm for fracture management following stabilization of life-threatening injuries.*

Care must be taken to prevent further soft tissue injury and compromise of blood supply. Regular re-examinations are essential to ensure that such complications, or the conversion of a closed fracture into an open one, have not occurred. Splints are usually only applied to fractures distal to the stifle or elbow, to the spine, or to the mandible. Humeral or femoral fractures are usually best left unsplinted, relying instead on restriction of movement of the animal and inherent muscle support to protect the damaged tissues. Splinting of such fractures often results merely in support of the lower limb and immobilization of joints distal to the fracture and places a fulcrum with increased motion at the fracture site, the very area at which one wishes to limit movement. Effective splinting of such fractures requires a spica splint or a correctly applied Thomas extension splint.

The presence of a fracture may not be in dispute, only the extent and type. Proper assessment and classification generally requires radiography but timing varies (see below). The area should be protected until radiography is deemed advisable or appropriate. Fractures are not always evident, though results of a careful clinical examination may increase the index of suspicion. This is especially so with undisplaced fractures or where only one of a pair or group of bones is injured (e.g. radius/ulna or tarsal bones) and adjacent structures give reasonable support. In such cases it is likely that subtle signs such as localized swelling or bruising or exquisite pain on examination/palpation will have to be relied on.

On identification or exclusion of grossly unstable fractures the remainder of the musculoskeletal system (as far as is practical) should be examined. Range of movement and stability of all joints, deep palpation of bones and soft tissues and assessment of the integrity of all structures – not just bone – should be performed. Where concurrent injuries allow, the patient should be examined at rest, on rising and at various forms of exercise. Multiple long bone fractures are likely to preclude such an examination but an undisplaced fracture may only become evident on a more critical evaluation following observation of a relatively mild lameness at exercise. The presence of such fractures in the presence of more severe injuries will always be a test of clinical ability but emphasizes the importance of a thorough evaluation of the entire patient.

The integrity of both neural (see above) and vascular structures require to be confirmed. Excellent fracture repair is of little value if the distal limb is avascular or acceptable limb function is not possible because of spinal or peripheral nerve injury. Uncertainties of tissue viability or future function may be extremely important factors in the owner's decision whether to pursue treatment.

Should the distal limb be warm and soft tissues bleed when pricked with a needle, the blood supply to the limb is generally assumed to be adequate. Shock and peripheral vasoconstriction, however, reduce the value of such tests. Correction of circulating blood volume and treatment of shock may make assessment easier but uncertainty as to tissue/limb viability may persist. Further investigation with arterial contrast studies, Doppler ultrasound or injection of intravascular fluoroscein dyes may assist detection of blood supply to a specific part of a limb. It would appear that even these tests have limitations and that the use of scintigraphy, where available, is a more reliable assessor of vascular integrity.

An increase in internal pressure within anatomically restricted regions (compartment syndrome) may require fasciotomy to prevent permanent vascular or neural damage.

RADIOGRAPHY OF THE FRACTURE REGION

High quality radiographs in at least two planes are required to confirm and further evaluate the extent of fractures. They provide information that is vital in producing definitive diagnosis and primary and secondary treatment plans. They therefore assist in formulating a prognosis as to expected return to function and estimating possible costs of therapy.

Heavy sedation or, more commonly, general anaesthesia is usually necessary to produce the quality of radiograph required for treatment planning. This is of little consequence when the intention is to proceed with definitive treatment under the same anaesthetic but often cannot be justified, on medical grounds, merely to confirm a provisional diagnosis knowing that surgery will be delayed, that further radiographs will be required and that information gleaned from interim radiographs is unlikely to alter the temporal management of the situation. In such cases radio-

graphs of lower quality (perhaps with regard to positioning and number of projections) taken of the conscious or lightly sedated animal may suffice, but unnecessary patient pain or discomfort should be avoided.

Such radiographs are of use in confirming the presence but not necessarily the absence of fractures. They should not be relied upon for formulation of the final pre-operative treatment plan as features such as fine cortical fissures or alterations in bone quality may be overlooked or may not be apparent, resulting in catastrophic fracture fragmentation at the time of surgery or inappropriate treatment of pathological fractures.

Delay in performing any fracture radiography until immediately prior to treatment may be justified in some instances on clinical, humane, ionizing radiation protection or financial grounds. If delay is to be of more than a day or so from the time of admission, good client communication and rapport are essential.

FRACTURE PLANNING

A treatment plan follows full clinical examination and fracture diagnosis. Repair technique decisions should not be delayed until fragments are exposed at surgery; neither should surgery be commenced with only one planned procedure. Complications may be encountered that will require modification of plan A or indeed change to plan B, C, or D, etc.

Depending on the complexity of the fracture and the methods of repair considered, the level of planning may vary. The AO/ASIF courses teach the value of tracing all fragments from both orthogonal views on separate sheets of clear acetate to allow reconstruction of the bone. By so doing it is possible to ascertain the size and number of implants required and how they relate to one another. This technique may seem rather laborious and time consuming but it is an excellent exercise in planning and often allows identification of potential problems, such as the proposed site of a plate screw coinciding with fracture lines.

Proper planning reduces both decision time and iatrogenic soft tissue injury at surgery. Surgical/anaesthetic times should be reduced and clinical results improved. It must be possible to alter technique according to circumstances (equipment and information must be available) but the better the pre-surgical assessment and planning, the less likely it is that unexpected surprises will be encountered at surgery.

CHAPTER SEVEN

Non-surgical Management of Fractures

Jonathan Dyce

INTRODUCTION

Historically, the management of long bone fractures using casts and splints pre-dates other means of repair. With appropriate case selection the results achieved by such rigid bandaging, otherwise known as external coaptation, could be very good. However, it should be appreciated that, with the advent of more sophisticated fixation techniques, optimal fracture management is now unlikely to involve primary coaptation. The aim of this chapter is to review the principles of non-surgical fracture management, with particular emphasis on casting. It does not give a comprehensive list of fractures suitable for non-surgical management, and the reader is directed to the chapters on specific fractures for guidance in the individual case.

CAST BIOMECHANICS

> **Cast management of fractures does not result in rigid immobility but should impart sufficient stability for fracture healing to occur.**

As rigid bone fixation is not achieved, healing will proceed by secondary bone union, with obvious callus formation. Therefore, aspects of the local fracture environment that favour callus formation will significantly influence selection for cast management.

The ability of a cast to immobilize a fracture depends on the stiffness of the cast, the intimacy of the cast layer to the bone, and the location of the fracture within the cast (Tobias, 1995).

The stiffness, or resistance to bending, is determined by the choice of cast material and the application technique. Of the forces acting at the fracture site, bending is neutralized well by a cylinder cast, but compressive, rotational, shearing and distractive forces are countered relatively poorly. Consequently, inherently unstable fractures (including avulsion fractures) are not suitable for coaptation. Casting materials are stronger in tension than compression, and so cast failure is likely to occur on the compression aspect of any angulation, but this vulnerable aspect may be reinforced by applying a spine moulded from the cast material.

The presence of large muscle masses about the humerus and femur precludes cast management of fractures proximal to the elbow and stifle, because of poor mechanical coupling between the cast and bone. Excessive cast padding will produce a similar effect.

The fracture should be located centrally within the cast as cast purchase on the proximal and distal limb is necessary for stabilization. The axiom that the joint proximal and distal to the fracture should be immobilized is a useful guide, but fractures with considerable intrinsic stability (e.g. isolated distal radial or ulnar fractures) may not require extension of the cast proximal to the elbow.

INDICATIONS FOR CASTING

The following criteria should be considered when assessing the suitability of a fracture for cast management.

Fracture configuration

Relatively stable fractures - for example, those with greenstick (incomplete) and interdigitating transverse configuration - are the most suitable for casting. If a fracture is minimally displaced, particularly in the immature animal, the periosteum is more likely to be intact, and to contribute to fracture stability.

Casting may be appropriate for those cases where one member of paired bones is fractured and the intact bone contributes significant support - for example, fracture of the radius with an intact ulna, or fewer than three metapodal fractures. Simple oblique or spiral fractures, which are stable on manipulation following reduction, may also be good candidates.

Comminuted fractures are rarely suitable for casting as subsequent deformation of the fracture plane is likely to occur.

Fracture location

The biomechanics of cast application and the difficulty of manipulative reduction preclude satisfactory coaptation of proximal limb fractures.

Intra-articular fractures proximal to the carpus and tarsus almost invariably dictate open reduction and internal fixation; coaptation should not be considered.

However, selected fractures of the carpus and tarsus can have a good clinical outcome without anatomical reconstruction, and coaptation may therefore be appropriate.

Growth plate fractures occur in young dogs with good osteogenic potential, but the advantage of an early return to weight bearing offered by internal fixation and the likelihood of complications of cast management of such juxta-articular fractures make cast management a poor option. Salter–Harris Type I fractures of the distal radius are a special case and may be managed by casting alone or by cross-pin fixation and adjunctive coaptation. The latter technique, where an intrinsically weak repair is protected by a secondary fixation, is referred to as adaptation osteosynthesis.

Fracture reduction

Reduction should be performed without an open surgical approach, to conserve the periosteal envelope and limit vascular compromise to the fracture site. The fracture is reduced with care, using a combination of linear traction and toggling of the bone ends. Following manipulation of transverse fractures, the fracture should appear more than 50% reduced in two radiographic planes. Although anatomical reduction is the ideal, it is rarely achieved and is certainly not a prerequisite for success.

Muscle masses in the proximal limb and soft tissue swelling may preclude fracture palpation and therefore adequate manipulative reduction.

If there is a delay to fracture management, muscle contracture and callus formation will progressively impede reduction. If adequate reduction is not possible then open reduction and alternative fixation must be considered.

Signalment

In general, limbs can be maintained comfortably in casts for 4 to 6 weeks. Candidates for coaptation should therefore produce adequate bridging callus within this period. Younger animals form callus more readily and on this criteria are good subjects for casting, but the rapidly growing juvenile is more likely to encounter complications associated with restricted limb growth within the cast.

The specific physiology of distal radial/ulnar fractures in toy breed dogs results in an unacceptably high incidence of failure following cast management. Such fractures dictate surgical intervention.

> **WARNING**
> **Distal radial/ulnar fractures should not be cast.**

Chondrodystrophic and obese dogs are difficult to cast effectively, because of limb conformation, and therefore alternative methods of fracture management are generally indicated.

Intended role of the patient

While casting is frequently possible, it is unlikely to be the optimal management for athletic and working animals. Expectations of function must be discussed with owners prior to fracture coaptation.

Cost

Economy is frequently cited as an indication for cast management of fractures. However, the cost of materials used in cast application is likely to exceed that of disposable materials used in simple external skeletal fixation. The incidence of complications leading to additional expense (e.g. cast replacement) should also be considered. The time commitment to fracture management and aftercare is similar for both treatment regimens.

CAST CONSTRUCTION

A cast typically comprises several layers: a contact layer (generally stockingette), a padding layer, a compression layer and the circumferential cast material.

Casting materials

For many decades, plaster of Paris (POP) was the only available casting material (Hohn, 1975). POP products are still produced, but are messy to apply, take many hours to reach weightbearing strength, deteriorate when wet, and are relatively heavy and brittle. Excellent conformability, radiolucency and economy are redeeming qualities, but a number of alternative casting materials are now available that are superior in key respects. Predictably, none is ideal (see below). For reviews of casting materials see Houlton and Brearley (1985) and Langley-Hobbs *et al.* (1996). Currently, the author uses resin-impregnated fibreglass for all small animal cast applications, and also finds this a versatile splinting material. This consistently makes well tolerated, strong and durable casts. Although such products are not cheap, the cost is justified by the likelihood of the initial cast delivering bone union without complication.

Properties of the ideal casting material include:

- High strength/weight ratio
- Easy to apply
- Short time to reach maximum strength after application
- Conformable
- Durable
- Radiolucent
- Water resistant but 'breathable'
- Easy and safe to remove
- Reusable
- Economical.

Cast application

If there is significant soft tissue swelling at the time of initial examination, casting should be delayed and a non-rigid compressive (Robert Jones) bandage should be applied to the reduced fracture, until this swelling has subsided. Typically, this will take 2 to 3 days.

Any skin wounds should be debrided and, when necessary, closed. The haircoat is clipped if it would interfere with cast application. The limb should be clean and dry. Following appropriate preparation, adhesive tape stirrups (e.g. zinc oxide tape) are applied to the limb to prevent distal migration of the cast (Figure 7.1a). Tapes placed on the dorsal and palmar aspects of the limb are preferred, as medial and lateral tapes may cause squeezing of the toes within the cast. The free

ends of the tapes are temporarily secured to a tongue depressor. Stockingette is rolled up the limb to incorporate any wound dressing, and is tensioned to eliminate creases (Figure 7.1b). Cast padding, such as Soffban (Smith & Nephew), is wound on to the limb with a 50% overlap on each turn. Two layers are generally indicated. Particular care is taken to ensure even padding over pressure points. Excessive padding about pressure points should be avoided and consideration should be given to increasing the padding in adjacent depressed regions with, for example, doughnuts of orthopaedic foam.

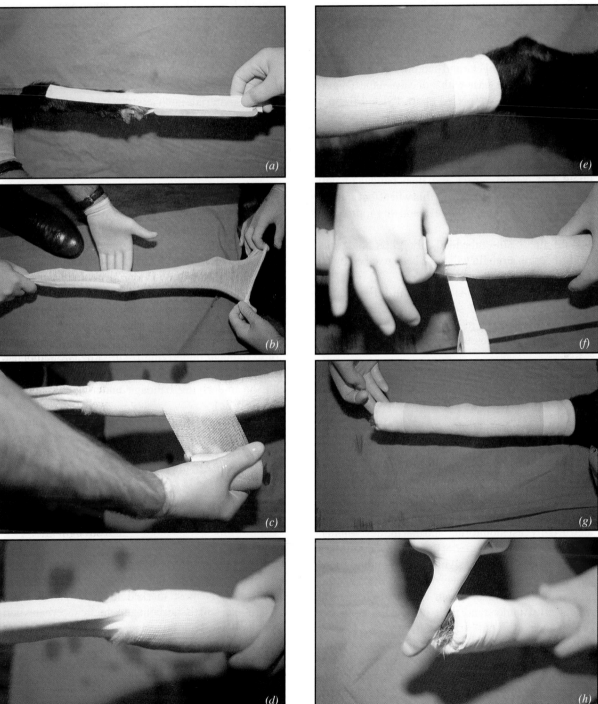

Figure 7.1: Cast application (see text for details).

Next, a compressive layer is applied in a similar manner to compact the padding.

The cast material is applied with appropriate tension, again with a 50% overlap on each turn (Figure 7.1c). Care is taken to maintain this overlap over the convex aspect of joints. A 1–2 cm margin of cast padding is left exposed proximal and distal to the cast (Figure 7.1d). Two or three layers of cast material are generally applied. Manufacturers' recommendations regarding wetting and handling should be followed. Tension is increased as the cast is applied proximal to the elbow or stifle to give a snug fit about the muscle masses and to prevent loosening.

It is important that an appropriate limb posture is maintained during casting and that indentations are not produced in the cast by the fingers. Once the cast has hardened, the stockingette and padding are rolled down and secured to the cast with adhesive tape (Figure 7.1e). The stirrups are peeled apart, twisted through 180° and bound to the distal cast (Figure 7.1f, g). The pads and nails of the axial digits should remain exposed (Figure 7.1h).

To facilitate removal, the cast may be cut along its cranial and caudal aspect and then bandaged with strong adhesive tape. However, this will affect some of the material properties of the cast, and this approach is not recommended.

With the resin-embedded fibreglass materials, weight-bearing strength will have been reached by the time of recovery from anaesthesia.

Medication with non-steroidal anti-inflammatory drugs is useful to limit soft tissue swelling and to provide analgesia. The requirement for ongoing treatment should be reassessed after 3 to 5 days.

CAST MAINTENANCE

> **WARNING**
> **Amputation may be the price paid for poor cast management.**

The majority of patients managed in a cast will be discharged to the care of their owners until cast removal. It is therefore essential that owners are educated in daily cast monitoring, and that the development of complications is reported at the earliest opportunity. It is a sobering fact that a significant amount of litigation arises from poorly managed casts. Written instructions should always be given out at discharge and owners must understand their responsibility in cast maintenance.

Points to monitor are swelling of the toes or proximal limb, toe discolouration and coolness, skin abrasion about the toes or proximal cast, cast loosening, angular deformity, damage, breakage, discharge or foul odour. Chewing at the cast may be a response to discomfort and should be investigated. In addition,

deteriorating weightbearing function of the cast limb and signs of general ill health (inappetence, dullness, etc.) may suggest the development of complications within the cast. It is sensible to schedule routine weekly appointments for cast assessment for the duration of casting. Rapidly growing dogs and other high-risk patients may require more frequent assessment.

Excessive exercise while cast will compromise cast survival and predispose to complications; therefore pen rest is recommended, with minimal leash exercise to toilet. The cast must be kept clean and dry. While outside, a polythene footbag is applied and secured using rubber bands or clothes peg.

> **WARNING**
> **The bag should be removed at all other times to prevent moisture build-up within the cast.**

Bedding materials such as straw can migrate between cast and skin, and should be excluded. Kennelled dogs can be successfully managed in casts provided that monitoring is diligent and hygiene good.

CAST REMOVAL

The time course for development of clinical union will be around 3 to 6 weeks, depending on individual patient and fracture factors. Radiography should be performed (Chapter 5) to confirm adequate fracture healing, prior to cast removal. Although plaster shears can be used to remove most casting materials, an oscillating circular saw is most suitable. Bilateral incisions are made in the cast (Figure 7.2a), taking care not to damage underlying tissue. The two halves are then prised apart using cast spreaders (Figure 7.2b), and the underlying bandage materials are removed (Figure 7.2c).

After cast removal it is important that a regimen of progressively increasing controlled exercise is enforced. The goal is stimulation of callus remodelling without jeopardizing fracture repair.

COMPLICATIONS

Joint stiffness
Limb immobilization will cause progressive joint stiffness and this is an inevitable consequence of cast management. It is most marked in those patients with periarticular soft tissue damage, which exacerbates periarticular fibrosis and adhesion. It is normal to cast joints in extension and, therefore, compromised joint flexion is to be expected following cast removal. The degree of compromise may be overcome (for example, in the carpus) by immobilizing the joint in a mild degree of flexion. At worst, fracture disease – a syndrome of stiffness, periarticular fibrosis, cartilage degeneration,

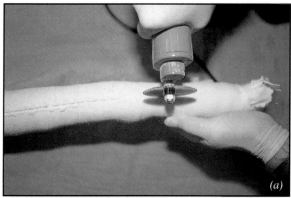

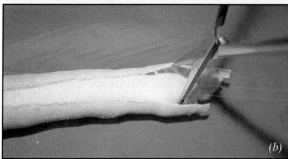

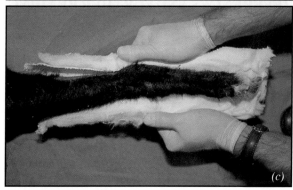

Figure 7.2: Cast removal.

muscle atrophy and osteoporosis – can occur. This is seen particularly following cast application to the proximal hindlimb in young dogs, where quadriceps contracture and the resultant genu recurvatum are devastating complications (Chapter 21).

> **WARNING**
> **Avoid stifle immobilization in skeletally immature animals.**

Joint laxity

Laxity is a particular complication in rapidly growing young dogs of large breeds. Carpal hyperextension, associated with palmar carpal ligament laxity is most commonly seen. Further coaptation is not appropriate and the majority of such cases will resolve spontaneously with controlled weightbearing.

Limb swelling

Excessive tension during cast application will cause attenuation of lymphatic and venous drainage and consequently distal limb oedema. This is likely to be seen within hours of cast application. It is therefore sensible to hospitalize the patient overnight to observe any early complications of casting. Ongoing soft tissue swelling within a properly pressurized cast will also cause distal limb oedema, but this will manifest later after application. Limb swelling is a potentially serious complication and requires diligent monitoring and appropriately rapid intervention.

Pressure sores

Bony prominences such as the olecranon, accessory carpal bone and calcaneus are particularly vulnerable to skin trauma. Two mechanisms are responsible: pressure necrosis and abrasion. Good application technique and appropriate cast monitoring will significantly reduce the incidence and severity of such complications. Direct skin trauma and a moist environment within the cast predispose to bacterial dermatitis. Staphylococcal organisms are generally responsible. The development of full thickness skin wounds can permit extension of infection to underlying tissues, and necrotizing cellulitis can become established. There may be few systemic clinical signs of deterioration and a purulent discharge staining the cast may be the first obvious sign. Unfortunately, amputation may be the only appropriate management in the severe case.

Abrasion of the toes caused by too short a cast should be managed by cast replacement rather than piecemeal reconstruction or local trimming.

Cast loosening

As the acute soft tissue swelling about the fracture subsides, the snug fit of the cast is lost. This will predispose to fracture instability and abrasion within and about the cast. Long-term casting will be inevitably associated with muscle atrophy and similar loosening.

Delayed union, malunion and non-union

Correct case selection and good casting technique should prevent fracture repair failure. Compromised fracture healing is more likely to be seen in association with any of the above complications. The frequent removal and reapplication of a cast may contribute to movement at the fracture plane and therefore failure of repair. Delayed union, malunion and non-union are discussed in detail in Chapter 24.

Refracture

Refracture rarely occurs following cast removal if there is radiographic evidence of bridging callus formation.

SPLINTED BANDAGES

Splinted bandages are useful in the management of fractures distal to the metacarpus/metatarsus as all toes are supported and not subjected to weight bearing. Ready-made plastic and metal 'metasplints' are available. Customized splints are readily made from casting materials and have the advantage of better conformability. Metacarpal fractures managed with non-mouldable splints are more likely to develop palmar bowing during fracture healing. The components of the splinted bandage are essentially the same as the cast, but without a rigid circumferential external layer. Padding is placed between the toes before bandaging to prevent interdigital sores. The splint is enclosed in the compressive layer and this is then covered with a flexible cohesive bandage. Splinted bandages are not as rigid as tubular casts and tend to be less suitable for fracture management. Phalangeal fractures are readily managed in splints.

Fractures of the tarsus may be immobilized by cranial or lateral half casts made from casting materials or thermally sensitive plastic.

OTHER BANDAGES

Support bandages such as the Spica splint and Schroeder–Thomas extension splint may be used for primary fracture management, but invariably they are not the first choice. Similarly, non-weightbearing slings such as the Velpeau, carpal and Ehmer should be considered only as adjunctive means to protect relatively fragile internal fixation, or reduced luxation.

In cases such as scapular and pelvic fractures that are not candidates for surgical intervention, it is rare that such bandage support will improve the prognosis or time of convalescence compared with more conservative management (see below). The likely incidence of complications of bandaging should also be considered.

EXTERNAL COAPTATION IN FRACTURES OF THE SKULL AND SPINE

Specific issues relating to the management of skull and spinal fractures are covered in Chapters 12 and 13, respectively.

CONSERVATIVE MANAGEMENT

A number of fractures – for example, of the pelvis caudal to the acetabulum – are best managed without any additional support beyond the local muscle bulk.

Management involves attention to ongoing analgesia, rest in an appropriately sized pen with flooring that offers a sure footing, and provision of comfortable bedding. In all cases in which ambulation is difficult, particular attention should be directed toward supervision of defaecation and urination. Consider the use of a belly band to support dogs when they are taken out to toilet.

REFERENCES AND FURTHER READING

Hohn RB (1975) Principles and application of plaster casts. *Veterinary Clinics of North America* **5**, 291.
Houlton JEF and Brearley MJ (1985) A comparison of some casting materials. *Veterinary Record* **117**, 55.
Langley-Hobbs SJ, Abercromby RH and Pead MJ (1996) Comparison and assessment of casting materials in small animals. *Veterinary Record* **139**, 258.
Swaim SF (1970) Body casts. Techniques of application to the dog. *Veterinary Medicine Small Animal Clinician* **65**, 1179.
Tobias TA (1995) Slings, padded bandages, splinted bandages, and casts. In: *Small Animal Orthopaedics*, ed. ML Olmstead. Mosby, St Louis.
Tomlinson J (1991) Complications of fractures repaired with casts and splints. *Veterinary Clinics of North America* **21**, 735.
Withrow SJ (1981) Taping of the mandible in treatment of mandibular fractures. *Journal of the American Animal Hospital Association* **17**, 27.

CHAPTER EIGHT

Instruments and Implants

John P. Lapish

Fracture repair in small animals using internal or external fixation is very dependent on corrosion-resistant materials for both instrumentation and implants. An understanding of stainless steel and its properties is one of the fundamentals of fracture management.

STAINLESS STEEL

Stainless steel is a generic term applied to a group of special steels containing varying amounts of chromium to improve corrosion resistance. All these steels will stain and corrode under certain conditions; the term stainless is, therefore, somewhat misleading. Veterinary surgery may involve the use of many types of stainless steel. Each will have a different composition dictated by the properties which are required.

Stainless orthopaedic implants must be very resistant to corrosion - all other properties are subordinate. Implant stainless steel contains high levels of chromium and nickel but low levels of carbon and as such belongs to a group of alloys called austenitic stainless steels. This type of steel cannot be hardened by heat treatment but can be hardened to a certain degree by 'working' the metal. Bone plate, for example, is rolled during manufacture, which makes it stiffer.

Surgical instruments, on the other hand, are required to have a certain degree of spring and be capable of taking and keeping a cutting edge. Surgical steels therefore contain relatively high levels of carbon and may be made hard by heat treatment. These steels belong to the martensitic group of stainless alloys, which are magnetic. Unfortunately this composition results inevitably in poor corrosion resistance - hence the requirement for a strict instrument care routine.

Stainless surgical instruments are protected from corrosion by a very thin coating of chromium oxide. Activities that encourage the production of chromium oxide (e.g. thorough cleaning of organic deposits, and dry storage) minimize corrosion and staining. Procedures that damage the protective layer (e.g. poor cleaning and rinsing, wet storage and certain chemical disinfectants) will encourage staining and rusting.

Manufacture of surgical instruments

The manufacture of a stainless surgical instrument from raw material to finished instrument involves some 30 different quality controlled processes.

The instrument maker is usually presented with a stainless steel blank which is roughly the same shape as the final instrument. The blank is machined to produce the relevant box joint, screw joint or ratchet. Hand and eye skills are required to grind and shape the blank into its final form. During forging, impurities accumulate on the surface of the blank. These are removed by abrasive wheels and belts during the process of glazing, the first of many stages designed to minimize corrosion.

The heat treatment process is of paramount importance in the manufacture of surgical instruments. The hardness of the steel is critical: if it is too soft, the scissors will not keep their edge; if it is too hard, the instrument will crack and break. Instruments that look right but fail to perform have often been hardened incorrectly.

Following hardening, the instruments are electropolished and passivated in special solutions to remove corrosive elements and to encourage the formation of chromium oxide. The final process is polishing, performed either by hand or, increasingly, by mechanical tumbling methods. The final polish may be bright or satin. A bright polished finish is most resistant to staining and corrosion. A satin finish is produced by microscopically roughening the surface, usually by blasting with small glass beads. This increase in surface area also increases the risk of staining.

The manufacture of surgical instruments remains very labour intensive, depending on the skills of craftsmen. This is particularly true of low volume production which does not justify mechanization. The durability of an instrument depends on strict quality control over all stages of manufacture together with equal attention to the use and maintenance of the instrument.

IMPLANTS AND INSTRUMENTS

Most veterinary orthopaedic instruments and implants are selected from the enormous range of human specialities. However, not all veterinary fractures have a comparable human fracture. Increasingly veterinary orthopaedic surgeons are demanding instruments and implants designed specifically for their needs.

Orthopaedic instrumentation may be classified under the following headings.

- Orthopaedic implants
- Implant insertion hardware
- Orthopaedic hand tools
- Orthopaedic power tools
- Bone manipulation instrumentation
- Bone cutting instruments
- Tissue retractors.

Orthopaedic implants

The range of available implants is enormous and their exact form will not be covered here in detail. The various shapes and sizes are illustrated in orthopaedic catalogues available from the major suppliers.

Four materials are currently employed for human implants: stainless steel, chrome cobalt molybdenum alloy, titanium and its alloys and high density polyethylene. All must meet British, US and international standards. Veterinary implants are not restricted in any way but, practically speaking, the available materials for implants meet the current human specifications.

Stainless steel

Very high purity austenitic materials are used for the production of bone plates, compression plates, bone screws, intramedullary pins etc. The current human specification for stainless steel in the UK is BS7252 composition 'D'. Equivalent international specifications include ISO 5832-1, ASTM F138-92 Grade 2 and DIN 17443-86. Components meeting these specifications may be mixed.

All these specifications are variants of stainless steel type 316L, which has no free ferrite stage – hence its very high corrosion resistance.

Chrome cobalt molybdenum alloy

This alloy is principally employed in the manufacture of total hip replacements.

Titanium and titanium alloys

This group of metals is primarily used in human orthopaedics in patients known to react to stainless steel. The component that usually causes the problem is nickel. Pure titanium is MRI-scanner compatible. Stainless steel implants must be removed prior to MRI scanning. Both these indications are very uncommon in veterinary orthopaedics.

Titanium has been used for canine total hip replacements. Although it has a very high strength to weight ratio, its wear characteristics are poor.

Titanium and its alloys should not be used with stainless steel components.

Ultra high molecular weight polyethylene

UHMWP is primarily used for acetabular components of total hip replacements but is compatible with all of the above.

> ### WARNING
> **To be safe for routine implants, use only stainless steel 316L type and UHMWP. For total hip replacement any combination of hard alloy and UHMWP is acceptable.**

Implant hardware

Most implants require dedicated instrumentation.

Intramedullary (IM) pins (hard wires)

IM pins may be inserted by a simple Jacobs chuck. Alternatively a power drill may be used. Driving trochar pins even by hand in a Jacobs chuck can produce enough heat to cause necrosis. Using power, heat necrosis followed by implant loosening is a significant risk.

Arthrodesis wires and K-wires (hard wires)

These may be inserted using a small Jacobs chuck if the bone is soft. Hard cortical bone is better penetrated by a power drill, preferably with a wire driver attachment (see section on power tools, below). The exposed section of wire should be kept short to minimize wobble and pin bending.

Orthopaedic/Cerclage wire (soft wire)

Where cerclage wire is cut from a roll, the ends of the wire must be twisted evenly around each other. To achieve this clinically it is important to twist under tension. Artery forceps or some kind of pliers will work but dedicated wire twisters which lock on to the wire are available (Figure 8.1).

Cerclage wire loop-ended lengths require a matching wire tightener (Figure 8.1) to pull the free end through the loop prior to locking and breaking. This system does not permit further tightening.

Rush pins

Rush pins are less commonly used in veterinary orthopaedics than previously; there has been a shift towards the use of arthrodesis wires and K-wires. A rush pin introducer is available to customize the bending and insertion of this implant.

Self-tapping screws

Self-tapping (Sherman) screws can be inserted with a minimum of special equipment:

- Drills equivalent to the screw core diameter (pilot) and outside diameter (clear):

3.5 mm (9/64 in)   pilot = 2.7 mm   clear = 3.5 mm
2.7 mm (7/64 in)   pilot = 2.4 mm   clear = 2.7 mm

- Depth gauge: it should be noted that self-tapping screws are measured from under the head to screw tip, i.e. thread length, whereas pre-tapped screws are measured as overall length. The appropriate gauge must be used or the difference compensated for.
- Screwdriver: self-tapped screws have slotted heads; 3.5 mm (9/64 in) screws have a cruciate head; 2.7 mm (7/64 in) and 2.0 mm screws have a single slot. Screwdrivers should be selected accordingly.

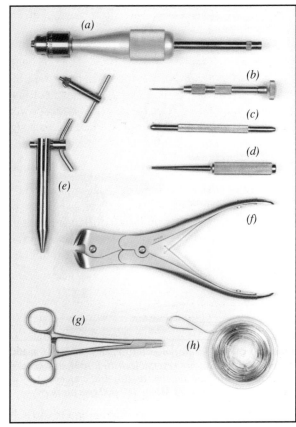

Figure 8.1: *Implant hand instruments: (a) Jacobs chuck; (b) small pin/tap vice; (c) K-wire bender; (d) K-wire punch; (e) wire loop tightener; (f) hard wire cutter (2.5 mm maximum); (g) soft wire twister/cutter; (h) soft orthopaedic wire.*

Pre-tapped screws (AO type)

Generally, but not exclusively, these are used with compression plates requiring a range of sophisticated instruments. Much of the specialized equipment is designed to place screw holes accurately with a minimum of soft tissue damage. The essential difference between the two types of screw is that the AO type will not cut their own threads in cortical bone. It is possible in certain circumstances to allow AO type screws to cut their own threads in cancellous bone. To pre-cut the threads, a tap is passed down the pilot hole.

- A tap is a threaded instrument possessing essentially the same thread form as the screw to be used. At right angles to the threads are three flutes (grooves) to allow removal of bone debris as the threads are being cut.

- Pilot drill equivalent to core diameter (clearance drill has the same diameter as the screw):

1.5 mm cortical	pilot 1.1 mm
2.0 mm cortical	pilot 1.5 mm
2.7 mm cortical	pilot 2.0 mm
3.5 mm cortical	pilot 2.5 mm
3.5 mm cancellous	pilot 2.0 mm
4.0 mm cancellous	pilot 2.0 mm
4.5 mm cortical	pilot 3.2 mm

- Screwdrivers. All screws have a recessed hexagonal head and the range of screws is covered by three different sizes (referring to the width across the flats of the hexagonal head):

  - 1.5 and 2.0 mm screws require a 1.5 mm hexagonal screwdriver
  - 2.7, 3.5 and 4.0 mm screws require a 2.5 mm hexagonal screwdriver
  - 4.5 mm screws require a 3.5 mm hexagonal screwdriver.

Orthopaedic hand tools

Jacobs chuck

This term has come to decribe an aluminium handle coupled to a stainless steel three-jawed device for holding pins. In fact only the stainless drill chuck made by the Jacobs Manufacturing Company should be described as a Jacobs chuck (Figure 8.1). Such chucks are fitted to virtually every orthopaedic drill available in the world today, as well as most intramedullary pin chucks.

The Jacobs (intramedullary) pin chuck is a simple tool widely used to insert intramedullary pins. It can, however, be used to hold and insert drills, external fixation pins, K-wires and arthrodesis wires. Control is good but it is difficult to produce the pure axial rotation necessary to obtain a perfectly round hole. It is difficult to cause heat necrosis using a hand-held chuck. Pin slippage is a frequent problem in all tools using a Jacobs chuck. At best this misleads the surgeon as to how deep the pin penetration is; at worst the pin can cause a serious injury to the surgeon.

- Always use the pin guard when driving long pins.
- Always lubricate the chuck mechanism. Stiff chucks do not tighten very well.
- Always replace worn chucks and keys. Having fewer teeth, the key wears first. Regular key renewal will prolong the life of the chuck.

Orthopaedic hand drill

Hand drills were widely used in veterinary orthopaedics prior to the more widespread use of power tools. The big disadvantage is that two hands are required to operate the drill, leaving the bone to be held by an assistant.

Orthopaedic power tools

Power drilling

Power drills remove much of the physical effort involved in many orthopaedic procedures. In addition they offer the surgeon more control than hand driven tools in that power drills may be held and controlled by a single hand, leaving the other hand free to hold the bone (or at least a drill guide connected to the bone). The major drawback of power drilling is that the heat produced by friction can cause heat necrosis and implant loosening.

Living bone is a difficult medium to drill. Twist drills are manufactured with flutes (grooves) spiralling along the length of the drill. As the subject material is drilled, the debris produced accumulates in the flutes and travels up and along the drill, appearing at and being discharged from the drill hole. When drilling bone, other than very dry bone, the bone debris clogs the flutes and is not removed from the drill tip. A build-up of debris reduces the cutting efficiency of the tip, increasing friction, which produces more heat, which coagulates any proteins in the bone debris, which then sets in the flutes – creating a vicious circle.

The net effect of the drilling properties of stainless steel and bone is the inevitable production of heat. The surgeon must take great care to deal with this.

- Use slow speed drilling, maximum 100 rpm.
- Use only sharp drill bits. Drilling 10 holes will dull orthopaedic drills. Any contact between drill tip and other implants will damage the drill tip.
- Clean bone drills very frequently, especially when drilling deep holes and when using AO type drill guides, which further limit debris clearance.
- Take care when drilling trochar tips, which are not designed for drilling. Some trochar tips are very poorly designed. Short stubby tips are the worst. Overall the length of the tip should be 2–3 times the diameter of the pin.
- Irrigate with sterile saline. To cool the drill tip, it must be removed from the hole!

Battery drills

Some very expensive surgical units will tolerate autoclaving but most units available to the veterinary surgeon are based on industrial designs and will be destroyed if autoclaved. For sterile use, therefore, battery drills (Figure 8.2) must be either gas sterilized

or shrouded before use. All are fitted with a stainless chuck which can be detached for separate autoclaving. Drill speed is controlled via the trigger and ideally should increase smoothly from zero to around 200 rpm. Most will in fact run at over 500 rpm so caution must be exercised.

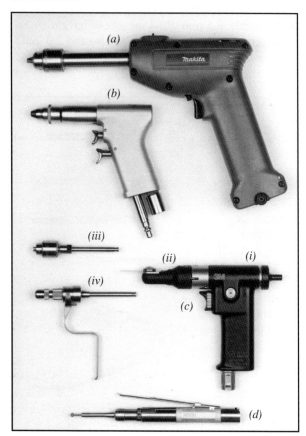

Figure 8.2: Orthopaedic power instruments: (a) rechargeable battery drill; (b) Synthes reversible drill; (c) 3M mini driver: (i) handpiece, (ii) saw attachment, (iii) drill attachment, (iv) K-wire driver; (d) 3M Minos 100 000 rpm air burr system handpiece.

Air drills

Generally speaking these are more expensive to buy and maintain than battery units but do have the advantage of being fully autoclavable. Compressed air is supplied by bottle or compressor. Single hose units venting at the table should use sterile bottled air. Units with double return hoses venting remotely are less demanding regarding air supply. The air and hose requirements make air drills more awkward to set up but they are usually lighter than their battery counterparts.

K-wire driver

This device (Figure 8.2) is available as a stand-alone unit or as an attachment for the modular drills. The instrument connects K-wires or arthrodesis wires to an air motor via a finger-operated clutch. Wires may be inserted incrementally, the wire being fed through the clutch, ensuring that at no point is a long vulnerable length of wire is exposed.

Power saws

Dedicated surgical saws are expensive. The mechanism to convert the rotating motion of drive systems into a to-and-fro saw system is difficult to manufacture in autoclavable materials. Surgical saws cut hard materials such as bone but leave soft tissues virtually undamaged. The cutting teeth move only a small distance. Bone, provided that it is held or has sufficient inertia, does not move and so the teeth will cut it. Soft tissues travel with the saw blade and the teeth are not drawn across the fibres. It should be understood, however, that if soft tissues are placed under tension the teeth of the saw will move across the fibres and will cut. This may be illustrated by oscillating cast cutters used over prominent bones or situations where the skin becomes tense.

Saws may be classified according to the direction of movement of the saw blade relative to the drive shaft:

Oscillating saws: These move in an arc of 5 or 6 degrees at right angles to the drive shaft. This type of action is also to be found in plaster saws. Indeed some 240 V cast cutters have been converted to surgical use by fitting surgical blades. The results can be satisfactory but compromises have to be made with respect to sterility and safety. The blades are arcs or segments of arcs and require that bone is either superficial or very well elevated (e.g. skull work or femoral head osteotomy).

Sagittal saws: These also move 5 or 6 degrees in an arc but in the same plane as the drive shaft. This action is the most useful in veterinary orthopaedics and is widely used for osteotomies. The cutting blade can be introduced deeply into surgical sites without fouling soft tissues with the drive system (e.g. for osteotomy of the ilium during the triple pelvic osteotomy procedure).

Reciprocating saws: These move to and fro along the line of the drive shaft in the manner of a hand-held wood saw. The distance of blade travel is very short. This type of action is rarely used but an example is the ischial cut in the triple pelvic procedure.

Burr systems

Ideally, orthopaedic or neurological burr systems should have high speed and low torque and be easy to sterilize. To obtain burr speeds in excess of 30 000 rpm requires an air-driven system.

Dedicated air systems: These systems (e.g. 3M Minos (Figure 8.2) and Halls Surgairtome) run at up to 100 000 rpm with a low torque. Using a range of burr guards to support the burr shaft it is possible to use burrs up to 70 mm long. Long burrs should not be used without a burr guard. The risk of shaft shatter in brittle carbide burrs is significant. The speed on both instruments is controlled by a lever on the handpiece. Generally speaking, air burrs are run at maximum speed. Some system of saline cooling will be required to avoid heat damage to tissues and coagulation of proteins on the burr.

Dental air drills: Neurological burrs fit the straight nose cone of the slow-speed handpiece (HP fitting burrs). The slow handpiece runs at a maximum of 20 000 rpm with relatively high torque. The high-speed handpiece will run at 400 000 rpm but the angle of the burr attachment severely limits its use. The handpiece can be autoclaved but the airline cannot, necessitating a shroud system.

Hobby type drills (electric): These drills have a maximum speed of 30 000 rpm to drive burrs either directly from the motor or via a flexible drive with a separate handpiece. The best-known system is the Dremmel, which has a variable speed via a foot control, a flexible drive shaft, and a separate handpiece which, with some modifications, will autoclave satisfactorily.

The non-dedicated systems (dental and hobby) give acceptable results but are much less satisfying to use. They are, however, approximately 15% of the cost of dedicated systems.

Bone manipulation instrumentation

A very large number of bone clamps are available to the human-orthopaedic surgeon. Many are appropriate for veterinary orthopaedics. Very few have been developed specifically for the veterinary field.

Bone is an unyielding substance. Holding instruments are usually adjustable over a range of positions and the adjustment may be locked in position by a long ratchet or, alternatively, by a threaded thumb screw. Locking clamps are particularly useful in general practice, where assistance is often lacking.

Fragment forceps

Fragment forceps (Figure 8.3) or pointed reduction forceps are single- or double-pointed clamps designed to maintain fragment reduction with a minimum of interference with implants and associated instrumentation. A range of sizes is available, covering most veterinary situations. A common application is the reduction of growth plate separations in the immature animal, e.g. distal femoral growth plate. Care must be exercised using fragment forceps on immature bone if one is to avoid excess trauma or a loss of reduction as the forceps points bite into the soft bone.

Single-pointed fragment forceps usually apply compression at the exact point where screw fixation is desirable, e.g. lagging bone fragments. Twin-pointed forceps are helpful in these situations. Gynaecological vusellum forceps may be used or twin-pointed forceps designed for orthopaedics are available. The advantage of the latter is that they will lock over a range of positions. Good examples of their use include fractures of the lateral condyle and fractures of the central tarsal bone in the racing Greyhound.

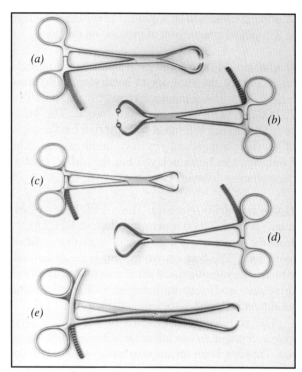

Figure 8.3: *Fragment or pointed reduction forceps: (a) twin-point fragment forceps; (b) plate-holding forceps; (c) small fragment forceps; (d) fragment forceps; (e) very large fragment forceps.*

Bone holding forceps

Bone holding forceps (Figure 8.4) are used to grip and manipulate large bone fragments. Sometimes large forces are required to overcome the forces of muscle

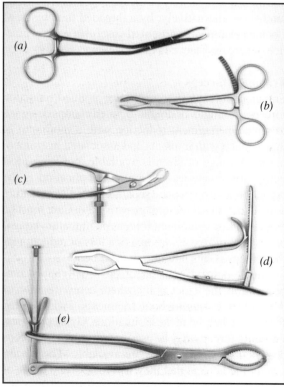

Figure 8.4: *Bone holding forceps: (a) Dingman forceps; (b) bone holding forceps; (c) self-centring forceps; (d) kern bone holding forceps; (e) Hey Groves forceps.*

contracture. These forces must be transmitted through the bone fragment without damaging bone or periosteum. Some older designs have a tendency to crush bone as pressure is applied (e.g. Fergusson 'Lion' bone forceps).

Bone cutting instruments

Bone cutters
Bone cutters (Figure 8.5) vary according to blade size, angle of cut and power of cut. The range for humans is enormous. The following is a selection of cutters found to be useful in veterinary orthopaedics.

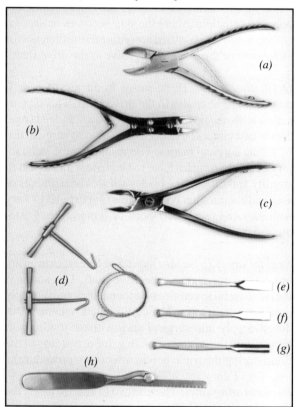

Figure 8.5: *Bone cutting instruments: (a) Liston bone cutters; (b) McIndoe bone compound cutters; (c) small angled cutters; (d) Gigli saw handles and wire; (e) osteotome; (f) chisel; (g) gouge; (h) adjustable bone saw.*

Liston cutters: Liston cutters are available in a large variety of sizes and blade cutting angles. Generally they are too heavy in construction for most veterinary procedures.

McIndoe compound cutters: McIndoe 7 in (175 mm) cutters are fine bladed and angled, and have a powerful compound action (double-jointed). A consequence of the compound action is that the jaws do not open very wide.

Small angled cutters: These cutters were developed as general purpose cutters for small animals. Applications include tibial crest transposition, and excision arthroplasty in small dogs.

Bone rongeurs

Bone rongeurs (Figure 8.6), or bone nibblers, are available in a range of sizes, angles and weights. A useful selection includes the following.

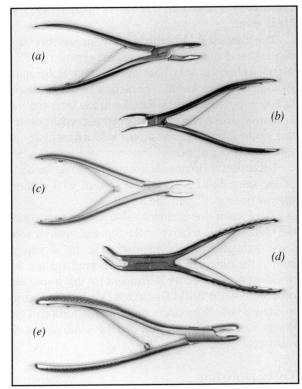

Figure 8.6: Bone rongeurs: (a) small angled rongeurs; (b) duckbilled Daniels rongeurs; (c) Daniels rongeurs; (d) compound action spinal rongeurs; (e) Luer rongeurs.

Luers: This is a heavy, simple action rongeur for rough work (e.g. removal of articular facets).

Jansen: This has a compound action with a smaller bite than Luers.

Daniels: The Daniels has a very small bite and a simple action.

Small angled rongeur: This is designed as a general purpose small animal rongeur.

Osteotomes

Osteotomes (Figure 8.5) possess a very fine, very sharp blade between 4 and 25 mm wide. They are used to slice through bone during elective osteotomies such as trochanteric osteotomy and excision arthroplasty.

Chisels and gouges

Chisels (Figure 8.5) are very much heavier than osteotomes in construction and have a bevelled blade. Their use is rare in veterinary orthopaedics. Gouges have curved blades of varying radii.

Bone curettes

Curettes will not cut cortical bone but may be used to scoop out cancellous bone or to scrape cartilage from joint surfaces during arthrodesis procedures. The Volkman (Figure 8.7) is the industry standard and is available as a single- or double-ended instrument; it will scoop diameters from 4 mm to 10 mm.

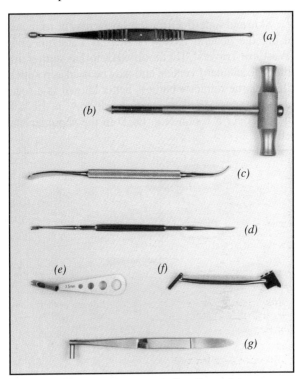

Figure 8.7: Curettes, elevators, drill guides and tissue protectors: (a) Volkman curette; (b) Michele's trephine; (c) periosteal elevator; (d) Freer periosteal elevator; (e) tissue protector; (f) drill guide; (g) ESF tissue protector.

Trephines

Trephines are used to cut windows in cortical bone, either to provide access for a bone scoop or to take a core of bone for biopsy. The most widely used type is the Michele's Trephine (Figure 8.7), usually 8 mm in diameter. Some authors suggest that this instrument may also be used to provide access to the spinal canal but this is not to be recommended.

Gigli saws

The gigli saw (Figure 8.5) is essentially a bone cutting wire with handles. This device can be threaded around bones which have limited access for conventional saws (e.g. excision arthroplasty and the ischial cut in the triple pelvic procedure). To-and-fro movement of the wire cuts through the bone. Unfortunately the 'teeth' on the wire are usually too coarse for medium-sized and small patients.

Periosteal elevators

These elevators (Figure 8.7) are used to reflect muscle from bone. They vary in tip shape, size and degree of sharpness. A double-ended general purpose instrument is available for most situations. A finer instrument, the Freer, is useful in spinal procedures.

Orthopaedic retractors

Retractors (Figure 8.8) are used in orthopaedics to maximize exposure and minimize soft tissue trauma. This in turn leads to faster surgery. Appropriate retraction can significantly reduce post-operative complications.

Skin and superficial muscle layers may be retracted using the general retractors such as Langenbeck's, West's or Travers'. The modified Gelpi has shorter tips than the standard version and may be used as a superficial tissue retractor but it is better known as a focal deep retractor used to create a window in the soft tissues over a lesion (e.g. OCD in the shoulder and elbow).

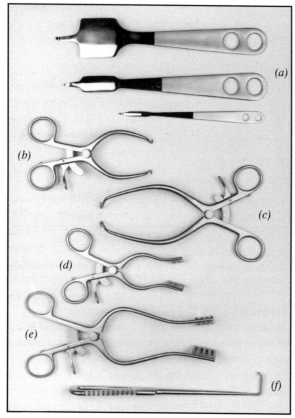

Figure 8.8: Retractors: (a) Hohmann; (b) small Gelpi self-retaining; (c) Gelpi self-retaining; (d) West's self-retaining; (e) Travers' self-retaining; (f) Langenbeck's.

Hohmann retractors

Over a dozen Hohmann variants are to be found in human orthopaedics. Only about four are found in regular usage in veterinary surgery. The spike part of the blade is placed at the posterior aspect of the bone to be exposed. The tip acts as a fulcrum for the rest of the blade. Downward pressure on the handle (the holes in the handle were originally designed for the attach-

ment of weights) brings the broad part of the blade into contact with overlying soft tissues, usually muscle masses, pushing them away and down. The overall effect is to appear to elevate the bone in the exposure. The degree of retraction will vary with tip length and blade width.

The most useful Hohmann in veterinary orthopaedics is the 18 mm blade with a short narrow tip. This variant is almost synonymous with the term 'Hohmann'. Examples of use include: retraction of tensor fascia lata to expose the lateral fabella in the over-the-top technique of anterior cruciate ligament repair; elevation of the femoral head and neck for arthroplasty or total hip replacement.

Other useful Hohmanns are smaller-scale versions of the same basic style of the 18 mm with a short narrow tip, e.g. 12 mm and 8 mm.

The 18 mm Hohmann may also be used to advance the tibial plateau relative to the femoral condyles for the examination of the menisci. The tip is placed behind the tibia and the blade is levered against the trochlea. A much better instrument for this important procedure is the Stifle Distractor (Veterinary Instrumentation) which produces much less distortion of the menisci. These distortions can be confused with menisceal tears.

Tissue protectors

Twist drills and the various types of threaded external fixator pin have a great tendency to attach themselves to soft tissues, which then become wrapped around the drill or pin. The consequences may be very severe if the tissues include nerves or blood vessels. In a large exposure (during plating, for example) it is possible to clear all soft tissue away from the drill site without causing extra soft tissue damage. In other procedures a limited dissection is desirable to minimize devascularization. In these situations a tissue protector (Figure 8.7) can be very useful.

The tissue protector is in essence a short stainless steel tube with small teeth at the distal end which can be introduced through the soft tissues and held on to the bone. The drill or pin is passed down the tube without contact with soft tissues. The tissue protector may also be used as a locating device for the drill or pin, ensuring that bone entry occurs at exactly the right point. Without such a device, drills (and to a lesser degree pins) tend to 'skate' over the bone surface. This results at best in incorrect positioning of the drill or pin. At worst the drill or pin slides off the edge of the bone, with consequent damage to patient or surgeon.

CHAPTER NINE

Principles of Fracture Surgery

Andrew Miller

PRE-OPERATIVE MANAGEMENT

Diagnosis

Diagnosis of fracture is usually relatively straightforward on clinical or radiographic grounds. Some fractures may be difficult to diagnose, e.g. non-displaced, incomplete or stress fractures. In some cases there may be multiple injuries in the same or different locations and it is easy to overlook more subtle lesions by concentrating on an obvious fracture. A complete diagnosis should include patient signalment, location and type of fracture; distal metaphyseal fractures of the radius and ulna in a 12-week-old Great Dane and a 7-year-old Poodle differ significantly.

Fracture classification systems have been discussed in Chapter 1.

Treatment options

A full diagnosis allows consideration of treatment options. Consideration must be given to:

- Fracture type and location
- Age, size and function of patient
- Type and quality of bone involved
- Involvement of joint surfaces
- Open or closed fracture
- Single or multiple fractures
- Single or multiple limb involvement
- Involvement of other tissues (e.g. neural tissue, pelvic canal contents)
- Magnitude and direction of forces acting at the fracture site
- Experience of surgeon
- Owner's requirements and resources
- Equipment available.

PRACTICAL TIP

It is usually good practice to have several treatment options available. In cases of difficult fractures or high owner expectations, consideration should be given to referral of the patient to a specialist surgical centre at the outset.

Estimation of prognosis/client expectations

Most fractures will heal. Some, however, will not heal or will heal in an inappropriate manner. In some cases healing of the fracture may not be accompanied by the return of full limb use or full athletic ability. It is helpful to be able to predict the chances of fracture treatment being successful in each case, whether in a sedentary pet or a racing Greyhound. Experience with a broad range of injuries, good recording of previous results and appreciation of the requirements of the patient's owner will assist in this.

Predicting complications

Some fractures are prone to particular predictable complications. Joint stiffness and osteoarthritis are possible following articular fractures. Distal radius and ulna fractures in toy breed dogs are predisposed to non-union. Constipation or obstipation may occur following non-surgical management of some pelvic fractures, particularly in cats. Any surgical fracture repair involves a certain risk of infection. Unanticipated complications can be difficult to explain and it is worth spending a few minutes discussing possible complications with clients prior to undertaking fracture treatment.

Estimation of costs

The cheapest fracture treatment is the one that works first time. Estimating the cost of fracture treatment is never easy. It is usually helpful to itemize anticipated costs prior to obtaining consent for treatment from the client and to explain whether the cost includes follow-up examinations or treatment of complications. The treatment that appears cheapest on paper may actually work out much more expensive (e.g. cast fixation of distal radius and ulna fracture if non-union results) and expected success rate and risk of complications should be taken into consideration. Consider also whether there might be any complicating factors as yet undiagnosed (e.g. pneumothorax, ruptured bladder).

Patient preparation

Patient stabilization

It is beyond the scope of this manual to describe critical care procedures in detail. Most fracture patients will have suffered major trauma and are very likely to require supportive treatment for shock and pain. Other relevant features might include respiratory compromise, haemorrhage, injury to vital organs and open wounds.

Patient assessment and minimum database
It must never be forgotten that every fracture is attached to a patient and the whole patient must be assessed prior to fracture treatment. A full physical examination should be undertaken, as well as selected radiographic and laboratory examinations. Factors to consider include:

· Presence of other injuries (bony or soft tissue)
· Presence of underlying pathology (e.g. neoplasia, nutritional bone disease).

Examinations indicated in particular circumstances might include:

· Rectal temperature and body weight
· PCV and total protein estimation
· ECG
· Radiographic examination of thorax and abdomen (e.g. trauma cases, possibility of neoplasia)
· Radiographic examination of contralateral limb, pelvis or spine (e.g. in animals with an obvious unilateral limb fracture that are non-ambulatory)
· Selected contrast radiographic procedures (e.g. retrograde urethrography in pelvic fractures, myelography in some spinal fractures).

Examinations may have to be repeated in some cases and results should always be recorded.

Temporary fracture support
Fractures distal to the elbow or stifle will usually benefit from temporary external support until definitive treatment is possible. A bulky bandage is ideal for this but must extend well proximal and distal to the fracture. Benefits to the patient include reduction in pain and prevention of further tissue injury, such as development of a closed fracture into an open wound. This is particularly important if the patient is to be transported. In addition, haemorrhage and swelling will be reduced, which aids the surgeon. Fractures proximal to the elbow and stifle can be difficult to immobilize satisfactorily and may be better left unsupported, as long as adequate provision is made for analgesia and confinement of the patient. If external support is desired, a bandage encircling the body may be applied. Definitive treatment of fractures using external support alone is discussed in Chapter 7.

> **PRACTICAL TIP**
> **It is important to make an effort to maintain normal joint angulation during bandage application.**

Anaesthesia and analgesia
All fracture patients must be provided with adequate analgesia throughout all phases of treatment. Useful drugs may range from non-steroidal anti-inflammatory drugs (NSAIDs) to morphiates. It is beyond the scope of this manual to describe general anaesthesia procedures in detail. The reader is referred to the standard texts.

> **WARNINGS**
>
> **Due to enhanced toxicity, combinations of NSAIDs and glucocorticoids should not be used.**
>
> **NSAIDs should be used with caution in the peri-operative period.**

Supportive therapy
Obvious supportive measures include:

· Intravenous fluid therapy (crystalloid, colloid, blood)
· Adequate analgesia
· Care of traumatic or surgical wounds
· Prophylactic antibiosis (see later)
· Adequate nutrition (nutritional requirements are often increased in the face of anorexia)
· Regular bladder emptying and prevention of decubitus sores in recumbent patients
· Assisted ambulation and physiotherapy.

Surgeon preparation

Theatre practice
It is good practice to aspire towards a completely clean operating environment. To this end, the following measures are recommended:

· Allow the minimum of air movement – avoid constant procession of casual observers, doors opening, etc.
· Clip hair and clean the patient's skin in a different room
· Empty patient's bladder and rectum prior to travelling to theatre.

Surgical attire
All operating theatre personnel should wear some type of theatre suit with surgical hood or cap and mask, as well as clean theatre shoes. Outdoor clothes and shoes are not acceptable. The surgeon and assistant(s) should wear sterile operating gowns. Surgical attire need not be expensive but it should be dedicated.

Good scrub technique for the surgeon and patient is essential and the surgeon and assistant(s) should wear surgical gloves.

PERI-OPERATIVE MANAGEMENT

Aseptic technique

Instruments
Instruments and implants are best autoclave sterilized, unless supplied sterile. Ethylene oxide is an acceptable substitute. It is important to check periodically that the sterilization process is working properly and to handle and store sterilized materials properly.

Drapes and draping techniques
Drapes may be traditional reusable cloth or disposable. They should be large, easy to handle and, ideally, impermeable to fluids in order to prevent 'strikethrough' infection by wicking of bacteria. Draping techniques are a matter of personal preference. Free-limb draping is often required to allow wide access to an injured limb and it is important to be able to drape the distal limb safely and effectively. Secondary draping following the initial skin incision is recommended, to reduce direct contact between surgeon and patient. Small towels or drapes may be clipped to the skin edges or adhesive plastic drapes may be applied, though these often loosen rapidly due to haemorrhage.

Prophylactic antibiosis
The use of prophylactic antibiotics is justifiable in fracture surgery. Fractures may be contaminated, tissues will certainly be severely traumatized, operating time may be prolonged and substantial amounts of foreign material may be inserted. All of these factors increase the risk of bacterial contamination or reduce the local host defence mechanisms. Infected fractures require therapeutic use of antibiotics.

Suitable drugs for antibiotic prophylaxis should be effective against anticipated contaminants and present at the operative site in effective concentrations for an appropriate period. This can be achieved by consideration of the following factors:

- Knowledge of the bacterial flora of the operating environment (e.g. by regular bacterial audit using strategically placed dishes of bacterial growth medium; recording results of bacteriological examination of post-operative infections)
- Administration of selected drug(s) by a suitable route at a suitable time (e.g. intravenously at the time of induction of anaesthesia)
- Maintenance of antibacterial concentration for an appropriate period (e.g. by repeated intravenous injection if duration of surgery exceeds 90 minutes; by systemic administration for 24–72 hours following surgery).

PRACTICAL TIP
The author's current empirical choice of antibiotic for routine use is clavulanate-potentiated amoxycillin.

WARNING
Use of prophylactic antibiotics will not compensate for poor preparation or surgical technique.

Surgical technique

Surgical anatomy and approaches
Familiarity with surgical anatomy and approaches is absolutely essential. It must always be borne in mind that anatomy may be severely deranged following trauma and surgical landmarks may have been altered or obliterated. Major surgical approaches and procedures should be practised on cadavers wherever possible before being attempted for the first time in the live animal. Reference to Piermattei (1993) is strongly recommended.

Instrumentation
There is no substitute for an adequate range of surgical instrumentation and implants. In particular, suitable retractors and bone holding instruments are required.

It is often helpful to pack particular sets of instruments together. Figures 9.1 to 9.3 show examples of such kits.

Tissue handling
Bone and soft tissues should be handled as atraumatically as possible. Surgical approaches that

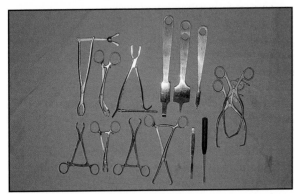

Figure 9.1: *Fracture kit instruments. Upper row (left to right): Hey Groves, Burns, Kern bone holding forceps; selection of Hohmann retractors; Gelpi self-retaining retractors. Lower row (left to right): small bone holding forceps (two); large and small pointed reduction forceps; small osteotome; periosteal elevator.*

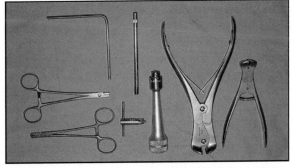

Figure 9.2: *Pin and wire kit instruments. Upper row: pin benders. Lower row (left to right): wire cutter/twisters (two); small chuck and key; large and small pin cutters.*

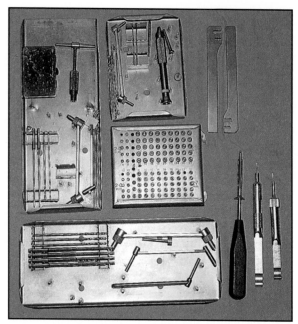

Figure 9.3: Range of drills, guards, depth gauges and taps for screw insertion.

allow separation rather than incision of muscles or tendons should be planned. Osteotomy is preferable to tenotomy. Sharp dissection and a 'no touch' surgical technique should be practised whenever possible. Important soft tissue structures (blood vessels, nerves) should be identified and protected. Penrose drains are ideal for gentle retraction of nerves.

Haemostasis and irrigation

Good haemostasis allows a clear surgical field and reduces the likelihood of post-operative wound infection due to bacterial strikethrough of blood-soaked drapes or the presence of an infected haematoma. Used surgical swabs or sponges should be counted and disposed of immediately into a bin or bucket rather than being deposited on drapes or instrument trays.

Tourniquets can be very helpful in minimizing intra-operative haemorrhage, especially in the distal limb, but must be applied with caution (Blass and Moore 1984). Electrocautery is very useful and bipolar cautery is usually more effective and controllable than monopolar. Surgical suction is very helpful for removal of gross haemorrhage or irrigating fluids.

The surgical field should be irrigated regularly using sterile saline or lactated Ringer's solution to refresh exposed tissues and wash away blood and bacteria. Dilution of bacterial populations helps to decrease the pathogen load at the end of surgery. Various antibacterial irrigating solutions are available but their value is unclear. Irrigation fluids should be aspirated promptly and completely from the surgical site and drapes should be kept dry.

Fracture planning

The importance of preparing a surgical strategy before commencing surgery cannot be over-emphasized (Fig-

ure 9.4). Operative time and soft tissue trauma should be kept to a minimum, so a precise plan of action should be made and followed. Surgical anatomy should be reviewed with consideration of approaches, positioning of retractors, etc. Radiographs taken in at least two orthogonal planes should be studied and fracture reconstruction rehearsed mentally or by the use of tracings of fracture fragments. Particular consideration should be given to potential locations for lag screws and bone plates, if plate fixation is planned. Reference to specimen bones can be very valuable for planning fragment reconstruction, reviewing anatomy and orientation and pre-bending of implants prior to sterilization in some cases (e.g. pelvis). Several options should be considered and ranked, so that there is at least one back-up plan if the original strategy must be discarded for whatever reason. The patient should be completely prepared and draped and all instrumentation should be assembled prior to the initial skin incision being made.

Multiple injuries

The presence of multiple orthopaedic injuries or involvement of more than one limb will influence choice of fixation method. In these situations the optimal (i.e. strongest) fixation method should always be selected as the repaired fracture(s) will be loaded to a far greater extent in the early stages of healing than in solitary injuries and fixation failure is significantly more likely to occur. In general, it is better to treat multiple injuries during a single operating session, assuming that the patient's condition and the surgeon's expertise allows for this.

Decision-making in fracture reconstruction

Fracture healing requires adequate fracture reduction, stability and vascularity and a balance between these must be achieved. Most fractures should be reconstructed as accurately as possible (as long as doing so does not compromise their vascular supply or the surrounding soft tissue envelope) and then stabilized as rigidly as possible, using the chosen method. Perfect anatomical reconstruction remains mandatory in articular fractures.

Some comminuted diaphyseal fractures cannot be anatomically reconstructed due to severity of comminution or small fragment size. Under these circumstances it may be advantageous to simplify the fracture by partial reconstruction and then perform osteotomy of bone ends to increase cortical contact (Figure 9.5).

Imperfect or even no reconstruction may be preferable to causing excessive further soft tissue damage in selected severely comminuted diaphyseal fractures. In such cases a minimally invasive strategy (MIS) may be adopted (see Chapter 10). This involves 'spatial realignment' (Aron *et al.*, 1995); that is, re-establishing normal bone length with less than five degrees of rotational or angular malalignment of the proximal and distal ends (or joints) and at least 50% axial overlap.

Spatial realignment may be achieved closed – for

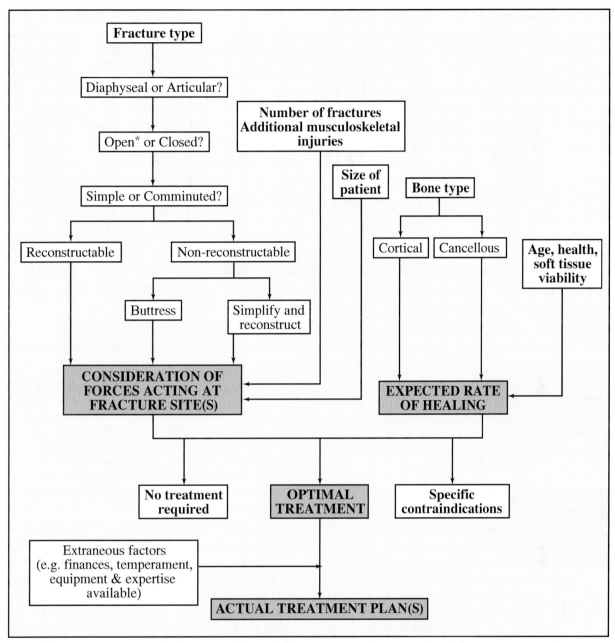

Figure 9.4: *Fracture treatment planning.* * *See Chapter 10 for management of open wounds and fractures.*

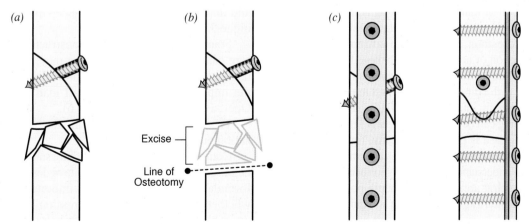

Figure 9.5: *Simplification of a comminuted diaphyseal fracture. (a) Comminuted diaphyseal fracture. (b) Partial reconstruction of major fragments using lag screws to produce interfragmentary compression. Small fragments are excised and osteotomy of major fragments is performed to mazimize bone to bone contact. (c) A neutralization plate is applied. The bone is inevitably shortened to some extent. This is rarely problematical in the femur or humerus.*

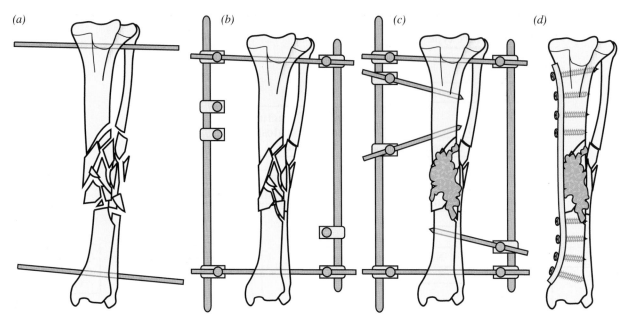

(a)   *(b)*   *(c)*   *(d)*

Figure 9.6: *(a-c) Severely comminuted tibial diaphyseal fracture treated by spatial realignment and buttressing by an external skeletal fixator. In the distal limb, spatial realignment may be achieved by suspending the limb vertically. A cancellous bone graft may be inserted if treatment is open. (d) Buttressing the same fracture using a plate and screws with cancellous bone graft.*

example, by traction on the bone (Johnson *et al.*, 1996) – or open, in which case an 'open but don't touch' (OBDT) approach is adopted towards fracture fragments. The intention is to minimize interference with fracture fragments and their envelope of organizing haematoma and soft tissue in the hope of reducing the likelihood of fragment sequestration.

Following spatial realignment, the fractured region must be buttressed rigidly to allow for weightbearing on the limb while the fracture heals and this can be achieved using an external skeletal fixator (+/– intramedullary pin +/– 'tie-in' configuration), a buttress plate (+/– intramedullary pin) or an interlocking nail (Figure 9.6).

It is important to realize that the minimally invasive strategy does not represent an abandonment of AO/ ASIF principles (see section below). Rather, this philosophy is derived from increased understanding of the relevance of interfragmentary strain on bone cells and fracture healing and depends upon rigid fixation. The combination of many large interfragmentary gaps and rigid fixation minimizes interfragmentary movement and therefore strain, optimizing the local environment for the production of new bone. It is believed that, in some cases, fracture healing can be by intramembranous ossification, i.e. the direct production and mineralization of osteoid without intervening cartilaginous tissue. This rapid healing can be coupled with early limb use, so that fracture disease is prevented. Clearly, rigid support by buttressing devices requires that they are extremely strong, and a clear understanding by the surgeon of biomechanical concepts such as area moment of inertia, polar moment of inertia and interfragmentary strain is required.

Compression, neutralization or buttressing?
Interfragmentary compression minimizes fracture gap and increases interfragmentary friction and stability.

Compression may be *dynamic*, i.e. dependent upon forces created by loading, or *static*, i.e. independent of loading, and may be created in a number of ways:

- Cerclage wires (static compression)
- Tension-band wires (dynamic compression)
- Lagged bone screws (static compression)
- Tension-band plates (dynamic compression)
- Dynamic compression plates (static compression unless used as tension band).

(See Operative Techniques 9.2, 9.3, 9.5 and 9.6.)

Static compression is often temporary due to the viscoelastic nature of bone and bone remodelling.

Following fracture reconstruction, forces acting at the fracture site may be neutralized using some device – usually a bone plate or external skeletal fixator that spans the fracture completely and transmits loading forces between proximal and distal intact fragments. There should be some degree of load sharing by bone and implant at the fracture site (see Operative Technique 9.6).

Fractures that cannot be reconstructed and therefore cannot share in load bearing may be buttressed using bone plates or external fixators. In this situation the implant is responsible for all load bearing (see Operative Techniques 9.4 and 9.6).

The interlocking nail is also applicable to neutralization or buttressing.

Compression is helpful in fracture stabilization and healing, but it is not always feasible or desirable. When formulating a treatment plan, it is important to identify whether interfragmentary compression is possible or desirable, or indeed whether the fracture can be reconstructed fully, partially or not at all.

Fracture fixation options are summarized in Table 9.1.

Fracture type	Ideal fixation*	Compromise fixation
Simple transverse diaphyseal	Compression plating	External coaptation External fixator Intramedullary pin plus external fixator Interlocking nail Non-compression plate
Oblique or spiral diaphyseal	Interfragmentary compression by lag screw(s) plus neutralization plating	Interfragmentary compression by cerclage wires and intramedullary pinning Interfragmentary compression by cerclage wires or lag screws and external fixator Interlocking nail Intramedullary pin
Comminuted diaphyseal†	Interfragmentary compression by lag screws plus neutralization plating	Partial reconstruction using interfragmentary lag screws followed by transverse osteotomy (simplification) and neutralization plating Partial reconstruction using interfragmentary lag screws or cerclage wires followed by buttressing using plate or ESF. Minimal or no reconstruction followed by buttressing using plate, pin and plate, interlocking nail, pin and external skeletal fixator, or external fixator alone (See Chapter 10)
Articular fracture	Anatomical reconstruction and rigid internal fixation with interfragmentary compression using lag screws ± plates	K-wire fixation if fragments small Fragment excision if very small Arthrodesis if severe derangement of articular surface Non-surgical management (e.g. selected acetabular fractures)
Open fracture	External fixator Plate and screws in selected fractures	Amputation if severe derangement of limb
Avulsion fracture	Tension-band technique	Lag screw fixation
Pathological fracture	No fixation Address underlying pathology	Depends upon pathology, necessity of fixation and type/location of fracture

Table 9.1: Fracture fixation options.

* Ideal fixation method is determined by the perceived balance between quality of fracture reduction, degree of rigidity of fixation and amount of soft tissue damage caused in achieving these for any given fracture and patient age or type. Other factors, including surgeon's experience, personal preferences and instrumentation available, must also be taken into account. These recommendations are based upon the author's preferences.
† Severely comminuted fractures can present a real challenge to the surgeon and serious consideration must be given to the value of reconstruction versus the risk of further iatrogenic trauma. Under these circumstances the ideal fixation method depends upon the morphology of the fracture and almost any of the methods listed may be regarded as appropriate alternatives.

Fracture reduction and stabilization

Methods of reducing fracture fragments include toggling, leverage and traction/counter-traction in simple fractures and the use of various fragment forceps in comminuted or small-fragment fractures. Pre-operative traction (e.g. by suspending the limb) may be useful in stretching or fatiguing muscles, thereby facilitating reduction.

Fragments may be stabilized temporarily using fragment or bone holding forceps. Temporary Kirschner wires (K-wires) may be driven across the fracture site or cerclage wires passed around it before definitive fixation is applied. Alternatively, fragments may be reconstructed using lag screws or cerclage wires to restore bone anatomy prior to the application of neutralizing or buttressing devices.

> **PRACTICAL TIP**
> **Many fractures require specific manipulations to effect reduction. These can often only be learned by experience or from more experienced colleagues, but wherever possible they have been described in appropriate sections of this manual.**

Fragment management

Bone fragments must be handled with care. Soft tissue attachments should be maintained if possible. Any fragment devoid of a substantial soft tissue attachment is dead bone and its potential value in reconstruction must be weighed against the risk of infection and sequestration. Free fragments that can be stabilized securely by interfragmentary compression and that contribute to reconstruction and overall stability may be retained. Others should be discarded. Alternatively, fragments may be left undisturbed and the fracture buttressed. The intention is that the fragments will then be incorporated in the healing process.

Bone grafting: types, indications and application

Three types of bone graft are used in fracture surgery; cancellous, cortico-cancellous and cortical. Bone grafts in small animal surgery are usually avascular, although vascularized bone grafting is possible (Szentimrey and Fowler, 1994; Szentimrey *et al.*, 1995). Bone autograft (derived from the same individual) or allograft (derived from a different individual of the same species) can be used. Zenograft (bone obtained from a different species) is not used in small animal surgery. Autogenous cancellous bone graft is by far the most useful. Bone grafts speed fracture healing in several ways:

- Osteoconduction: provision of a scaffold for neovascularization and new bone formation (Elkins and Jones, 1988)
- Osteoinduction: provision of factors that recruit local pluripotential cells to differentiate into

osteoblasts and induce formation of new bone (BMP; bone morphogenetic proteins). BMP is now produced synthetically (Kirker-Head, 1995)
- Filling of interfragmentary defects and/or provision of structural support.

Bone grafting is indicated in any situation where it is anticipated that healing could be delayed:

- Comminuted fractures
- Presence of bony defects
- Delayed or non-union fractures
- Elderly patients
- Arthrodesis.

> **WARNING**
> **Bone graft, usually being dead tissue, should be used with caution in the face of infection. Cortical bone graft is contraindicated in this circumstance.**

Bone for grafting can be obtained from a number of sites:

- Cancellous bone: proximal humeral or tibial metaphysis, wing of ilium
- Cortico-cancellous bone: wing of ilium, rib, ulna
- Cortical bone: ulna (autogenous), most long bones (allograft).

The most commonly used site is the proximal humeral metaphysis, as a large volume of cancellous bone can be obtained with least donor site morbidity (Penwick *et al.*, 1991). Use of long bones carries the risk of iatrogenic fracture. As an alternative, cortico-cancellous bone sludge can be obtained from the wing of the ilium using a power reamer (Culvenor and Parker, 1996; Stallings *et al.*, 1997).

Solid cortical or cortico-cancellous bone grafts must be rigidly stabilized. Soft cancellous or cortico-cancellous grafts are simply packed around fracture sites and maintained in position by surrounding soft tissues.

Drains

Drains are used only rarely following fracture surgery, probably due to concern over the risk of ascending infection. Closed suction drainage can be useful for 12–24 hours post-operatively if major fluid accumulation is anticipated.

Post-operative external support

Bandaging can be useful for a few days following surgery to limit post-operative swelling and thereby reduce patient discomfort, protect the surgical wound and optimize tissue perfusion. In certain circumstances, external support may be necessary to supplement internal fixation devices.

Principles of use of pins and wires

The advantages and disadvantages of different types of pin are shown in Tables 9.2 to 9.4, and indications and contraindications are given in Tables 9.5 to 9.7.

Kirschner wires

K-wires are solid steel pins of 0.9–2 mm diameter. They may have trocar or bayonet tips. Arthrodesis wires are the most useful, having a trocar tip at each end.

Steinman pins

These pins are solid steel rods, circular in cross-section. They are available in sizes from 1.6 to 8 mm in diameter and 300 mm in length and generally have trocar tips at each end. One end may be threaded, which may reduce pin migration.

Rush pins

Rush pins are a form of dynamic intramedullary cross-pinning, most often used for the fixation of distal femoral condylar fractures (Lawson, 1959; Campbell, 1976). They are best manufactured as required, using appropriately sized K-wires or small Steinman pins according to the following guidelines.

- Pins should not exceed one-third of the width of the medullary canal
- Pins should be approximately 3 times the length of the smaller fragment
- One end should have a sledge-runner tip
- The other end should be hooked
- The whole pin is slightly curved.

The use of Rush pins is illustrated in Chapter 18.

Interlocking nails

An interlocking nail (ILN) is a solid steel rod 6 or 8 mm in diameter, with a number of holes in it through which bone screws can be inserted to fix the rod within the bone and eliminate rotational and axial movement (See Chapter 3). The screws are inserted using either a specially designed jig or fluoroscopy. The 8 mm ILN appears to provide superior resistance to bending and torsion than comparable plate or external fixator repairs (Dueland *et al.*, 1996). Interlocking nails are used increasingly in humans and their use is becoming accepted in veterinary surgery (Muir *et al.*, 1993).

Kuntscher nails

These are hollow trefoil (cloverleaf) or V-shaped nails, usually with a taper at one end and a slot used for removing the nail at the other. They are available in greater widths than Steinman pins, but are of little use in small animal orthopaedics.

Eliminating rotational instability

Rotation in long bone fractures is a major problem with

Advantages	Disadvantages
Resist bending forces well due to location at neutral axis of bone	Resist rotation, distraction and shearing very poorly
Quick and easy to insert and remove	Rarely provide adequate stability alone
Little special equipment or training required	May allow wicking of bacteria along medullary canal
Fracture healing relatively easy to assess	

Table 9.2: Advantages and disadvantages of intramedullary pins.

Advantages	Disadvantages
Resist bending forces well due to location at neutral axis of bone	Insertion technique requires practice
Resist rotation well due to spring-loaded effect	Limited usefulness other than distal femur
Fracture healing relatively easy to assess	

Table 9.3: Advantages and disadvantages of Rush pins.

Advantages	Disadvantages
Resist bending forces well due to location at neutral axis of bone	Difficult to insert and remove
Resist rotation, distraction and shearing well due to interlocking function	Special equipment and training required
Fracture healing relatively easy to assess	

Table 9.4: Advantages and disadvantages of interlocking nails.

Indications	Contraindications
Completely reducible, intrinsically stable simple transverse* or short oblique interlocking diaphyseal fractures in animals with good healing potential	Irreducible fractures with significant rotation, distraction or shearing
Completely reducible long oblique or spiral fractures with cerclage wires	Open or infected fractures
Irreducible severely comminuted fractures if used in conjunction with ESF or plate and screws as part of a minimally invasive strategy	Metaphyseal or articular fractures
	Any fracture where the pin cannot be inserted safely (e.g. radius)
Cats	Avulsion fractures

* Many transverse fractures are poor candidates for intramedullary pinning due to lack of resistance to rotation

Table 9.5: Indications and contraindications for intramedullary pins.

Indications	Contraindications
Distal femoral condylar fractures	Open or infected fractures
Selected other metaphyseal fractures	Avulsion fractures
	Comminuted fractures

Table 9.6: Indications and contraindications for Rush pins.

Indications	Contraindications
Diaphyseal fractures of the long bones	Open or infected fractures
Irreducible severely comminuted fractures	Metaphyseal or articular fractures
	Avulsion fractures
	Any fractures where the pin cannot be inserted safely (e.g. radius)

Table 9.7: Indications and contraindications for interlocking nails.

intramedullary pins as, in general, they are very poor at resisting it. Rotation within the developing callus is a major obstacle to healing and a common cause of delayed or non-union. Rotational instability can be minimized by the following measures:

- Select transverse or short oblique interlocking fractures with good intrinsic rotational stability (NB: rotational stability is often poor in such fractures)
- Select fractures with potential for rapid healing, e.g. simple fractures in young healthy dogs or cats
- Use cerclage wires in appropriate long oblique or spiral fractures
- Use external fixator as auxiliary fixation
- Use plate and screws as auxiliary fixation
- Use interlocking nail
- Use external support judiciously.

Use of multiple intramedullary pins (stack pinning) is of little value, as pins tend to loosen and migrate.

Biodegradable rods
Metallic implants may have theoretical and practical disadvantages relating to potential for sarcoma induction and relative mismatch between rigidity of bone and implant. Rods formed from self-reinforced polygalactide or polylactide have been described for use in cancellous bone and, more recently, in the diaphysis (Axelson *et al.*, 1988; Räihä *et al.*, 1993a,b). Suggested benefits include a gradual transfer of stress from implant to bone during the healing phase and avoidance of a second surgery for implant removal.

These implants are inserted into slightly smaller pre-drilled bone tunnels using specially designed applicators. They are difficult to remove once inserted and are radiolucent, although this latter attribute may facilitate assessment of the fracture line. Biodegradable implants have, to date, gained little popularity in the UK other than for the reattachment of intra-articular osteochondral fragments to the canine tibial tarsal bone, presumably due to relatively high costs of implants and applicators and limited range of sizes available.

Orthopaedic wire
Orthopaedic wire should always be monofilament steel and should be obtained from the same source as pins. Useful diameters range from 0.8 to 1.2 mm. Wire nar-

rower than 0.8 mm or thicker than 1.2 mm cannot be tightened adequately. Wire may be tightened using combined cutter/twisters, parallel pliers, or various special wire twisters or tighteners. AO/ASIF wires have looped ends to permit tensioning using a special device.

Indications and principles of cerclage wire

Full cerclage wires encircle the bone completely. Hemi-cerclage wires pass through a tunnel in the bone at some point, which may provide more secure fixation but can be challenging to apply. Cerclage wires may be used to supplement intramedullary pins by applying interfragmentary compression in long oblique or spiral fractures, or completely reducible mildly comminuted fractures, but are inappropriate for sole fixation of long bone fractures. There is no detrimental effect upon the bone (Wilson, 1987).

Principles for use of cerclage wire are as follows:

- Fracture should be fully reconstructable
- Length of fracture should be at least 2 times diameter of bone
- At least two cerclage wires should be used
- Wires should be not less than 1 cm apart
- All wires must be tight.

Tension-band wire

A tension-band is an inelastic device positioned in a location whereby it is placed under tension. The tension-band, which may be a wire or a plate, converts tensile force to compression (Figure 9.7). This is termed dynamic compression. Tension band wires are generally indicated for treatment of avulsion fractures,

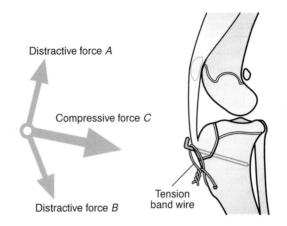

Figure 9.7: *Tension-band effect: the sum of two forces (A, B) exerted at different angles will result in a compressive force (C). The example shows tension-band wiring in the treatment of tibial tuberosity avulsion.*

where a relatively small fragment of bone is detached by tensile forces generated by soft tissues to which it is attached (e.g. tibial tuberosity separation, distal tibial malleolar fracture, osteotomy of the greater trochanter of the femur). The wire is used in conjunction with one or two small pins, whose function is to aid in fragment stability by resisting the comparatively small angular or rotational forces.

Principles of use of external skeletal fixation

Definitions

External skeletal fixators (external fixators, fixators, ESFs) consist of a series of percutaneous transosseous

Size	Transfixing pin*	Connecting bar
Small	2 mm (1/16-3/32″)	3 mm (1/8″)
Medium	3 mm (3/32-1/8″)	4 mm (3/16″)
Large	4 mm (5/32-3/16″)	8 mm (5/16″)
Extra Large	5 mm (3/16-1/4″)	10 mm (7/16″)

* Core diameter of pin

Table 9.8: *External fixator sizes.*

Advantages	Disadvantages
Minimal instrumentation required	Soft tissue problems possible
Certain components recyclable†	Application technique requires practice
Minimal disruption of local soft tissues	Premature pin loosening common
Minimal foreign body at fracture site	Perception as panacea has led to abuse
Open wound management easy	Difficult to apply to proximal limb
Easy to combine with other implants	
Rigidity and alignment easily adjustable	
Gradual linear and angular traction possible, allowing progressive correction of deformities	
Assessment of fracture healing easy	
Easy to remove	

† Clamps and (possibly) bars may be reused. Pins may not.

Table 9.9: *Advantages and disadvantages of external skeletal fixation.*

Indications	Contraindications
Diaphyseal fractures Highly comminuted fractures Open or infected fractures Mandibular fractures Auxiliary fixation Corrective osteotomy Transarticular immobilization	Sole fixation method in proximal limb Situations where anatomical fixation is required

Table 9.10: Indications and contraindications for external skeletal fixation.

transfixing pins that penetrate both cortices of the bone to which they are applied but may or may not penetrate soft tissues on both sides of the limb, connected by some type of external bar(s). The pins may be smooth in outline, or may be centrally or terminally threaded.

Connecting bars may be steel rods to which the transfixing pins are connected by clamps or may be acrylic resin (e.g. polymethylmethacrylate bone cement, dental acrylic, etc.). Clamps may be single, to connect pins to bars, or double, for connecting a number of bars to one another in the assembly of more complex configurations.

Fixators are extremely versatile devices and are very well tolerated, but it is prudent to counsel owners regarding their appearance, or to show photographs of previous cases.

External fixators are available in a range of sizes (Table 9.8). The advantages and disadvantages of external skeletal fixation are shown in Table 9.9, and the indications and contraindications for its use are in Table 9.10.

APEF system
The acrylic pin external fixator (APEF) system uses corrugated tubing that is attached to traditional transfixing pins before being filled with pre-packaged polymethylmethacrylate. This system is used in an identical manner to traditional systems, but it has the advantage that all pins may be inserted prior to application of the connecting bar. Hence, greater versatility in multiplanar pin insertion and more inventive configuration design are possible (Figure 9.8). Acrylic appears to be strong enough to satisfy its role as a connecting bar (Willer *et al*., 1991) and APEF systems appear to perform well in small animals (Okrasinski *et al*., 1991).

Configurations
To allow fracture healing, the fixator must fulfil the biomechanical demands of the particular fracture over the required period of time. Frame configuration and properties are, therefore, important considerations. One advantage of fixators is the ability to vary the characteristics of the frame, changing the number, size and orientation of its components to suit the needs of any particular fracture. An infinite number of varia-

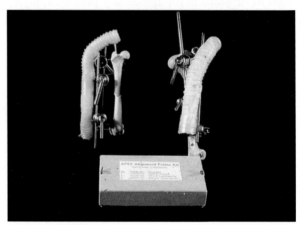

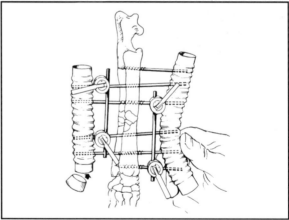

Figure 9.8: (a) APEF system comprising traditional transfixing pins and plastic tubing containing acrylic cement. (b) Temporary fracture stabilization using removable clamps and steel bars. Plastic tubing is pushed over pin ends following fracture reduction and bottom-plugged. Acrylic is mixed in self-contained packets and poured into tubing while still in the liquid phase. The steel clamps and bars are removed once the acrylic is set.

Courtesy of J.P. Lapish

tions on the basic external fixator could be constructed, but a good philosophy is to apply the simplest configuration that will provide sufficient strength for the job in hand. With current hardware, unilateral systems are satisfactory for most situations and have a lower complication rate than more complex systems. External fixator configurations are described as uniplanar or biplanar and unilateral or bilateral (Carmichael, 1991). In addition, ring fixator systems exist (e.g. Ilizarov). Useful configurations are illustrated in Figure 9.9.

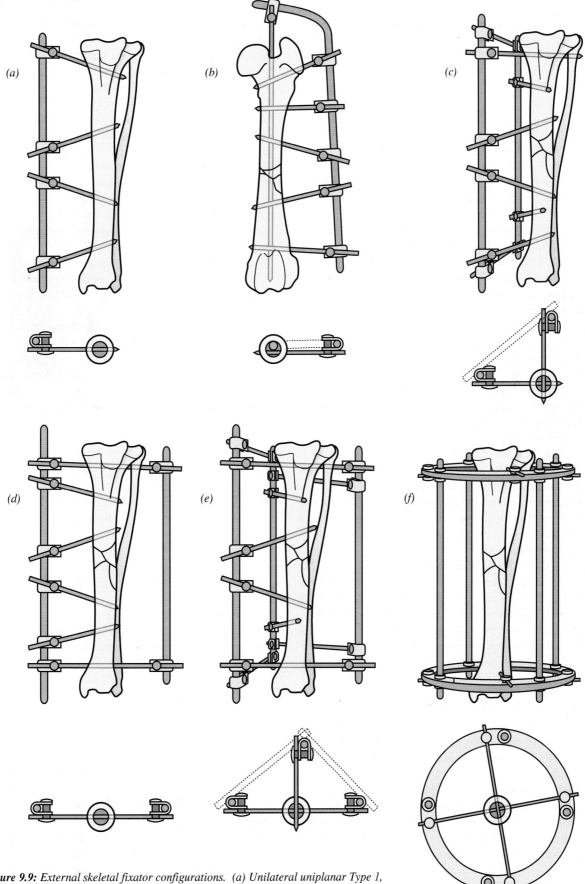

Figure 9.9: *External skeletal fixator configurations. (a) Unilateral uniplanar Type 1, half frame. (b) Unilateral uniplanar external skeletal fixator and intramedullary pin tie-in. (c) Unilateral biplanar; quadrangular, delta frame. (d) Bilateral uniplanar (modified) Type 2. (e) Bilateral biplanar Type 3. (f) Ilizarov ring.*

Altering rigidity of the external skeletal fixator
The following measures will increase the stiffness of a unilateral frame.

- Apply frame in a mechanically advantageous position
- Increase the number of transfixing pins (up to four per main fragment)
- Increase the diameter of transfixing pins (up to 20–30% of bone diameter)
- Increase the spread of transfixing pins
- Increase the rigidity of the connecting bar (Pollo *et al.*, 1993)
- Increase the number of connecting bars
- Decrease the distance between clamp and skin or contour the connecting bar to the limb (Bouvy *et al.*, 1993)
- Use a biplanar configuration
- Use intramedullary pin 'tie-in' configuration (Aron *et al.*, 1991).

The opposite measures can clearly be used to decrease frame stiffness.

Ilizarov and ring fixators
The ring fixators, of which the Ilizarov system is one example, offer a different philosophy. These devices use a number of very small pins (in effect K-wires) that are inserted through the limb in whichever plane is most appropriate and connected to an encircling or hemicircumferential connecting bar. Crucially, these pins are tensioned before tightening, making them disproportionately strong in much the same way as the spokes of a bicycle (Thommasini and Betts, 1991). Ring fixator systems offer tremendous versatility in constructing frames to deal with almost any situation. Complicated fractures, filling bone defects (Lesser 1994), correction of angular deformities and limb lengthening procedures using distraction osteogenesis (Elkins *et al.*, 1993) can be undertaken. Their main disadvantages relate to the greater difficulty in application and their cumbersome nature as compared with bar fixator systems.

External fixator boot
On occasion, in the distal limb, it is necessary to apply an external skeletal fixator to the metacarpals or metatarsals. This is often a transarticular external skeletal fixator. The arched structure of the bones and their relatively small size may make pin selection and placement challenging. A 'boot' of cast material may be applied to the distal limb and pins incorporated into it rather than being driven into the metatarsals or metacarpals (Gallacher *et al.*, 1990, 1992).

Pin design and insertion technique
The pin–bone interface is the weakest link in any external fixator configuration and the point of maxi-

mal stress concentration during loading, especially on the *cis* cortex when unilateral systems are used (*cis* refers to the near cortex; *trans* is the distant cortex). Excessive strain causes bone resorption and replacement with fibrous, synovial-like and cartilaginous tissue around the pin, with consequent pin loosening. Loose pins do not contribute any stability to the fixation, but do cause periosteal and soft tissue pain, leading to poor limb use and predisposing to pin tract infection.

The holding power of pins depends largely on their design, the insertion method and the nature and quantity of the involved bone (Clary and Roe, 1995). Pin-bone purchase is less critical in situations of rapid healing or good load sharing between bone and fixator. The use of threaded pins increases holding power. Threads may be cut into the pin (negative profile, e.g. Ellis pin), or may be rolled on during manufacture (positive profile, e.g. IMEX pin) (See Operative Technique 9.4). Negative profile pins have the disadvantage that a stress riser exists at the thread/non-thread junction. This region must be protected by being located within the medullary canal, or else there is a risk of the pin breaking (Palmer and Aron, 1990). Hence, Ellis pins have a fairly short threaded section. Positive profile pins do not have this weakness, but do have the disadvantage that they cannot be inserted through fixation clamps. Whatever pin type is selected, it should not exceed 20–30% of the diameter of the bone in question.

Recommended methods of pin insertion include slow-speed drilling and insertion into slightly smaller pre-drilled holes, especially for positive profile pins (Clary and Roe, 1996). High-speed drilling leads to thermal necrosis of bone and poor fixation; manual insertion is prone to lead to mechanical damage to the bone due to hand wobble (Egger *et al.*, 1986).

Post-operative management
Despite the presence of percutaneous pins, infection is rare and antibiotic therapy is not necessary other than in the peri-operative period. Pin tracts require no specific treatment and are best left to heal by second intention. The patient should be restricted to the house and to controlled activity, as fixators can get tangled in trees, bushes, etc. and could be avulsed prematurely. Follow-up radiographs should be taken at regular intervals. The progression of fracture healing is easy to assess as there is minimal hardware at the fracture site to obscure this on radiographs.

Staging down
As healing progresses and callus formation increases, it is advantageous to decrease the strength of the fixator as the strength of the bone increases. This can be done by reversing the measures taken to increase the strength of the fixator outlined above. This is usually appropriate around 6 weeks after surgery (Egger *et al.*, 1993).

If done too soon, there will be insufficiently strong callus and healing will be retarded due to instability.

Fixators are generally removed piecemeal, firstly by removal of additional connecting bars (if present), then by removal of centrally located transfixing pins. This can be done without general anaesthesia if desired, although this is usually necessary for radiographic evaluation in any case. There will often be haemorrhage from empty pin tracts, but this rarely requires specific treatment other than a light bandage.

Dynamic external fixators exist that allow strictly controlled axial micromovement, which increases callus formation and maturation, accelerating clinical union (Lanyon and Rubin, 1984). Note that this micromovement is very strictly controlled, being purely axial in nature, and this situation is fundamentally different from one of unstable fixation or staging down. These devices are currently prohibitively expensive for the veterinary market.

Principles of use of plates and screws

Bone plates act as internal splints, stabilizing fracture fragments while healing occurs. Plates are contoured to fit the bone and fixed to it by screws. They depend upon friction between plate and bone for their grip. Plates are generally good at resisting distraction and rotation, but are weaker than intramedullary devices with respect to angulation.

Types of plate

Bone plates have undergone considerable evolution since their development and some examples are illustrated in Figure 9.10.

WARNING
The Sherman and Burns style plates and semi-tubular plate are not recommended.

Various special plates also exist for use in particular situations (e.g. curved plates for acetabular fractures, T-plates for metaphyseal fractures) and custom-made plates can be manufactured if required for specific awkward situations.

Types of screw
Screws can be divided broadly into:

- Cortical and cancellous
- Self-tapping and non self-tapping (ASIF-type).

Cortical screws have a relatively fine thread pitch and are designed for use in thin but hard cortical bone, although they may also be used in cancellous bone. Cancellous screws have a much coarser pitch and are designed for use in cancellous bone only; they have a smaller core diameter and therefore a lower AMI than corresponding cortical screws. They may be fully threaded or partially threaded. Partially threaded screws can be difficult or impossible to remove following healing, as bone fills the space left around the non-threaded portion.

Self-tapping screws have a cutting tip and a 'triangular' thread. These cut their own thread in bone, inevitably damaging it to some extent. If the screw must be removed during surgery, the thread will often strip, necessitating the insertion of a larger screw. The screw head is of the traditional slotted type. Non-self-tapping screws have a rounded tip and a 'buttress' thread (Figure 9.11) and require the use of a tap to cut a thread in the bone prior to their insertion. The tap damages the bone much less, so screws can be removed and replaced if required. The tap should always be used, even in soft bone. The screw head has a hexagonal recess to receive the screwdriver and allows significantly better purchase and less chance of damage to the head as compared with the slotted type. The underside of the head is semi-circular, allowing greater versatility in directing the screw through the plate hole.

Screws may be used with flat steel washers to prevent the screw head from sinking into soft bone.

Screw sizes and appropriate drill sizes are listed in Table 9.11.

PRACTICAL TIP
The DCP is the most versatile plate for routine use.
The most useful screws are non-self-tapping (ASIF-type) cortical screws.

Screw size	Thread hole	Gliding hole	Tap
1.5 mm cortical	1.1 mm	1.5 mm	1.5 mm
2.0 mm cortical	1.5 mm	2.0 mm	2.0 mm
2.7 mm cortical	2.0 mm	2.7 mm	2.7 mm
3.5 mm cortical	2.5 mm	3.5 mm	3.5 mm
3.5 mm cancellous	2.0 mm	3.5 mm	3.5 mm
4.0 mm cancellous	2.0 mm	4.0 mm	4.0 mm
4.5 mm cortical	3.2 mm	4.5 mm	4.5 mm
6.5 mm cancellous	3.2 mm	6.5 mm	6.5 mm

Table 9.11: Appropriate drill and tap sizes for various screws.

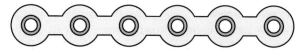

Figure 9.10: *(a) Sherman, Burns style plates: Round holes; plate narrows considerably between holes, resulting in significant weakening.*

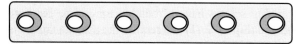

(b) Semi-tubular plate: Weak plate, designed for minimal loading. Screw holes may be oval, allowing eccentric screw placement and a degree of axial compression.

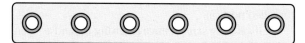

(c) Venables plate: Stronger plate. Screw holes round and often insufficient number. Modern variant is thicker and stronger than traditional design.

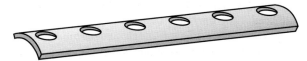

(d) Dynamic compression plate (DCP) AO/ASIF type: Strong plate, specially engineered self-compressing screw holes use 'rolling ball' principle to allow axial compression using special 'load' drill guide to position screw hole eccentrically in plate hole. Enormous range of sizes available. The best plate for routine use.

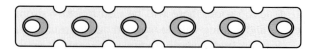

(e) Reconstruction plate: DCP-style plate that is notched between screw holes to allow for more versatile three-dimensional bending, at the cost of some strength. Useful for pelvic (Dyce and Houlton, 1993) or distal femoral condylar fracture repair (Lewis et al., 1993) where very complex plate contouring may be required.

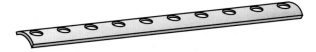

(f) Veterinary cuttable plate: Semi-tubular, round hole plate. Purchased as very long plate, from which the required length is cut. High screw density is useful when bone stock is limited e.g. buttressing severely comminuted long bone fractures. May be stacked one on top of another in order to increase strength (McLaughlin et al., 1992). Useful in smaller bones (Gentry et al., 1993).

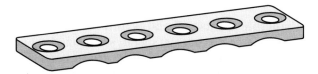

(g) Limited contact dynamic compression plate (LC-DCP): Plate with specially-designed undercuts that reduce impairment of osseous blood flow by limiting contact area between plate and bone and eliminate stress concentration at screw holes. Screw holes are bevelled to allow axial compression in either direction.

(h) The DCP screw hole. When the semi-circular screw head contacts the 'shoulder' in the specially-designed plate hole the screw slides towards the fracture site.

(i) The DCP drill guide has 'neutral' and 'load' functions; the 'load' guide normally has an arrow that should point towards the fracture site. Axial compression is produced by positioning the screw eccentrically within the screw hole i.e. distant from the fracture site.

(j) Tightening the screws results in compression of the fracture as the screws slide towards one another.

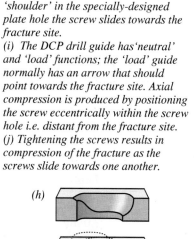

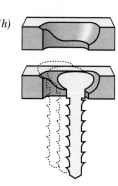

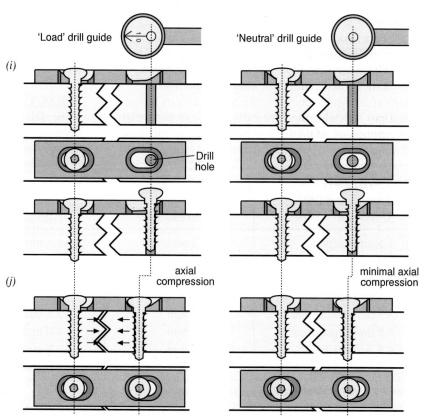

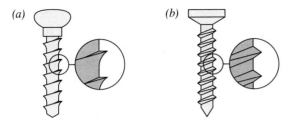

Figure 9.11: Screws. (a) Non-self-tapping AO-type screw. (b) Self-tapping screw.

AO/ASIF principles and instrumentation

The formation of the Arbeitsgemeinschaft für Osteosynthesefragen / Association for the Study of Internal Fixation group (AO/ASIF) in Switzerland in the 1950s was in reaction to an unacceptable incidence of fracture disease associated with contemporary fracture fixation methods. The group defined a number of aims and principles for a rapid return to full function following fracture treatment (Prieur and Sumner-Smith, 1984):

- Anatomical reduction of fracture fragments, especially with respect to articular surfaces
- Preservation of blood supply to bone fragments and soft tissues by delicate atraumatic surgery
- Stable internal fixation, satisfying the biomechanical requirements
- Early active pain-free movement and full weight bearing of the traumatized limb, avoiding fracture disease.

The AO/ASIF group also designed novel implants and instrumentation to achieve these goals, the prime amongst which is the dynamic compression plate.

It can be seen that, currently, two of the AO/ASIF principles (i.e. anatomical reduction and internal fixation) are not invariably the surgeon's aim. Other principles (i.e. rigid fracture fixation, atraumatic technique and early mobilization) are still paramount. For a full description of AO/ASIF philosophy and techniques, refer to the excellent manual of Brinker *et al.* (1984).

WARNING
The development of AO principles still represents one of the most important advances in the history of orthopaedic surgery and the surgeon would be ill advised to ignore them.

Interfragmentary compression

Compression between fracture fragments reduces the fracture gap and, by increasing interfragmentary friction, increases stability. Both these factors help to optimize conditions for healing in the presence of rigid stability. Note that the size of the fracture gap(s) can have a crucial bearing on interfragmentary strain if there is interfragmentary movement (see Chapter 3).

Interfragmentary compression may be *dynamic* (i.e. it is produced by axial loading or muscle forces) or *static* (i.e. it does not depend on the above forces).

Interfragmentary compression using lag screws: Insertion of a *lagged* screw across a fracture gap will result in interfragmentary compression (see Operative Technique 9.5).

Lag screw fixation may be the sole method of fixation (e.g. lateral distal humeral condylar fracture) or may be used to reconstruct comminuted fracture fragments. In the latter situation, lag screws may be used through the plate, or separate from it. Note that lag screws generate *static* compression.

WARNING
Only lag screws should cross fracture lines, unless this causes fracture collapse.

Axial compression using plates: Plate fixation with axial compression is a good way of repairing simple transverse or short oblique fractures but is not appropriate for comminuted fractures. Plates can generate axial compression in several ways and more than one of these may act in any given situation:

- Application of the plate to the tension surface of the bone will allow the tension-band effect to apply and will result in axial compression of the bone under the plate. This is *dynamic* compression (Figure 9.12)

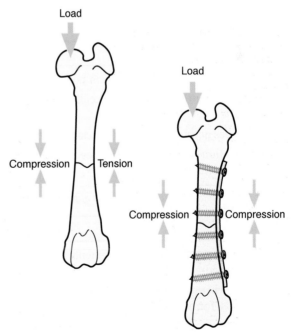

Figure 9.12: Tension-band effect using plate. Most bones (e.g. femur) are loaded eccentrically and have tension and compression surfaces. Fractures will therefore also tend to have tension and compression surfaces. Application of an inelastic device (plate) to the tension surface will convert tensile forces generated by loading to compression at that surface. This need not be a DCP-style plate.

- Use of a tensioning device at the end of the plate can produce *static* axial compression
- Use of a DCP can allow generation of *static* axial compression by eccentric screw positioning in the oval plate hole using a special drill guide (see Operative Technique 9.6).

Neutralization and buttressing

Axial compression in comminuted fractures is not desirable. Fracture fragments may be reconstructed using lag screws, so that interfragmentary compression is present. Axial compression subsequent to this would disrupt interfragmentary compression. Instead, plates are used to protect the repaired fracture from loading when weightbearing occurs.

- Neutralization plates span the reduced fracture and transmit loading forces past the fracture (see Operative Technique 9.6). Variable amounts of load-sharing between fracture and implant occur. Very accurate plate contouring is essential so that unwanted forces are not created within the repaired fracture as the screws are tightened.
- Buttress plates (see Operative Technique 9.6)

PRACTICAL TIP
Compression, neutralization and buttress are descriptions of plate application and function rather than design. The DCP is most commonly used in all these roles, although custom-made plates are very useful in buttressing roles.

span fractures that are not reduced and bear fully the forces generated by weight bearing. It is obvious that the plate is extremely vulnerable in this situation. Implant strength and healing rate should be maximized.

Application of plate and screws

The basic guidelines for plate and screw application are as follows:

- Use as long a plate as possible and contour it accurately to the bone
- Engage at least six cortices proximal and distal to the fracture
- Fill all screw holes
- All screws must be tight and should engage both cortices
- Only lag screws may cross fracture lines (in some situations lagging a screw across a fracture line may cause fragment collapse; in this situation a position screw may be inserted, thread cut in both cortices – i.e. no lag effect)
- Avoid cortical defects, especially on the compression surface
- Learn to plan fixation carefully and work quickly.

Clearly, it is not always possible to fulfil all these guidelines. Some fractures (for example, metaphyseal or articular fractures) do not allow for six cortices to be engaged on either side. These guidelines should, however, form a useful checklist to apply to most plate fixations.

Advantages	Disadvantages
Anatomical fracture reconstruction possible	Specialist equipment and training required
Healing with little or no external callus formation possible	Wide exposure of bone required
Most forces acting at the fracture resisted well	Large foreign body inserted at fracture site
Rigid fixation allows early pain-free mobility and prevents fracture disease	Substantial investment in materials

Table 9.12: Advantages and disadvantages of plate and screw fixation

Indications	Contraindications
Fractures involving sizeable fragments that can be reconstructed	Inadequate screw purchase in bone possible (e.g. very young patient, osteopenia)
Fractures where anatomical reconstruction and minimal callus formation are required (e.g. articular fractures)	Selected comminuted fractures in which alternative buttressing methods apply.
Any fracture requiring compression (e.g. non-union)	
Buttressing non-reconstructable fractures	
Arthrodesis	

Table 9.13: Indications and contraindications of plate and screw fixation

The advantages and disadvantages of plate and screw fixation are listed in Table 9.12, and the indications and contraindications in Table 9.13.

Combining fixation system: maximizing rigidity of fixation

Chemical and physical compatibility

As a rule, different implant systems should not be mixed, due to possible small differences in chemical composition that could cause galvanic effects or variances in dimension that could lead to mismatches, e.g. between tap and screw sizes (Baumgart, 1991). Practically speaking, all reputable instruments and implants should be of identical chemistry and construction and incompatibility should be unlikely (see Chapter 8).

Combining different fixation methods can be enormously helpful in situations where maximum strength or rigidity of fixation is required, e.g. for buttressing non-reconstructable severely comminuted fractures. This approach is generally combined with a minimally invasive 'open but don't touch' (OBDT) philosophy (see Chapter 10) and allows considerable inventiveness.

Pin–ESF systems

Combining an intramedullary device with an external fixator produces a very strong fixation, but significant complications can be associated with the use of such a combined device in the proximal limb (Foland *et al.*, 1991). The intramedullary pin may be allowed to protrude through the skin and be clamped to the connecting bar of the external fixator. This is a 'tie-in' configuration (see Figure 9.14). The flaring of the bone towards the metaphysis usually allows sufficient room for insertion of transfixing pins.

Pin–plate systems

Combining an intramedullary pin with a plate is even more rigid (Hulse *et al.*, 1994). To facilitate screw insertion, the pin should be 50–70% of the diameter of the medullary cavity (Figure 9.13). Monocortical screws may be used with success.

POST-OPERATIVE MANAGEMENT

Client education

Rest requirements

Requirements for post-operative care of fracture surgery patients must be explained clearly to their owners and documented on case notes. Written directions should be provided for owners wherever possible. The traditional view that cage rest should be advocated following fracture surgery is out-dated and in most cases detrimental to fracture healing and patient con-

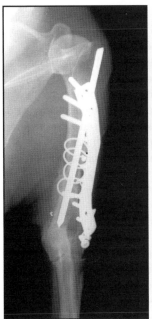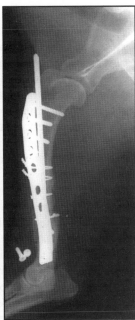

Figure 9.13: *Radiograph of healing comminuted humeral fracture treated by cerclage wiring and pinplate buttressing 6 weeks earlier. There is moderate bridging callus formation (the so-called bio-buttress). The pin had migrated proximally and was removed. The free and broken screw are remnants of a failed surgical repair.*

valescence/rehabilitation. Modern fracture fixation methods allow rigid immobilization of the fracture without immobilization of the limb, and controlled limb use should be allowed along with provision of analgesia, in order to minimize fracture disease. Vigorous or uncontrolled activity should be avoided until fracture healing has occurred. Short bouts of leash exercise (for example, 10–15 minutes two to three times a day) are generally appropriate for the first 3–4 weeks, after which time this may be increased, pending the results of follow-up radiography.

Physiotherapy

Physiotherapy is difficult to use to any great extent in dogs and cats for reasons of practicality and expense. In most cases, however, owners can be instructed in a few simple flexion–extension exercises if appropriate. Controlled or even assisted ambulation is useful and swimming can be particularly beneficial once skin wounds have sealed, allowing full limb mobilization and maintaining muscle bulk without excessive loading of repaired fractures. Many equine rehabilitation units are happy to allow dog owners to use their facilities and a few swimming pools specifically for dogs now exist. Experienced supervision is required for swimming in order to eliminate violent uncontrolled movement in the early stages of healing.

> **PRACTICAL TIP**
> **Frequent short bouts of exercise or physiotherapy are superior to infrequent long bouts.**

Following up

Critical appraisal of fracture repair

Constant self-appraisal is essential to maintain and improve standards. Radiographs of fracture repairs should always be taken at the end of surgery and at intervals until fracture healing has been documented. The result of surgery should be assessed and compared with the original fracture plan. The fracture plan itself should also be reviewed and appraised once its result is known.

Record keeping

Detailed records should be kept and reviewed regularly in order to assess the results of fracture treatment and to compare these with the experiences of other surgeons and published results. If results of fracture repairs appear unusually poor, possible reasons for this should be sought and treatment protocols amended accordingly. If results appear unusually good, reasons for this should be identified and published in order to disseminate the increased knowledge and improve quality of care generally.

Assessment of fracture healing (see Chapter 5)

Fracture healing should be assessed physically and radiographically at regular intervals, usually monthly or bimonthly. Functional union will usually occur prior to radiographic union. Healing is easier to assess with some fixation systems than others. Fractures treated by plate and screw application can be particularly difficult to assess as the fracture line may be difficult or impossible to visualize immediately following repair and therefore assessment of healing, which may occur with little or no visible callus formation, may be challenging. Conversely, fractures treated using external skeletal fixation will usually be fairly visible and there will usually be appreciable amounts of callus formation, which facilitate assessment.

Recognizing and dealing with complications

It is important to realize and accept that not all fracture fixations will be without complications. Problems noted on post-operative radiographs (e.g. inappropriate implant placement) should not be tolerated, but should be remedied by immediate revision surgery. Evidence of infection or of delayed or non-union should be treated aggressively. Complications will always occur, but their frequency can be minimized by attention to good planning and surgical technique. Anticipating complications will allow their early detection and treatment.

Implant removal

Surgical implants may be removed following complete fracture healing if required. This can be beneficial in terms of removing any shielding effect from the bone, which could result in disuse atrophy of the bone ('stress protection'), though this may be less important than previously believed (Glennon *et al.*, 1994; Muir *et al.*, 1995). Implants will also occasionally loosen, especially pins, and may cause discomfort if they are loose or other problems if they migrate. If there has been infection of the fracture site, this may become associated with the implant ('cryptic infection') and lead to recurrent lameness or, possibly, predispose to fracture-associated sarcoma, although a definite link between metallic implants and cancer in dogs has not been shown (Li *et al.*, 1993). Persistence of bacteria at a significant proportion of metallic implants has been documented (Smith *et al.*, 1989). Implants in some sites, e.g. pelvis and humerus, are rarely removed. It must be remembered that open screw holes left after implant removal will concentrate stress and predispose to fracture, so restricted exercise or even external support should be advised especially after plate removal. The perceived benefits and possible risks of implant removal must always be weighed up against one another.

REFERENCES

Aron DN, Foutz TL, Keller WG and Brown J (1991) Experimental and clinical experience with an IM pin external skeletal fixator tie-in configuration. *Veterinary and Comparative Orthopaedics and Traumatology* **4**, 86–94.

Aron DN, Johnson AL and Palmer RH (1995) Biologic strategies and a balanced concept for repair of highly comminuted long bone fractures. *Compendium of Continuing Education for the Practising Veterinarian* **17**, 35.

Axelson P, Räihä JE, Mero M, Vainionpää S, Törmälä P and Rokkanen P (1988) The use of a biodegradable implant in fracture fixation: a review of the literature and a report of two clinical cases. *Journal of Small Animal Practice* **29**, 249–255.

Baumgart F (1991) The 'mixing' of implant systems. *Veterinary and Comparative Orthopaedics and Traumatology* **4**, 38–45.

Blass CE and Moore RW (1984) The tourniquet in surgery: a review. *Veterinary Surgery* **13**(2), 111–114.

Blass CE, Piermattei DL, Withrow SJ and Scott RJ (1986) Static and dynamic cerclage wire analysis. *Veterinary Surgery* **15**(2), 181–184.

Bouvy BM, Markel MD, Chelikani S, Egger EL, Piermattei DL and Vanderby R (1993) *Ex vivo* biomechanics of Kirschner–Ehmer external skeletal fixation applied to canine tibiae. *Veterinary Surgery* **22**(3), 194–207.

Brinker WO, Hohn RB and Prieur WD (1984) *Manual of Internal Fixation in Small Animals*. Springer-Verlag, Berlin.

Campbell JR (1976) The technique of fixation of fractures of the distal femur using Rush pins. *Journal of Small Animal Practice* **17**, 323–329.

Carmichael S (1991) The external fixator in small animal orthopaedics. *Journal of Small Animal Practice* **32**, 486–493.

Clary EM and Roe SC (1995) Enhancing external skeletal fixation pin performance: consideration of the pin–bone interface. *Veterinary and Comparative Orthopaedics and Traumatology* **8**(1), 1–8.

Clary EM and Roe SC (1996) *In vitro* biomechanical and histological assessment of pilot hole diameter for positive-profile external skeletal fixation pins in canine tibiae. *Veterinary Surgery* **25**, 453–462.

Culvenor JA and Parker RJ (1996) Collection of corticocancellous bone graft from the ilium of the dog using an acetabular reamer. *Journal of Small Animal Practice* **37**, 513–515.

Dueland RT, Berglund L, Vanderby R and Chao EYS (1996) Structural properties of interlocking nails, canine femora and femur-interlocking nail constructs. *Veterinary Surgery* **25**, 386–396.

Dyce J and Houlton JEF (1993) Use of reconstruction plates for repair of acetabular fractures in 16 dogs. *Journal of Small Animal Practice* **34**, 547–553.

Egger EL, Histand MB, Blass CE and Powers BE (1986) Effect of fixation pin insertion on the bone–pin interface. *Veterinary Surgery* **15**(3), 246–252.

Egger EL, Histand MB, Norrdin RW, Konde LJ and Schwarz PD (1993) Canine osteotomy healing when stabilized with decreasingly rigid fixation compared to constantly rigid fixation. *Veterinary and Comparative Orthopaedics and Traumatology* **6**, 182–187.

Elkins AD and Jones LP (1988) The effects of Plaster of Paris and autogenous cancellous bone on the healing of cortical defects in the femurs of dogs. *Veterinary Surgery* **17**(2), 71–76.

Elkins AD, Morandi M and Zembo M (1993) Distraction osteogenesis in the dog using the Ilizarov external ring fixator. *Journal of the American Animal Hospital Association* **29**, 419–426.

Foland MA, Schwarz PD and Salman MD (1991) The adjunctive use of half-pin (type 1) external skeletal fixators in combination with intramedullary pins for femoral fracture fixation. *Veterinary and Comparative Orthopaedics and Traumatology* **4**, 77–85.

Gallacher LA, Rudy RL and Smeak DD (1990) The external fixator boot: application, techniques and indications. *Journal of the American Animal Hospital Association* **26**, 403–409.

Gallacher LA, Smeak DD, Johnson AL, Boone RJ and Rudy RL (1992) The external fixator boot for support of surgical repairs of injuries involving the crus and tarsus in dogs and cats: 21 cases. *Journal of the American Animal Hospital Association* **28**, 143–148.

Gentry SJ, Taylor RA and Dee JF (1993) The use of veterinary cuttable plates: 21 cases. *Journal of the American Animal Hospital Association* **29**, 455–458.

Glennon JC, Flanders JA, Beck KA, Trotter EJ and Erb HN (1994) The effect of long-term bone plate application for fixation of radial fractures in dogs. *Veterinary Surgery* **23**, 40–47.

Hulse D, Nori M, Hyman B and Slater M (1994) Clinical, *in vitro* and mathematical analysis of plate/rod buttressing for biological fracture stabilisation. *Veterinary Surgery* **23**, 404 (ACVS abstract 40).

Johnson AL, Seitz SE, Smith CW, Johnson JM and Schaeffer DJ (1996) Closed reduction and type-II external fixation of comminuted fractures of the radius and tibia in dogs: 23 cases (1990–1994) *Journal of the American Veterinary Medical Association* **209**, 8, 1445–1448.

Kirker-Head, C.A. (1995) Recombinant bone morphogenetic proteins: novel substances for enhancing bone healing. *Veterinary Surgery* **24**, 408–419.

Lanyon LE and Rubin CT (1984) Static versus dynamic loads as an influence on bone remodelling. *Journal of Biomechanics* **17**, 897–905.

Lawson DD (1959) The technique of Rush pinning in fracture repair. *Modern Veterinary Practice* **40**, 32–36.

Lesser AS (1994) Segmental bone transport for the treatment of bone deficits. *Journal of the American Animal Hospital Association* **30**, 322–330.

Lewis DD, van Ee RT, Oakes MG and Elkins AD (1993) Use of reconstruction plates for stabilisation of fractures and osteotomies involving the supracondylar region of the femur. *Journal of the American Animal Hospital Association* **29**, 171–178

Li XQ, Hom DL, Black J and Stevenson S (1993) Relationship between metallic implants and cancer: a case-control study in a canine population. *Veterinary and Comparative Orthopaedics and Traumatology* **6**, 70–74.

Marti JM and Miller A (1994a) Delimitation of safe corridors for the insertion of external fixator pins in the dog. 1: Hindlimb. *Journal of Small Animal Practice* **35**(1), 16–23.

Marti JM and Miller A (1994b) Delimitation of safe corridors for the insertion of external fixator pins in the dog. 2: Forelimb. *Journal of Small Animal Practice* **35**(2), 78–85.

McLaughlin RM Jr, Cockshutt JR and Kuzma AB (1992) Stacked veterinary cuttable plates for treatment of comminuted diaphyseal fractures in cats. *Veterinary and Comparative Orthopaedics and Traumatology* **5**, 22–25.

Muir P, Parker R, Goldsmid SE and Johnson KA (1993) Interlocking intramedullary nail stabilisation of a diaphyseal tibial fracture. *Journal of Small Animal Practice* **34**, 26–30.

Muir P, Markel MD, Bogdanske JJ and Johnson KA (1995) Dual-energy Xray absorptiometry and force-plate analysis of gait in dogs with healed femora after leg-lengthening plate fixation. *Veterinary Surgery* **24**, 15–24.

Okrasinski EB, Pardo AD and Graehler RA (1991) Biomechanical evaluation of acrylic external skeletal fixation in dogs and cats. *Journal of the American Veterinary Medical Association* **199**(11), 1590.

Palmer RH and Aron DN (1990) Ellis pin complications in seven dogs. *Veterinary Surgery* **19**(6), 440–445.

Pardo, AD (1994) Relationship of tibial intramedullary pins to canine stifle joint structures: a comparison of normograde and retrograde insertion. *Journal of the American Animal Hospital Association* **30**, 369–374.

Penwick RC, Mosier DA and Clark DM (1991) Healing of canine autogenous cancellous bone graft donor sites. *Veterinary Surgery* **20**(4), 229–234.

Piermattei DL (1993) *An Atlas of Surgical Approaches to the Bones and Joints of the Dog and Cat*, 3rd edn. WB Saunders Co.

Pollo FE, Hyman WA and Hulse DA (1993) The role of the external bar in a 6-pin type 1 external skeletal fixation device. *Veterinary and Comparative Orthopaedics and Traumatology* **6**, 75–79.

Prieur WD and Sumner-Smith G (1984) In: *Manual of Internal Fixation in Small Animals,* ed WO Brinker, RB Hohn and WD Prieur, pp 6–7. Springer-Verlag, Berlin.

Räihä JE, Axelson P, Rokkanen P and Törmälä P (1993a) Intramedullary nailing of diaphyseal fractures with self-reinforced polylactide implants. *Journal of Small Animal Practice* **34**, 337–344.

Räihä JE, Axelson P, Skutnabb K, Rokkanen P and Törmälä P (1993b) Fixation of cancellous bone and physeal fractures with biodegradable rods of self-reinforced polylactic acid. *Journal of Small Animal Practice* **34**, 131–138.

Roe SC, Johnson AL and Harari J (1985) Placement of multiple full pins for external fixation. Technique and results in four dogs. *Veterinary Surgery* **14**(3), 247–252.

Smith MM, Vasseur PB and Saunders HM (1989) Bacterial growth associated with metallic implants in dogs. *Journal of the American Animal Hospital Association* **195**, 765–767.

Stallings JT, Parker RB, Lewis DD, Wronski ThJ and Shiroma J (1997) A comparison of autogenous cortico-cancellous bone graft obtained from the wing of the ilium with an acetabular reamer to autogenous cancellous bone graft obtained from the proximal humerus in dogs. *Veterinary and Comparative Orthopaedics and Traumatology* **10**, 79–87.

Szentimrey D and Fowler D (1994) The anatomic basis of a free vascularised bone graft based on the canine distal ulna. *Veterinary Surgery* **23**, 529–533.

Szentimrey D, Fowler D, Johnston G and Wilkinson A (1995) Transplantation of the canine distal ulna as a free vascularised bone graft. *Veterinary Surgery* **24**, 215–225.

Thommasini MD and Betts CW (1991) Use of the 'Ilizarov' external fixator in a dog. *Veterinary and Comparative Orthopaedics and Traumatology* **4**, 70–76.

Willer RL, Egger EL and Histand MB (1991) Comparison of stainless steel versus acrylic for the connecting bar of external skeletal fixators. *Journal of the American Animal Hospital Association* **27**, 541–548.

Wilson JW (1987) Effect of cerclage wires on periosteal bone in growing dogs. *Veterinary Surgery* **16**(4), 299–302.

OPERATIVE TECHNIQUE 9.1
Insertion of intramedullary pin

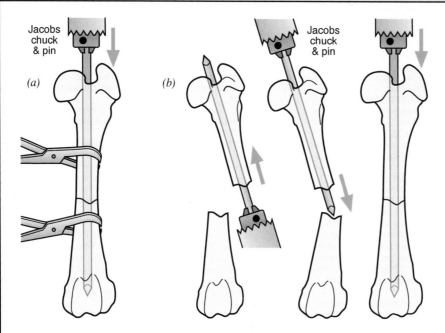

Figure 9.14:
Pin insertion:
(a) normograde;
(b) retrograde.

Pins may be inserted normograde or retrograde.

Tray extras
Gelpi retractors; bone holding forceps; pointed reduction forceps; Jacob's chuck or motorized pin driver; small and large pin cutters; appropriate pin(s)

Surgical approach
Appropriate for bone involved

Selection of pin size
Pin diameter slightly less than diameter of medullary cavity at its narrowest point (isthmus).

Length of pin best determined from pre-operative radiograph of same bone in contralateral limb: tip should impact in (distal) metaphysis; free end should protrude approximately 5–10 mm (proximally) to allow removal.

Pin may be cut to appropriate length pre-operatively (best option), or notched pre-operatively and broken *in situ*, or cut following insertion (very robust pin cutters may be required; hacksaw is inappropriate)

Reduction and fixation
The fracture is exposed if required and the fragment ends are examined for fissuring. Any fissures present should be protected using cerclage wires. The fracture should be reduced and temporarily stabilized using suitable bone holding forceps.

Normograde pin insertion
The pin is driven into the medullary canal at some point distant from the fracture and advanced along the medullary canal, traversing the fracture site and impacting in the metaphysis of the opposing fragment.

The pin is then cut (unless pre-cut) leaving 5–10 mm protruding to allow for removal.
It is sometimes possible to perform normograde insertion closed.

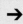

OPERATIVE TECHNIQUE 9.1 (CONTINUED)
Insertion of intramedullary pin

Retrograde pin insertion

The pin is inserted into the medullary canal at the fracture site and driven along the medullary canal until it exits the bone at some appropriate distant site.

The chuck is reversed and the pin is then drawn out of the exit site until only the tip is visible at the fracture.

The fracture is reduced and the pin is driven across the fracture site and impacted in the metaphysis of the opposing fragment.

Open pin insertion is always required and double-pointed pins are advantageous.

Most long bones are suitable for either normograde or retrograde pinning.

Landmarks for normograde pinning:
- **Humerus**
  Craniolateral metaphysis proximally
- **Femur**
  Intertrochanteric fossa, immediately medial to greater trochanter
- **Tibia**
  Craniomedial aspect, immediately caudomedial to insertion of straight patellar ligament.

PRACTICAL TIP
The tibia should be pinned normograde (Pardo 1994).

WARNING
The radius should never be pinned.

PRACTICAL TIP
Remember to allow for radiographic magnification (10–15%). Small changes in pin diameter produce large changes in AMI and pin strength.

OPERATIVE TECHNIQUE 9.2
Application of cerclage wire

Tray extras
Gelpi retractors; bone holding forceps; pointed reduction forceps; parallel pliers and wire cutters or combined cutter/twisters; assorted wire (0.8, 1.0 and 1.2 mm diameter); wire passer.

Reduction and stabilization
The fracture is reduced and stabilized using bone holding forceps or temporary K-wire.

Application of cerclage wire
For full cerclage wire (Figure 9.15a), the wire is passed around the bone, avoiding soft tissue entrapment (a wire passer may be helpful), or through bone tunnel for hemicerclage (Figure 9.15b)

The ends are twisted tight (tension must be placed on the wire as it is tightened to ensure that even and secure twisting occurs) and cut short (two or three twists should remain). The free end may be twisted and bent flat if desired.

As an alternative, ASIF type wire loop or 'dynamic' double loop cerclage may be used (Blass *et al.*, 1986).

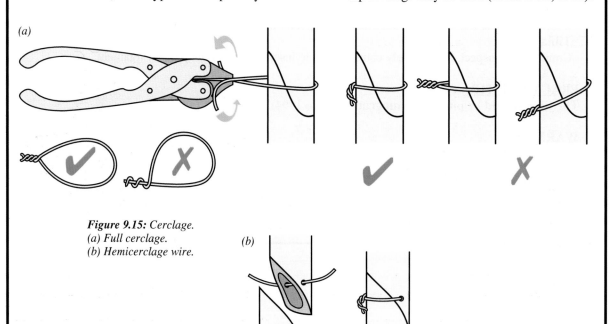

(a)

Figure 9.15: *Cerclage.*
(a) Full cerclage.
(b) Hemicerclage wire.

(b)

OPERATIVE TECHNIQUE 9.3
Application of tension band wire

Tray extras
Pointed reduction forceps; Jacob's chuck or motorized pin driver; small pin cutters; assorted small pins; pin bender; parallel pliers and wire cutters or combined cutter/twisters; assorted wire (0.8, 1.0 and 1.2 mm diameter).

Reduction and stabilization
The fracture or osteotomy is reduced using one or two K-wires or arthrodesis wires.

A transosseous tunnel is drilled distant from the fracture site in the main fragment (distance = approximately 2.5 x length of smaller fragment).

A piece of wire is passed through the bone tunnel and the ends are crossed over.

A second length of wire is passed around the ends of the pins (ensure that local soft tissues, e.g. tendons, are not entrapped) or through a bone tunnel adjacent to the pins.

The ends of the pins are bent over and the wires are twisted tight evenly (tension must be placed on wire as tightened to ensure that even and secure twisting occurs).

The wires are cut short and the ends are bent down.

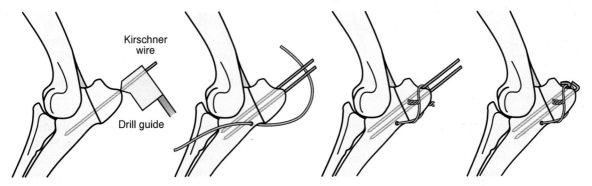

Figure 9.16: Tension band wire.

PRACTICAL TIP
Use small pins and heavy tension-band wire. Ensure the wire tension-band is of adequate length.

OPERATIVE TECHNIQUE 9.4
Application of external skeletal fixator

Tray extras
Appropriate retractors and bone-holding forceps for open reduction; Jacob's chuck or motorized pin driver; small and large pin cutters; appropriate drills, transfixing pins, clamps and connecting bars; spanner or socket for tightening clamps.

Reduction and stabilization
The fracture is reduced. Reduction may be open or closed and may involve the use of cerclage wires, lag screws or intramedullary pins.

Application of unilateral uniplanar (Type I) external fixator (Figure 9.17)

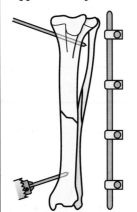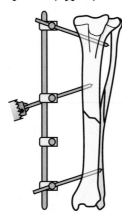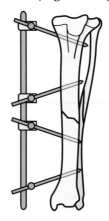

Figure 9.17: Application of Type I external fixator.

The appropriate size of system is selected. Transfixing pins should not exceed one-third of the diameter of the narrowest part of the bone involved.

Stab incisions are made through the skin on the appropriate aspect of the limb as far distant from the fracture proximal and distal as possible, without interfering with adjacent joints or vital soft tissue structures (Marti and Miller, 1994a, b). The incisions should be large enough (0.5 to 1 cm) to prevent any tension in the skin after pin insertion, as this will result in skin necrosis. Stab incisions should ideally be distant from any surgical incision.

Proximal and distal pins are inserted either directly, using a low speed drill, or into slightly smaller pre-drilled holes if the bone is hard. These pins should be inserted at converging angles of around 60°–70° to the bone axis and should be threaded (Figure 9.18) (positive profile is best). All pins must penetrate both cortices of the bone.

Ellis pin (negative profile)

Terminal thread positive profile pin

Central thread positive profile pin (for bilateral fixators)

Figure 9.18: Types of fixator pin.

→

OPERATIVE TECHNIQUE 9.4 (CONTINUED)
Application of external skeletal fixator

The connecting bar, with all the required clamps attached, is connected to these transfixing pins and their clamps are tightened, leaving a gap of around 1 cm between skin and clamp to allow for swelling. Clamps may be positioned with the nut 'inside' or 'outside' the bar according to personal preference. 'Outside' is probably better as the length of pin from bone to clamp is less and therefore the fixation is stronger.

A second connecting bar may be attached in the same way, external to the first, if increased strength of fixation is required.

Fracture reduction is checked and the remaining pins are inserted as above, using their loose clamps as guides. This is essential to ensure proper alignment of all the pins. It is not possible to insert all the pins and then apply the bar. In general, sets of pins within major fragments should converge. Positive profile pins cannot be inserted through the clamps, so smooth or negative profile pins should be used. All pins must penetrate both cortices.

The remaining clamps are tightened and fracture alignment checked again.

Application of unilateral biplanar external fixator
Proceed as above.

A second fixator is applied using the same principles within an arc of 90° to the first (e.g. primary fixator applied along medial aspect of the radius with the second applied cranially).

The two fixators are connected using small connecting bars and double clamps.

When both devices lie within a 90° arc the system is regarded as unilateral. If the arc is greater than 90°, it is bilateral.

Application of a bilateral uniplanar (Type II) external fixator
Proximal and distal pins should be inserted perpendicular to the bone axis. These should penetrate the soft tissues on both sides of the limb and should be connected to a connecting bar on either side of the limb. These pins should have a centrally located positive profile thread.

Additional pins are placed as before. It is difficult to maintain alignment of the transfixing pins through the limb and to engage the clamps on the far side properly. It is helpful to attach a second connecting bar on the operator side and to use this as a drill guide in order to improve planar alignment of the pins (Roe *et al.*,1985). The supplementary connecting bar on the operator side is subsequently removed. Alternatively, further pins may be unilateral (modified Type II).

Application of bilateral biplanar (Type III) external fixator
Use principles described above.

Radiographs in at least two planes should be taken to assess fracture alignment prior to the pins being cut short. Sharp pin ends should be covered by cohesive tape (adhesive tape is very difficult to remove later) and the fixator may be protected by a small bandage. It is sometimes helpful to apply a padded bandage around the limb for 2–3 days to reduce post-operative swelling.

OPERATIVE TECHNIQUE 9.5
Application of lag screw

Tray extras
Appropriate retractors and bone-holding instruments; appropriate drills, guides and taps; appropriate screw sizes.

Reduction and stabilization
The fracture is reduced and stabilized temporarily using pointed reduction forceps. A hole the same diameter as the screw threads is drilled in the *cis* cortex (gliding hole) and an insert guide is passed through this. A drill the same diameter as the screw core is inserted through the guide to ensure central placement and a hole is drilled in the *trans* cortex (thread hole). The hole in the *cis* cortex may be countersunk if required, although this can be risky in the very thin cortices of canine and feline bone.

The necessary length of screw is measured using a depth gauge. The *trans* cortex only is tapped and the screw is inserted. Approximately 2 mm is added to the measured length. (The length of the screw is measure from the head to the tip, which tapers and does not grip the bone well. Adding 2 mm ensures adequate thread contact in the *trans*-cortex.)

Tightening the screw generates axial compression along its length and compresses the *trans* cortex towards the screw head, where it engages the *cis* cortex or the plate. For maximum function, the lag screw should be inserted midway between the perpendicular to the fracture line and the perpendicular to the longitudinal axis of the bone. A lag effect can be created using a partially threaded cancellous screw, although it may be difficult to ensure that the threaded portion of the screw is of an appropriate length.

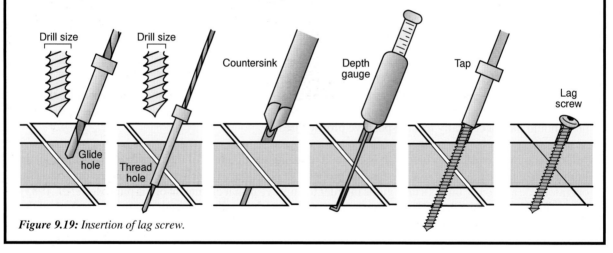

Figure 9.19: *Insertion of lag screw.*

OPERATIVE TECHNIQUE 9.6
Application of plate and screws

Tray extras
Appropriate retractors and bone-holding instruments; appropriate drills and taps; appropriate sizes of plate and screws.

Reduction and stabilization of a simple transverse diaphyseal fracture using a compression plate (Figure 9.20)
The fracture and most or all of the involved bone should be exposed. The bone ends must be examined for occult fissuring. (If fissuring is present, axial compression should be avoided. Secure the bone ends using cerclage wire to prevent further fissuring and proceed with neutralization plate fixation.)

The fracture is reduced, usually by toggling or traction, and reduction is maintained using bone holding forceps or temporary K-wire(s).

The plate is contoured to fit the bone. A small gap may be left between plate and bone over the fracture (pre-stressing) to produce compression of the *trans* cortex (Figure 9.21). An appropriately sized thread hole is drilled close to one fracture end (Figure 9.20a), the hole is measured through the plate and the thread is tapped. The plate is applied to the bone and a screw is inserted but only tightened until the underside of the screw head contacts the 'shoulder' of the screw hole (Figure 9.20b).

The plate is slid proximally or distally so that the screw contacts the side of the screw hole distant from the fracture site and clamped or held in that position. Using the 'load' drill guide, the screw hole on the opposite side of the fracture is drilled, ensuring that both ends of the plate contact bone (Figure 9.20c). This hole is measured and tapped as before. The screw is inserted and both screws are fully tightened in turn, compressing the fracture (Figure 9.20d).

Further screws are inserted on either side, using the 'neutral' drill guide (Figure 9.20e), progressively moving away from the fracture. All screws are checked for tightness prior to closure.

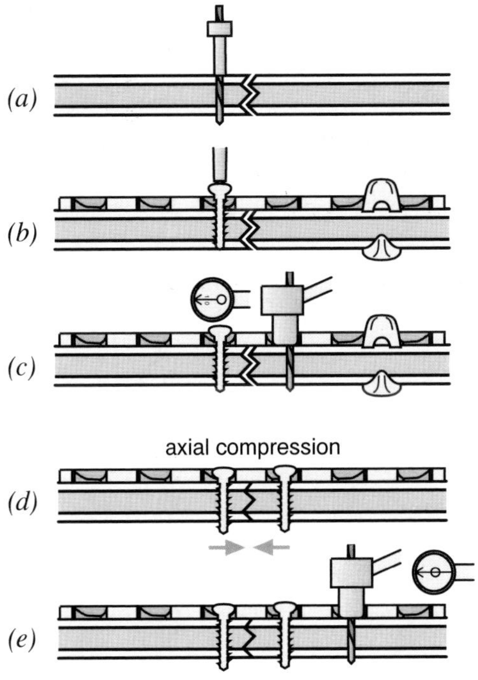

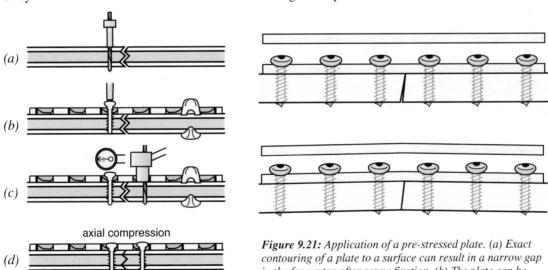

(a)

(b)

(c)

(d) axial compression

(e)

Figure 9.20: Application of a compression plate.

Figure 9.21: Application of a pre-stressed plate. (a) Exact contouring of a plate to a surface can result in a narrow gap in the far cortex after screw fixation. (b) The plate can be pre-stressed to create a curve in the part that will lie above the fracture. The far cortex is now compressed when the screws are tightened.

→

OPERATIVE TECHNIQUE 9.6 (CONTINUED)
Application of plate and screws

Reduction and stabilization of a comminuted diaphyseal fracture using lag screws and a neutralization plate (Figure 9.22)
The fracture is approached as above and stepwise fragment reconstruction is commenced from either main fragment. Fragments are stabilized temporarily using pointed fragment forceps or K-wires. Any fragments that cannot be securely fixed must be discarded.

Interfragmentary compression is achieved using lag screws and the fracture is rebuilt until only two main fragments remain. These are reduced with care, and lag screw fixation may again be used. Consideration must be given to the location of lag screw heads in relation to the position of the plate. Lag screws may be inserted through the plate if required. The plate is contoured to the bone without pre-stressing.

Plate screws are inserted using the 'neutral' drill guide and the steps detailed above. The order of screw insertion is not critical; it may be advantageous to insert the terminal plate screws first to ensure that the ends of the plate are located over bone. All screws are tightened prior to closure. The repair, especially the compression surface, is examined for cortical defects and these are packed with cancellous bone if present.

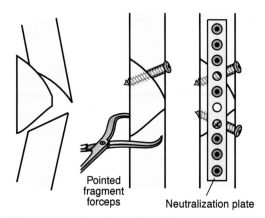

Figure 9.22: Application of a neutralization plate using lag screws.

Pointed fragment forceps

Neutralization plate

Reduction and stabilization of a severely comminuted diaphyseal fracture using a buttress plate (Figure 9.23)
Little or no attempt is made to reconstruct the fracture, although large fragments may be reconstructed using lag screws or cerclage wires if wished.

A pre-contoured plate is applied to the major proximal and distal fragments to regain normal bone length and alignment. The 'load' guide should be used with the arrow pointing away from the fracture to ensure that there is no axial compression.

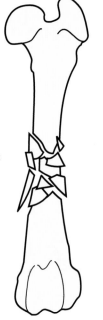
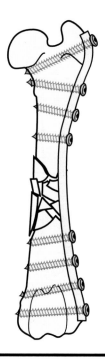

Figure 9.23: Application of a buttress plate.

CHAPTER TEN

Complex, Open and Pathological Fractures

Chris May

COMPLEX FRACTURES

This first section considers the management of severely comminuted diaphyseal fractures (see definition of complex fractures in Chapter 1). Comminution occurs because of a high energy impact and is usually associated with considerable damage to local soft tissues and other body systems. Careful and complete evaluation of the whole patient is essential.

One major challenge with these fractures arises from the need to provide rigid fixation and early return to function for an inherently unstable fracture site. There may also be devitalized bone fragments and extensive soft tissue damage. In some situations, anatomical reconstruction with plate and screws will be appropriate (Chapter 9). In other cases, attempts at anatomical reconstruction may be considered unfeasible or even undesirable because:

- Reconstruction may be impossible due to small fragment sizes
- Reconstructive surgery would be prolonged and/ or would result in excessive tissue dissection. This would damage local blood supply to the fracture site, compromising fracture healing and predisposing to infection.

In these circumstances, a shift to a *minimally invasive strategy (MIS)* is advantageous. Such strategies have also been called 'biologic' in American literature, but this terminology is avoided here because the author regards all fracture healing as biological.

A minimally invasive strategy for repairing complex fractures

The principles of this strategy are:

- Use closed alignment, or minimal exposure alignment of the two major fracture fragments to achieve spatial reconstruction (see below)
- Aim for *maximum* preservation of blood supply to the bone fragments
- Provide sufficient stability to allow for the lack of load sharing by the non-reconstructed bone.

Spatial reconstruction has been defined by Aron *et al.* (1995) as:

- Reconstruction of normal bone length
- Adjustment of the two main bone fragments to within 5° of normal torsion or angulation
- At least 50% overlap, in the mediolateral and

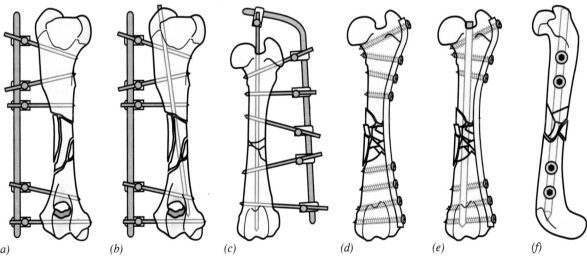

(a)   *(b)*   *(c)*   *(d)*   *(e)*   *(f)*

Figure 10.1: *Techniques, compatible with a minimally invasive strategy, for stabilizing complex fractures: (a) external fixator; (b) external fixator + intramedullary alignment pin; (c) external fixator + 'tied-in' intramedullary alignment pin; (d) bridging plate; (e) plate and 'rod' (intramedullary pin) technique; (f) interlocking nail.*

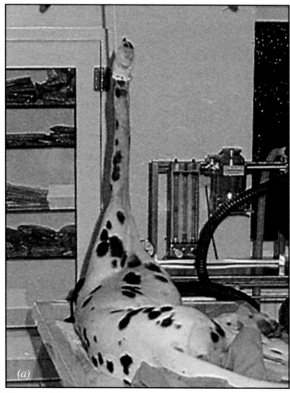
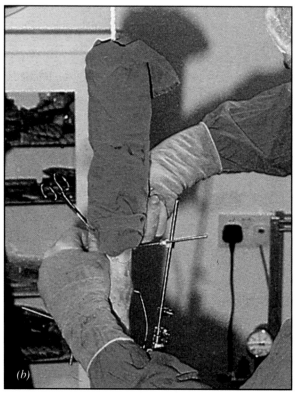

Figure 10.2: (a) 'Hanging limb' preparation prior to closed reduction of a radius and ulna fracture in a dog. (b) Application of an external fixator to the limb shown in (a).

craniocaudal planes, of the two main bone fragments.

For adhering to these principles, the author's preference is the use of external skeletal fixation (ESF). Alternative methods include bridging plates with or without an intramedullary pin and interlocking intramedullary nails (Figure 10.1) (see Chapter 9).

Minimally invasive strategy for fractures of the antebrachium and crus

Spatial reconstruction can be achieved by suspending the patient in the hanging limb position routinely used to overcome fragment overriding. Reduction is confirmed by closed palpation, or by a minimal exposure of the fracture site, and the fixator is placed with the animal maintained in the suspended position (Figure 10.2). In most cases a modified type II fixator is indicated (Chapter 9). However, more rigid configurations may sometimes be required initially because of the lack of load sharing by the bone. As fracture healing progresses, the ESF is usually removed by staged disassembly, typically beginning 4 to 6 weeks after the initial repair.

Minimally invasive strategy for fractures of the femur and humerus

Both the femur and the humerus can be repaired by a minimally invasive approach. However, these are more challenging than distal limb fractures, because there are no safe corridors for ESF pin placement

(Marti and Miller, 1994a,b) and it is more difficult to achieve a rigid construct because of the proximity of the torso.

Closed alignment is often not possible with these bones and the hanging limb position does not complete spatial reconstruction. The alternative is to make a minimal surgical approach between muscle bellies to accomplish alignment of the two main fragments and positioning of the fixation device whilst leaving the intervening minor fragments undisturbed (*minimal exposure alignment*).

Minimal exposure alignment

- Only expose the main proximal and distal fragments – do not handle individual intervening cortical fragments as this may deprive them of blood supply
- Only remove those fragments that are totally devoid of soft tissue attachments
- Achieve spatial alignment of the two main fracture segments by minimal manipulation
- In some cases, alignment can be achieved through fascia or muscle, thus avoiding complete exposure of the fracture site and further damage to soft tissues and blood supply.
- If ESF is used for stabilization, there should be minimal pin penetration of surrounding muscle masses.

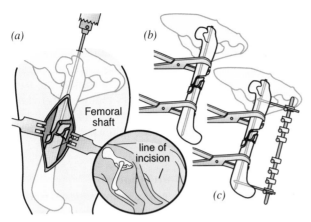

(a)

(b)

Femoral
shaft

line of
incision

(c)

Figure 10.3: Schematic view of a complex femoral fracture to illustrate placement of an intramedullary alignment pin and external fixator: (a) minimal exposure of the main fragments to facilitate pin positioning (see text for details); (b) use of bone holding forceps to 'slide' the fragments along the pin, thus restoring limb length; (c) application of the external fixator (see text for details).

In both the humerus and the femur, reduction may be facilitated by the use of a narrow intramedullary alignment pin (Figure 10.3). Typically, a 3–4 mm pin is used for a 30 kg dog and a 1–1.5 mm K-wire for a cat. Larger pins are unnecessary and may hinder fixator pin placement. Theoretically, normograde placement of the alignment pin is less likely to disturb the local blood supply. However, the author finds accurate pin positioning to be easier via retrograde placement. Provided the ends of the two major fragments are exposed through a small incision in the overlying fascial plane (MIS!) and the intervening fragments are not disturbed, retrograde placement of the alignment pin does not appear to affect fracture healing adversely in practice.

The alignment pin maintains axial alignment and helps to minimize the number of fracture manipulations necessary before application of ESF, thus helping to preserve blood supply. The pin is generally left in place as it increases the rigidity of the construct. It may also be 'tied in' to the fixator (Figure 10.1), and is then removed as part of the staged disassembly during fracture healing.

When ESF is used, a rigid construct is created to cope with the non-load sharing and the excessive muscle tensions in the proximal limb. This may be by an enhanced bi-planar configuration (Aron *et al.*, 1995) but the author has success with double bar type I fixation using threaded pins and ensuring *a minimum of six (preferably eight) cortices* gripped by the fixator pins in each segment (Figure 10.4). An alternative to traditional ESF devices is the use of polymethylmethacrylate to form the connecting bars, with either pins or bone screws for transfixation (Dew *et al.*, 1992; Ross and Matthiesen, 1993). This allows more creative formation of the connecting bars, which can help in constructing a rigid device despite the confines of limited transfixation pin positioning.

Although placement of autogenous cancellous bone grafts is simple and recommended in most comminuted fracture repairs (Chapter 9), the author does not routinely graft when using a MIS, particularly if it involves disturbing fracture fragments.

Cortical autografts and allografts

In fractures with severe bone loss, replacement of large sections of diaphysis may prove necessary. This may be achieved with an autograft (rib or distal ulna) or with a cortical allograft from banked bone. In either case, fixation is by rigid bone plating with strict adherence to the principles of fixation and of asepsis.

For further discussions of bone grafting and bone banking see Weigel (1993) and Parker (1993).

OPEN FRACTURES

In open fractures, the amount of energy absorbed by the limb at the time of fracture has important prognostic implications. High energy impacts cause greater soft tissue devitalization and may have a higher risk of infection. Wound size may not be a major consideration in prognosis, as severe soft tissue crushing can occur even with small puncture wounds. The classification of open fractures is discussed in Chapter 1.

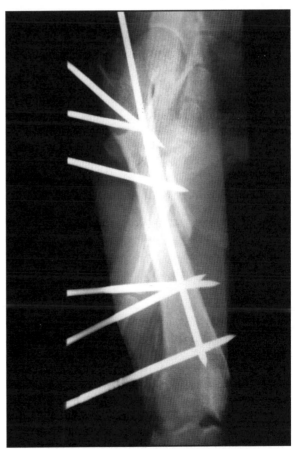

Figure 10.4: Post-operative radiograph showing the use an an intramedullary alignment pin and external fixator for managing a complex femoral fracture in a dog.

The goals in the treatment of open fractures are:

- To stabilize the fracture and allow wound management
- To prevent contamination progressing to infection
- To achieve bone union and restore limb function as soon as possible.

Open fracture management can be considered in four phases:

- First aid care
- The rational use of antibiotics
- Wound management
- Fracture stabilization.

First aid care
Primary consideration must always be given to the basics of acute care for trauma patients.

> **WARNING**
> **Approximately 30% of patients with open fractures have significant injuries to other body systems.**

Open fractures have a high association with compromised neurovascular function. This should be fully assessed as early as possible, as it will have a major bearing on fracture management. Severe compromise of the soft tissue envelope may be an indication for early amputation.

Immediate first aid considerations for the open fracture site include the following.

- *Do not* obtain samples for bacterial cultures at this stage. Recent studies suggest that such cultures are not helpful in planning fracture therapy (Moore *et al.*, 1989).
- *Do not* probe or manipulate the fracture site.
- *Do* cover open wounds with sterile, soaked compression dressings. The dressings may be soaked in any of the following:
- Sterile normal saline
  Chlorhexidine diacetate solution (0.05%)
  Povidone–iodine solution (0.5-1%).

The dilution and composition of these solutions is critical and the author prefers to use only sterile saline. The use of compression dressings helps to control haemorrhage from the site.

> **WARNING**
> **The hospital environment is the major source of contaminating organisms that produce subsequent infection in open wounds.**

- *Do* provide limb splint support for the fracture sites (e.g. Robert Jones bandage, gutter splint or Zimmer splint). The dressings should stay in place until the animal reaches an operating suite. If they must be removed (e.g. for evaluation of the soft tissue envelope, or for radiography), they should be replaced as soon as possible.
- *Do* obtain appropriate radiographs as soon as possible.

The rational use of antibiotics
Antibiotic use in open fracture management is a complex and controversial topic more thoroughly covered in other publications (Patzakis *et al.*, 1974; Worlock *et al.*, 1988; Patzakis and Wilkins, 1989; Robinson *et al.*, 1989; Gustilo *et al.*, 1990).

Antibiotic therapy should be instituted as soon as possible in all open fractures. An intravenous bactericidal antibiotic is preferred, such as clavulanate potentiated amoxycillin or a cephalosporin. Tissue samples (Figure 10.5) are submitted for aerobic and anaerobic culture and antibiotic sensitivity testing. Antibiotics are discontinued after 5 days unless there are positive findings on culture or if the patient's condition indicates frank infection. Sensitivity testing may dictate a change in the antibiotic being used and antibiotic therapy should continue for at least 3 weeks if culture is positive.

An exception to these general guidelines is in very severe type III open fractures, in which there may be merit in a continuous antibiotic course.

Wound management
The principles of wound management in open fractures are no different from those for other open wounds. Good wound management hinges on haemostasis, copious irrigation, debridement of devitalized tissues, drainage and wound closure or reconstruction (Figure 10.5).

Fracture stabilization
Fracture stabilization occurs simultaneously with management of the open wound. Indeed, stability at the fracture site contributes significantly to combating local infection because:

- Restoration of limb length minimizes dead space.
- Stabilization of the fracture secondarily stabilizes the neighbouring soft tissues and facilitates revascularization. Oxygenation via a healthy blood supply is the single most important factor in re-establishing tissue resistance to infection.
- Stabilization of tissues assists white blood cell infiltration of the contaminated tissues by providing a constant chemotactic gradient, not found in unstable tissues.
- Early stability provides for muscle and joint mobility, which helps to encourage both venous and lymphatic drainage and reduce oedema.

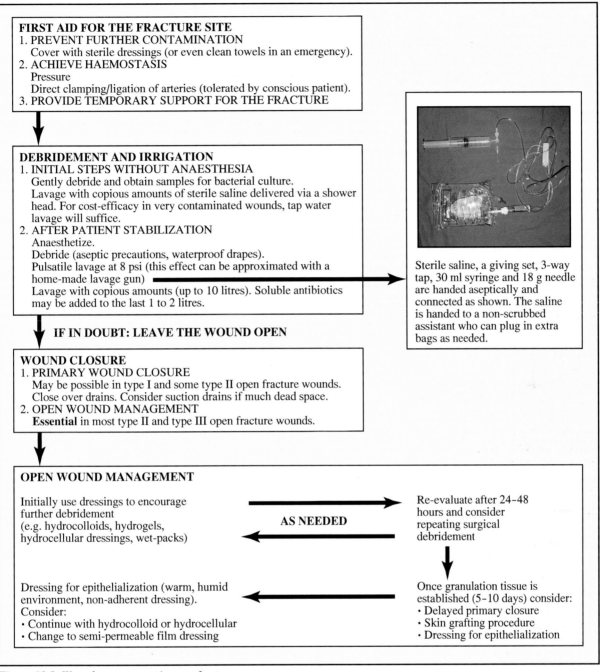

FIRST AID FOR THE FRACTURE SITE
1. PREVENT FURTHER CONTAMINATION
   Cover with sterile dressings (or even clean towels in an emergency).
2. ACHIEVE HAEMOSTASIS
   Pressure
   Direct clamping/ligation of arteries (tolerated by conscious patient).
3. PROVIDE TEMPORARY SUPPORT FOR THE FRACTURE

DEBRIDEMENT AND IRRIGATION
1. INITIAL STEPS WITHOUT ANAESTHESIA
   Gently debride and obtain samples for bacterial culture.
   Lavage with copious amounts of sterile saline delivered via a shower
   head. For cost-efficacy in very contaminated wounds, tap water
   lavage will suffice.
2. AFTER PATIENT STABILIZATION
   Anaesthetize.
   Debride (aseptic precautions, waterproof drapes).
   Pulsatile lavage at 8 psi (this effect can be approximated with a
   home-made lavage gun)
   Lavage with copious amounts (up to 10 litres). Soluble antibiotics
   may be added to the last 1 to 2 litres.

Sterile saline, a giving set, 3-way tap, 30 ml syringe and 18 g needle are handed aseptically and connected as shown. The saline is handed to a non-scrubbed assistant who can plug in extra bags as needed.

IF IN DOUBT: LEAVE THE WOUND OPEN

WOUND CLOSURE
1. PRIMARY WOUND CLOSURE
   May be possible in type I and some type II open fracture wounds.
   Close over drains. Consider suction drains if much dead space.
2. OPEN WOUND MANAGEMENT
   Essential in most type II and type III open fracture wounds.

OPEN WOUND MANAGEMENT

Initially use dressings to encourage further debridement (e.g. hydrocolloids, hydrogels, hydrocellular dressings, wet-packs)

AS NEEDED

Re-evaluate after 24–48 hours and consider repeating surgical debridement

Dressing for epithelialization (warm, humid environment, non-adherent dressing).
Consider:
• Continue with hydrocolloid or hydrocellular
• Change to semi-permeable film dressing

Once granulation tissue is established (5–10 days) consider:
• Delayed primary closure
• Skin grafting procedure
• Dressing for epithelialization

Figure 10.5: Wound management in open fractures.

In most cases, rigid fixation will be required and this is most readily achieved by either lag screws and bone plates or by external skeletal fixation (ESF).

> **WARNING**
> **Whichever technique is chosen, the surgeon must pay meticulous attention to the principles of fracture fixation as the risks of infection and/or non-union are high if the stabilization is anything less than optimal.**

Internal fixation
The role of internal fixation in open fractures is controversial, but appropriate use of the technique in fresh,

open fractures is associated with good results and a reasonably low complication rate. In humans, complication rates as low as 8.2% for acute osteomyelitis, 0.5% for chronic osteomyelitis and a 2.2% incidence of salvage by amputation have been reported following fixation by bone plating or intramedullary nailing with reamed or locking nails (Clancey and Hansen, 1978; Chapman and Mahoney, 1979; Rittman *et al.*, 1979). Most complications were associated with type III open fractures.

Steinmann pins, commonly used for intramedullary nailing in veterinary surgery, cannot be routinely recommended for the more severe types of contaminated fracture as they often fail to provide appropriate stability and may contribute to the intramedullary spread of infection. In most veterinary cases, rigid internal stabilization of open fractures will comprise lag screw and bone plate fixation. Specific indications for primary internal fixation of open fractures include:

- Fractures in multiple injury patients when early mobilization is essential and ESF is impractical
- Articular fractures
- Open fractures of the long bones of elderly animals in which ESF may be inadvisable.

Plate application should ideally be through the open wound or by extension of the open wound after debridement (Chapman, 1993). This may not always be practical but it does minimize the additional soft tissue trauma inherent in a second, elective incision. Whenever possible, soft tissue cover should be provided for the plate. In gaining access through the open wound and endeavouring to place the plate under healthy soft tissue cover, it may prove necessary to apply the plate in a non-traditional location.

External skeletal fixation

ESF is the author's first choice for most open fractures, unless a specific indication exists for internal fixation. It is undoubtedly the method of choice for stabilizing open fractures below the stifle in the pelvic limb or below the elbow in the thoracic limb. Correctly applied, ESF provides suitable stability and has a number of advantages over internal fixation for the management of open fractures:

- The device is relatively easy to apply and may even be adjusted during the fracture healing process
- There are no metal implants at the fracture site and ready access is usually gained for open wound management.

Disadvantages of ESF, specific to open fractures, include:

- The pins may interfere with plastic reconstruction procedures
- There is a risk of pin loosening and pin tract infection adding to contamination problems
- The physical bulk of the more complex devices may be awkward and interfere with attempts at early limb mobility, particularly in patients with multiple limb injuries.

Shearing injuries

Shearing injuries of the distal extremities are particularly amenable to transarticular ESF. The injuries are often complex and comprise 'degloving' of soft tissues and abrasion of bones, ligaments and other articular structures, usually over the tarsus or carpus (Chapter 20). Historically, these have been repaired by ligament

substitution with a variety of artificial prostheses anchored around screws placed into the residual bone. However, in many cases, the extremity can be stabilized by ESF throughout the period of wound management and without addition of prosthetic implants. *Subsequent fibrosis is often sufficient to stabilize the injured joints.*

Bone grafting

The high risk of non-union associated with open fractures makes grafting of autogenous, cancellous bone desirable in almost all cases.

WARNING
Large cortical allografts or autografts are contraindicated in the face of infection.

Particular indications for using autogenous cancellous bone grafts in open fractures include:

- Comminution
- Bone loss
- Internal fixation by plates and screws.

Grafting may be performed early, when adequate soft tissue cover exists, or at the time of delayed primary closure of the wound if initial soft tissue cover is inadequate to retain and revascularize the graft. In type III injuries it may be appropriate to delay grafting for several weeks to allow for adequate soft tissue recovery first.

Amputation

In some injuries, early amputation may be the treatment of choice. Indications include:

- *Reduction of morbidity.* Early amputation can provide a rapid return to acceptable function, and, for many dogs and cats, a return to pre-injury life style. This may be judged preferable to a prolonged clinical course and the associated risk of complications inherent in managing complex open fractures.
- *Severe type III injuries.* The severe vascular compromise in such injuries makes amputation the only viable procedure in many cases. Removal of large amounts of poorly vascularized tissues may even be essential to preserve life.
- *Financial considerations.* The combined requirements of open wound management and complex fracture management are potentially expensive in labour and materials. In open fractures it is a matter of financial realism that early amputation may be the only option for many owners.

PATHOLOGICAL FRACTURES

A pathological fracture is fracture of a bone without excessive trauma as a consequence of pre-existing bone disease reducing the ultimate strength of the bone.

Local disease that may result in pathological fracture (Figure 10.6):

- Neoplasia
- Osteomyelitis
- Bone cysts
- Local bone atrophy (e.g. disuse).

Generalized diseases that may result in pathological fracture (Figure 10.7) are:

- Hyperparathyroidism (alimentary, renal or primary)
- Hyperadrenocorticism
- Rickets (now rare in pets in the UK)
- Generalized neoplasia (e.g. myeloma).

The prognosis and treatment of pathological fractures are ultimately governed by the primary disease process and also by the site of the pathological fracture. Pathological fractures of the vertebral column giving rise to significant neurological injury frequently have a poor prognosis.

Neoplasia
Consider amputation or a limb salvage procedure.

Osteomyelitis
Appropriate treatment of the inciting infection is combined with rigid fixation (Chapter 25).

Bone cysts
Treat with reduction, rigid fixation and packing of deficits with autogenous bone grafts. Consider corticocancellous grafts if large structural defects exist.

Alimentary hyperparathyroidism
Often these cases present with folding fractures and the bone is already too soft to withstand fixation. The best strategy is usually to provide analgesia and cage rest. The nutritional disease is corrected immediately but definitive treatment of bone deformities is delayed. Several weeks later, once bone density has improved, corrective osteotomies can be planned as needed.

Stress riser effect
When load sharing between a fracture fixation device and the bone is spread along the longest length of bone possible, the risk of a stress riser effect is minimized.

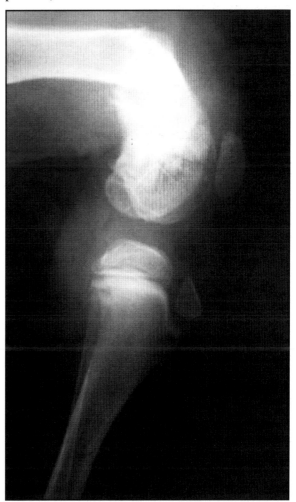

Figure 10.7 Pathological fracture secondary to nutritional secondary hyperparathyroidism in a puppy.

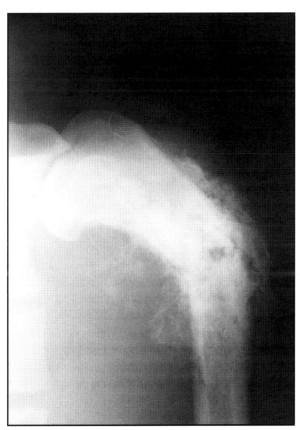

Figure 10.6 Pathological fracture secondary to a primary bone tumour.

Thus, when internal fixation is used on bone of reduced strength, the longest possible bone plate should always be applied. Similarly, if ESF is used, pin placement should be distributed along the greatest possible length of bone.

REFERENCES AND FURTHER READING

Aron DN, Palmer RH and Johnson AL (1995) Biologic strategies and a balanced concept for repair of highly comminuted long bone fractures. *Compendium of Continuing Education* **17**, 35-49

Brinker WO, Hohn RB and Prieur WD (eds) (1984) *Manual of Internal Fixation in Small Animals*. Springer-Verlag, Berlin

Chapman MW (1993) Open fractures. In: *Operative Orthopaedics*, 2nd edn, ed. MW Chapman. JB Lippincott Co., Philadelphia

Chapman MW and Mahoney M (1979) The role of internal fixation in the management of open fractures. *Clinical Orthopaedics* **138**, 120

Clancey GJ and Hansen ST Jr (1978) Open fractures of the tibia: a review of 102 cases. *Journal of Bone and Joint Surgery* **60-A**, 118

Dew TL, Kern DA and Johnston SA (1992) Treatment of complicated femoral fractures with external skeletal fixation utilizing bone screws and polymethylmethacrylate. *Veterinary and Comparative Orthopaedics and Traumatology* **5**, 170-175

Gustilo RB, Merkow RL and Templeman D (1990) The management of open fractures. *Journal of Bone and Joint Surgery* **72-A**, 299

Harari J (ed.) (1992) External skeletal fixation. *Veterinary Clinics of North America* **22:1**

Marti JM and Miller A (1994a) Delimitation of safe corridors for the insertion of external fixator pins in the dog 1: Hindlimb. *Journal of Small Animal Practice* **35**, 16-23

Marti JM and Miller A (1994b) Delimitation of safe corridors for the corridors for the insertion of external fixator pins in the dog 2: Forelimb. *Journal of Small Animal Practice* **35**, 78-85

Moore TJ, Mauney C and Barron J (1989) The use of quantitative bacterial counts in open fractures. *Clinical Orthopaedics* **248**, 823

Parker RB (1993) Establishment of a bone bank. In: *Disease Mechanisms in Small Animal Surgery*, ed. MJ Bojrab. Lea and Febiger, Philadelphia

Patzakis MJ and Wilkins J (1989) Factors influencing infection rate in open fracture wounds. *Clinical Orthopaedics* **243**, 36

Patzakis MJ, Harvey JP and Ivler D (1974) The role of antibiotics in the management of open fractures. *Journal of Bone and Joint Surgery* **56-A**, 532

Rittman WW, Schibli M, Matter P and Allgöwer M (1979) Open fractures: long term results in 200 consecutive cases. *Clinical Orthopaedics* **138**, 132

Robinson D, On E, Hadas N *et al.* (1989) Microbiologic flora contaminating open fractures: its significance in the choice of primary antibiotic agents and the likelihood of deep wound infection. *Journal of Orthopaedics and Traumatology* **3**, 283

Ross JT and Matthiesen DT (1993) The use of multiple pin and methylmethacrylate external skeletal fixation for the treatment of orthopaedic injuries in the dog and cat. *Veterinary and Comparative Orthopaedics and Traumatology* **6**, 115-121

Weigel JP (1993) Bone grafting. In: *Disease Mechanisms in Small Animal Surgery*, ed. MJ Bojrab. Lea and Febiger, Philadelphia

Worlock P, Slack R, Harvey L and Mawhinney R (1988) The prevention of infection in open fractures. An experimental study of the effect of antibiotic therapy. *Journal of Bone and Joint Surgery* **70-A**, 1341

CHAPTER ELEVEN

Fractures in Skeletally Immature Animals

Stuart Carmichael

INTRODUCTION

When a fracture occurs in an immature animal, both bone healing and fracture management will be markedly influenced by the growing process taking place in the skeleton. This presents an additional set of considerations and challenges for the orthopaedist. The active anabolic state of the skeleton produces rapid fracture healing and, as a result, non-union fractures are extremely rare in immature animals. Malunion or the production of excessive amounts of callus around the fracture site are more realistic problems. Growth may be altered as a result of abnormal activity at the growth plates leading to shortening or progressive deformity of the affected long bone. If implants are used to stabilize the fracture they may impair the growth process or be engulfed by newly formed bone during healing, making removal of these implants a complicated procedure.

Therefore, when facing a fracture problem in an immature animal, the orthopaedist not only needs a good working knowledge of the best way to stabilize the bone but also has to understand the growth process fully and how it will influence the outcome of fracture repair. The dynamic state of growth during this period is also important since a three-month-old patient with a fracture will present a very different set of problems to one in a patient of seven months of age.

Structural weakness present at the metaphyseal growth plate, particularly in the newly formed bone, predisposes to failure at this site.

The range of fractures seen in young animals is therefore very different from those in the adult and demands an entirely different approach to management.

INCIDENCE OF FRACTURES IN YOUNG ANIMALS

A very high proportion of all fractures in dogs and cats are found in animals less than one year of age. In a four-year retrospective study of long bone fractures in dogs, 452 of 844 (54%) were present in animals less than one year old (Marretta and Schrader, 1983). In a similar study in dogs and cats by Phillips (1979), 123 fractures

out of a total of 283 fractures were in dogs of under one year. This represents almost 50% of the total. In cats, 121 out of 244 fractures were presented in animals less than one year old, representing 49% of all fractures seen. Many of these fractures are found affecting the metaphyseal growth plate, as a direct result of the structural weakness in this area. In Marretta and Schrader's study, 135 of the 452 (30%) fractures reported in juveniles in the study were described as epiphyseal.

SPECIAL CONSIDERATIONS WHEN MANAGING FRACTURES IN YOUNG ANIMALS

Growth

The successful management of fractures in immature animals depends on a good working knowledge of the growth process. It is outside the remit of this chapter to consider all aspects of growth, which are well documented elsewhere (Brighton, 1978; Ham and Cormack, 1979; Herron, 1981) but it is worth reviewing some important points which may influence decision-making processes when dealing with these fractures.

The growing process is taking place at all parts of the skeleton but is concentrated at certain points:

- The metaphyseal growth plates
- The periosteum
- Subchondral area in the epiphysis.

As bone is produced in these specific areas, the shape of the skeleton is defined and the long bones achieve their adult proportions. When a fracture occurs, bone development must be altered. The objective of management is to restore the situation to normal as quickly as possible.

The metaphyseal growth plate ('growth plate' or 'physis')

The most important area of growth is the metaphyseal growth plate. Bone is formed very rapidly in this location by the process of endochondral ossification (Figure 11.1). Any disturbance to this area by fracture or by fixation methods will have a profound effect on

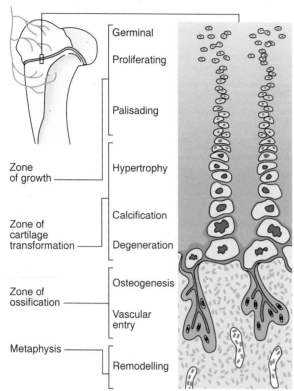

Figure 11.1: *Metaphyseal growth plate showing the different regions of cartilage differentiation and bone formation.*

bone growth and development. The growth plate is mechanically weaker than the adjacent bone or articular structures, and so a high incidence of growth plate fractures are seen in immature animals compared with a corresponding low number of ligamentous or soft tissue disruptions of the adjacent joints. The weakness of this area is due to the presence of cartilaginous matrix and newly formed bone (Figure 11.1).

A fracture occurring in a long bone inevitably leads to some disturbance of growth. Fortunately there seem to be good compensatory mechanisms which act to preserve limb length. General stimulation of growth of the affected long bone in the period after fracture has been described in children (Reynolds, 1981). In addition, compensatory increase in length of adjacent long bones has been observed experimentally (Wagner *et al.*, 1987) and in healed fracture cases (Alcantara and Stead, 1975; Denny, 1989). These processes will allow some compensation for initial disruption in growth and act to preserve total limb length provided the growth plates remain functional.

When planning fracture repair, it is important to consider the time at which a particular growth plate loses function naturally and closes. The average time of closure of commonly involved growth plates in the dog and cat is detailed in Table 11.1.

Periosteum and subchondral areas

New bone can be produced in both of these areas to augment fracture healing and remodelling. The periosteum is of particular interest in young animals as it is

Bone	Average closure time (months)	
	Dog	Cat
Scapula		
Tuber scapulae	6	4
Hemipelvis		
Multiple junction (Acetab)	3.6	
Tuber ischii (secondary)	10	
Femur		
Femoral head	10.5	8
Greater trochanter	10.5	7.5
Distal	11	15
Fibula		
Proximal	10	13
Distal	9.5	12
Humerus		
Proximal	12.5	21
Lateral/medial condyle	6	3
Lateral epicondyle	7	3
Metacarpals/tarsals		
Distal epiphysis II–V	7	9
Phalanges		
Proximal II–V	6	4.5
Radius		
Proximal	8.5	7
Distal	10.5	16.5
Tibia		
Proximal	11	15
Tibial crest	8	15
Distal	10.5	10.5
Medial malleolus	4.5	
Ulna		
Proximal	10	10
Distal	8.5	18
Carpus		
Carpal bones	3.5	
Accessory	4.5	4
Tarsus		
Tarsal bones	5	
Fibular tarsal	3	9
Skull:	Individual bones are joined at birth by cartilaginous or fibrous sutures. These stay physiologically open until 11–14 months of age, after which they may become fused by calcification	
Vertebrae:	The primary centres have fused to form a complete neural arch at birth. The epiphyseal plates stay open for varying periods up to 11 months	

Table 11.1: *Average time of radiographic growth plate closure: dog and cat.*

very thick and easily stripped from the bone. As a result of its mechanical strength it is able to hold fragments in the vicinity of the fracture, allowing reincorporation during the rapid healing process. This may allow anatomical healing in the absence of surgical reassembly of fracture fragments in comminuted fractures and is one of the major factors supporting a more conservative approach to fracture surgery in immature dogs. Needless to say, the periosteum must be preserved and handled with care during surgery.

Bone strength and structure

Juvenile bone is markedly different in composition from that found in the adult, resulting in softer more pliable bones. The bone structure itself is more porous, with an increased number of Haversian canals. Immature bone is much more resistant to fracture than adult bone because of these properties (Sharrard, 1993). Nevertheless fractures in immature animals are common and constitute a considerable proportion of all fractures seen in small animal patients (see above).

Incomplete fractures

A higher percentage of incomplete or greenstick fractures are seen in young animals, as a result of their more pliable, less rigid skeleton. In incomplete fractures part of the cortex fails while the remainder remains intact and can act as a support for the damaged bone (Figure 11.2).

Poor mineralization of bone

The demands of the growing skeleton for calcium can result in weakness as a result of poor mineralization if dietary deficiency is present. Secondary nutritional hyperparathyroidism is the common underlying cause and multiple folding fractures of poorly mineralized bone may result (Figure 11.3).

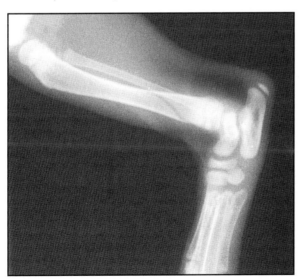

Figure 11.2: A greenstick fracture of the lower tibia in a young cat. The fracture can be seen as a spiral line traversing the distal third of the bone. The cortex is still part intact and the fracture remains undisplaced.

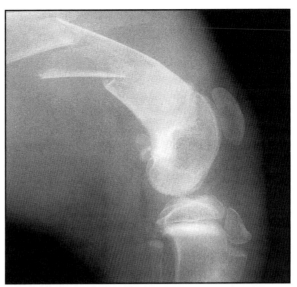

Figure 11.3: Pathological fracture of the femur in a dog suffering from nutritional secondary hyperparathyroidism. The bone gives the appearance of folding, hence the term 'folding fracture'.

Poor holding potential for implants

The soft nature and thin cortices of immature bone have significance for the placement of implants such as bone screws, which achieve the best grip in hard material like mature cortical bone. The same security cannot be obtained in immature bone and this must be considered in the selection of implants, especially when the use of bone plates is considered. Conversely, the large medullary canal present in juveniles, with its high proportion of trabecular or cancellous bone, is significant when intramedullary devices are considered.

Other considerations

Prompt diagnosis

Rapid identification of the fracture and prompt decision making with regard to fracture management are vital to ensure a successful outcome in young animals, as the healing process can be extremely fast. Since most growth stops at about nine to ten months of age, this identifies the time scale during which these conditions apply.

Radiographic interpretation

Early diagnosis depends on a thorough clinical examination and pertinent radiographic investigations. Radiographic interpretation poses problems itself in immature animals as a result of incomplete calcification of the young bones and the presence of open physes, both of which can produce a confusing picture and disguise fractures.

Fracture manipulation

The rapid healing process in immature animals is an obvious biological advantage but can cause problems if fracture management is delayed for any reason. Callus already formed may have to be broken down to reset the fracture. This can produce difficulty in achieving proper fracture reduction, especially when closed fracture reduction is employed, and can result in longer operating times and additional soft tissue traumatization if surgical reduction is selected. In many cases imperfect reduction may be preferred to additional traumatic manipulation and a reliance may be placed on the compensatory mechanisms present in young bone to produce a functional result in the absence of complete anatomical reduction.

Post-fracture patient management

Additional problems are posed by the activity of the patient during the healing period. Puppies and kittens are by nature very active and extremely difficult to rest. Any fixation method must take account of this problem and allow the owners a reasonable chance of adhering to management instructions. At the same time the low body weight of young puppies and kittens reduces the load on the bones and so the mechanical challenge on the healing fracture. This improves the overall success of fixation.

GROWTH PLATE FRACTURES

When trying to identify or assess fractures in this location, it is important to understand the different loads being applied through the area. Epiphyses can be broadly divided, by function, into pressure and traction epiphyses. The forces applied through the growth plate often dictate the type of fracture produced and the management regime necessary to resolve the problem.

All injuries of the epiphyseal region must be investigated carefully so that fractures are not overlooked. Fractures have to be dealt with rapidly and often require surgical intervention to preserve fully the function of the adjacent joint. Involvement of the articular surface and/or impairment of growth by damage to the growth plate are important complications of fractures in this area and significantly affect prognosis. The Salter–Harris classification of growth plate injuries (Figure 11.4) is often used to describe and attempt to comment on prognosis of individual fractures. In reality, all fractures involving the growth plates must be regarded as having an adverse effect on long bone growth and a prognosis must be given accordingly. In the same way, if surgical fixation is attempted due

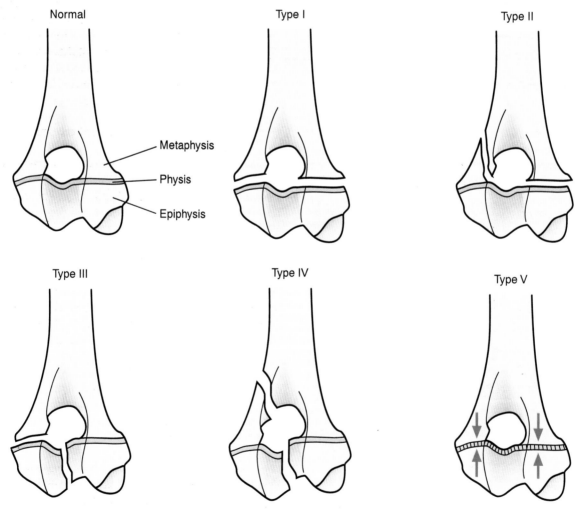

Figure 11.4: The Salter–Harris classification of growth plate fractures.

consideration must be given to the effect on continued growth from the surgical intervention and from any implants employed.

Growth plate fractures adjacent to pressure epiphyses

When faced with these fractures at pressure epiphyses, it is convenient to review Salter types I and II separately from Salter types III and IV.

Fractures involving the growth plate without involvement of the articular surface (Salter I and II)

Fractures falling into this classification form the largest group of physeal fractures occurring in cats and dogs. In the series described by Marretta and Schrader (1983), 65.5% of the fractures were identified as either Type I or II. Fractures can be found at various sites (Figure 11.5) but the most common locations involve the distal and proximal femoral epiphyses, respectively. Fractures in both of these sites present different problems for management (Chapter 18). The majority of distal femoral fractures are classified as Salter type II while most proximal femoral fractures are classified as Salter type I. General considerations for dealing with this type of fracture are outlined in Table 11.2. Recommendations are as follows:

- Secure the epiphysis with the least invasive method possible
- Preserve soft tissues around physis
- Use parallel, small K-wires if possible
- Place the implants to avoid impairing joint function
- Aim for early limb use.

Fractures involving the growth plate with involvement of the articular surface (Salter III and IV)

The most common site of occurrence is the distal humerus, though other sites have been reported. In the series described by Marretta and Schrader (1983), 25.5% of the fractures were identified as either type III or IV.

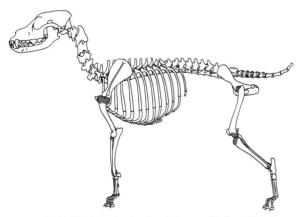

Figure 11.5: *The location in the skeleton of Salter–Harris type I and II fractures.*

Factors	Type	
	I/II	**III/IV**
Positive		
Potential for rapid healing	+	+
Negative		
Small fracture fragments	+	+
Proximity of joint	+	+
Soft cancellous bone	+	+
Possibility of further damage during fracture manipulation	+	
Involvement of the articular surface	–	+

Table 11.2: *General considerations in management of fractures involving the growth plate without (Salter types I and II) and with (Salter types III and IV) involvement of the articular surface in skeletally immature animals.*

Type IV fractures predominated (24%). The involvement of the articular surface alters the priorities in dealing with these fractures. It is imperative that the fracture is reduced accurately to allow the articular surface to heal well and avoid the possibility of debilitating joint disease later in life. Compression fixation has been demonstrated to lead to improved articular surface healing and so fractures are often stabilized using lag screw fixation. Early mobilization is also encouraged, to protect the function of the joint. General considerations are detailed in Table 11.2. Recommendations are as follows:

- Accurate anatomical reduction of the articular surface is a priority
- Stabilize the articular fracture with compression fixation if possible
- Place the implants to avoid impairing joint function
- Preserve soft tissue structures
- Plan early limb use.

The application of all of these recommendations will obviously depend on the site involved, the age and size of the patient and the details of the fracture. Impaired growth is a much more important consideration in animals under 6 months of age. Similarly, problems with small fragments and soft bone are more likely in very young animals. However, the important principles outlined for each fracture type must be applied for any chance of good success in any patient.

General guidelines for management of growth plate fractures

- Early recognition and treatment is important
- Surgical intervention is usually indicated
- Handle fracture fragments carefully to avoid further damage

- Take special care in manipulating epiphyseal fracture surface to avoid damaging germinal layer
- Implant selected should occupy < 20% of the physeal diameter
- Avoid fixing cortical bone on both sides of the growth plate, which would prevent longitudinal expansion
- Complete and accurate reduction of articular fractures is necessary
- Aim for early removal of implants once fracture has healed.

Implants used in the management of growth plate fractures

It is worth considering the relative merits of different implant systems commonly used to stabilize physeal fractures. The systems include:

- Parallel pins
- Rush pins
- Crossed pins
- Biodegradable pins
- Bone screws.

It is common to use small diameter smooth pins (K-wires) to stabilize the Salter I and II fractures (Figure 11.6). To give rotational stability, two or three wires are usually used. Careful positioning allows them to be placed so that they do not interfere with joint function during the healing process. The manner in which they are positioned determines the effect they will have on continued physeal function. The optimal position seems to be parallel pins running perpendicular to the growth plate. This method is simple, minimally invasive and ideal for very young animals. Migration of pins may occur but this is not a major problem as early removal is planned.

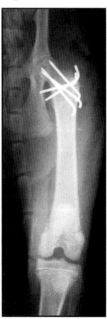

Figure 11.6: Proximal femoral physeal fracture (Salter–Harris type I) in a cat. The fracture was stabilized using three K-wires. A concomitant fracture of the greater trochanter was repaired with two K-wires.

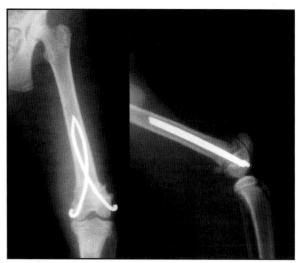

Figure 11.7: Craniocaudal and lateral post-operative radiographs of a cat with Rush pins used to stabilize a distal femoral fracture.

Rush pins (Figure 11.7) achieve better seating in the epiphyseal fragment and should allow longitudinal expansion, as their bodies lie within the intramedullary canal. However, studies have shown that impaired growth is common even after this type of fixation.

Crossed pins are popular for dealing with physeal fractures but they can be difficult to position in the epiphyseal fragment to allow good purchase. They can also bridge the growth plate and theoretically impair longitudinal development while in position, especially if placed almost perpendicular to the long axis of the bone.

Biodegradable pins are commonly used in a parallel fashion and have the advantage of not requiring a second surgical procedure for removal. Reported success has been good.

Fractures involving the articular surface (Salter III and IV) are best stabilized using a lag screw. The use of bone screw fixation or the use of any threaded implants to span the fracture is not commonly indicated to stabilize physeal fractures, because of the possible effect they may have on growth plates (Newton and Nunamaker, 1985). The possible exceptions are fractures in animals reaching the end of their growing period.

Managing growth plate fractures adjacent to traction epiphyses

Avulsion fractures are common and are a direct result of the force applied from the attached muscle mass resisting movement of the adjacent joint: the epiphysis is literally pulled free from the area of endochondral ossification, resulting in an avulsion fracture. Any site where a major muscle mass attaches to a traction epiphysis is a potential site for fracture (Figure 11.8), but these injuries most commonly involve the tibial tuberosity (Chapter 19) or the greater trochanter of the femur (Chapter 18). Such fractures pose a serious technical challenge because of the small size of the

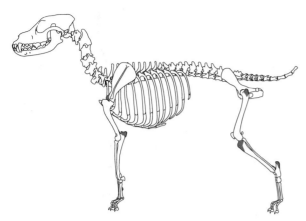

Figure 11.8: Location in the skeleton of common sites of avulsion fractures at traction epipyses.

bone and the large forces generated by the attached muscle. Surgical intervention is necessary to reappose the fracture surfaces and allow healing to take place. Stabilization of the fracture is achieved using combinations of pins and wires.

In most cases the safest way to deal with this fracture separation is to apply a tension-band wire. This will produce secure fracture stabilization with minimal compromise to the surrounding soft tissues. Using small pins to secure the fragment reduces the possibility of iatrogenic fracture while allowing two fixation points for rotationary stability. Very fine pins can be used as they are protected by the tension wire. The wire must be of sufficient diameter to develop tension when tightened to resist the distractive pull of the muscle involved.

In very young dogs a compressive force across the growth plate will cause the plate to fuse, with possible undesirable effects. The most common example of this is seen in young Greyhounds with avulsion injuries of the insertion of the straight patellar ligament. The tibia may continue to grow, leaving the tibial tuberosity fused below the plate and so in an anatomically incorrect position (Chapter 19). For this reason two pins inserted either parallel or in a convergent or divergent fashion without a tension wire may be preferred, avoiding direct compression across the growth plate in very young animals. An alternative approach is to remove the tension wire earlier in the healing period, leaving the pins in position, but this necessitates an additional surgical procedure.

DIAPHYSEAL FRACTURES

Fractures affecting the diaphysis of immature patients are usually low energy type and are typically incomplete or simple fractures. This is due directly to the pliable nature of immature bones. High energy fractures (typically comminuted fractures) are not as frequently found as in adults. When they do occur they are usually found in young, large or giant breed dogs 6–9

months of age nearing the end of growth and they often involve the bones of the upper limb.

Fractures resulting from bone weakness due to pre-existing bone disease must always be considered in the juvenile fracture patient as a result of possible congenital or hereditary disorders or, more commonly, nutritional imbalances affecting the bones (Figure 11.3). These so-called pathological fractures usually occur with a history of minimal trauma and there may be evidence of multiple site involvement.

General considerations

In general management, strategies should be simple and involve stabilization systems that can be removed early and easily. Rapid biological healing means that many of these fractures can be managed using external coaptation. However, each individual case must be considered carefully before a choice of fixation is made, taking into account both positive and negative factors.

Positive factors

- Rapid healing
- Production of large callus
- Low mechanical loading compared with adult
- Thick periosteum can act to support fragments of bone.

Negative factors

- Soft bones with relatively thin cortices
- Poor purchase for implants
- Variable length and shape of diaphysis
- Impairment of continued growth
- Implants engulfed by new bone, making removal difficult
- Exuberant callus with soft tissue entrapment.

Specific recommendations for fracture management

Incomplete (greenstick) fractures

These are often found on the tension surface of the bone, while the compression side bends or folds instead of breaking. Diagnosis can be difficult in the absence of recognizable deformity. The patient may present with an acute lameness, with focal pain over the site of the incomplete fracture. Definitive diagnosis depends on positive identification of the cortical break, using radiography. Primary management, once the diagnosis has been established, is aimed at preventing the fracture line propagating further and producing a complete fracture, and at preventing angulation at the fracture site as the bone heals.

A dressing, cast or external fixator in the lower limb will protect the bone and provide support while the fracture heals. In the upper limb the bone is less accessible and an external fixator may be the surest method of providing the necessary support. The fracture will heal very quickly and early removal of the support in 3–4 weeks should be planned.

Simple fractures

Simple fractures tend to occur in the mid-diaphyseal area. They will heal quickly if reapposed and stabilized. The simplest methods of stabilization should be considered because of the biological advantage these fractures have. For fractures of the lower limb a tubular cast may allow good, uncomplicated healing, provided the normal conditions for selecting a cast as the method of stabilization are satisfied (Chapter 7). Otherwise surgical fixation with an external fixator will allow stabilization. For the upper limb, intramedullary pins and external fixators used alone or in combination will allow healing to occur. Fracture healing should be checked at regular intervals and the support removed as soon as it is redundant.

Comminuted fractures

When comminution is present different mechanical and biological circumstances exist, producing a more complicated picture. The simplest way to approach these situations is to make full use of the biological potential of the comminuted fragments to heal together: provide rigid splinting across the fracture site. In the lower limb this can be best achieved by applying an external fixator, which is ideally designed to maintain limb length and position without involving the area of the fracture. It will also permit early limb use, which is an important factor since these fractures may take longer to stabilize than simple fractures. The use of external coaptation methods is far from ideal in many of these cases. Cast fixation will not easily preserve limb length; in circumstances where prolonged healing time is anticipated, immobilization of joints and muscles (especially when exuberant callus is being produced) may lead to fracture disease (Chapter 23).

In the upper limb, the bone is once again less accessible, due to the surrounding muscle mass, and this produces a dilemma when considering the best option to give a good result. Often external fixators can be used, despite the fact that their use is less ideal as a result of the increased muscle mass. If they are placed carefully they will produce good stability with minimum invasion of the fracture site. Combining these with intramedullary pins can give better alignment of the main fragments and enhance the stability by 'tying in' the fixator (Langley-Hobbs et al., 1996).

Bone plates have been used to provide a biological bridge across the fracture with good success (Drape, personal communication). In these cases no attempt is made to reconstruct the fracture. The plate is attached proximally and distally. Plates with low mechanical strength, such as cuttable plates, have been used in small dogs and cats.

All of these methods rely on a good biological response and short fracture healing time so that dependence on the implant is only required for short periods of time.

Fractures as a result of pre-existing bone disease

Secondary nutritional parathyroidism arising from dietary imbalance is the most common cause of bone disease in juveniles, resulting in poor skeletal mineralization and weak bones. There may be pathological folding fractures (Figure 11.3), which can be difficult to diagnose since the bones may be difficult to visualize on radiographs because of poor calcification. The radiographs need to be inspected carefully as multiple fractures may be present. Diagnosis is made from the history, radiographic evidence of poor mineralization and the characteristic appearance of the fractures. Management is primarily aimed at preventing further fractures and ensuring pain relief for the patient. It is often a mistake to use external or internal fixation devices, due to the poor mechanical state of the bone. The devices may produce additional fractures and complicate the situation even more. The patient is cage rested to try to prevent further fractures occurring while the dietary problem is reversed.

General guidelines for dealing with diaphyseal fractures in skeletally immature animals

- Eliminate bone disease as a cause of fracture
- Use minimally invasive technique if surgery is required
- Complete anatomical construction of fracture is unnecessary
- Casts may be considered, due to rapid healing requiring short support period
- Check stability weekly and remove implant or cast as soon as practical.

Implants used in diaphyseal fracture management

No single fixation technique will overcome all the problems that can be encountered in the juvenile fracture patient. The surgeon should understand the benefits and disadvantages of using each type of implant in order to make a correct selection in any given situation.

Bone plates

Often the most predictable and dependable implant in orthopaedic surgery in adults, bone plates produce both mechanical and biological difficulties in juveniles. The soft cortical bone does not provide good screw purchase for stability and the strong rigid bone plates and screws are mismatched with the more flexible diaphyseal bone in young animals. Biological problems may be produced by the extensive surgical exposure and dissection required to place the plate, and the large contact area with bone. Growth may be compromised if it is necessary to fix the plate in the proximity of the growth plate. Early removal of a bone plate necessitates a second major surgical procedure.

Intramedullary pin or nail

The medullary canal of growing bone is relatively larger in diameter than an adult bone and contains more cancellous bone. Intramedullary pins are useful, producing good mechanical and biological environments in suitable fractures. Early removal can be achieved easily with a minor surgical procedure.

External fixators

The external fixator is disadvantaged by poor purchase of pins in cortical bone in much the same way as bone plates. However, the short duration of dependence on the implant, the flexibility possible in designing and applying frames and the relative ease of removal makes the fixator a versatile and useful method of stabilizing fractures in young animals.

REMOVAL OF FIXATION SYSTEMS

This should be planned in every fracture. This is more important in young animals since problems may occur as a direct result of the implant's presence as the animal ages. The longer the implant remains in position, the more likely it is to produce a problem. Implants should be removed when their presence is no longer essential to the stability and function of the bone. This can be at the time of clinical union of the fracture but the point of radiographic union is more often selected as a safer option. In very young dogs removal of the implant may ensure continued longitudinal growth.

The ideal method of fracture repair in immature animals would incorporate the following points:

- Allow rapid healing by callus formation
- Allow weight bearing and limb use throughout healing

- Be simple to apply and remove
- Allow growth to continue unimpaired
- Allow assessment of clinical union on different occasions
- Allow radiographic assessment of healing
- Be well tolerated and produce no problems that might complicate healing.

REFERENCES AND FURTHER READING

Alcantara PJ and Stead AC (1975) Fractures of the distal femur in the dog and cat. *Journal of Small Animal Practice* **16**, 649–659

Berg RJ, Egger EL, Konde LJ and McCurrnin DM (1984) Evaluation of prognostic factors for growth following distal epiphyseal injuries in 17 dogs. *Veterinary Surgery* **13**, 172–180

Brighton C (1978) Structure and function of the growth plate. *Clinical Orthopaedics* **136**, 22–32

Denny HR (1989) Femoral overgrowth to compensate for tibial shortening in the dog. *Veterinary and Comparative Orthopaedics and Traumatology* **1**, 47.

Ham AW and Cormack DH (1979) *377, Histophysiology of Cartilage, Bone and Joints.* JP Lippincott, Philadelphia, PA

Herron AJ (1981) Review of bone structure, function, metabolism and growth. In: *Pathophysiology in Small Animal Surgery*, PP. 791–801. Lea and Febiger, Philadelphia, PA.

Langley-Hobbs S, Carmichael S and McCartney W (1996) Use of external skeletal fixators in the repair of femoral fractures in cats. *Journal of Small Animal Practice* **37**, 95–101.

Lawson DD (1958) The use of Rush pins in the management of fractures in the dog and the cat. *Veterinary Record* **70**, 97–172

Marretta SM and Schrader SC (1983) Physeal injuries in the dog. A review of 135 cases. *Journal of American Veterinary Medicine Association* **182**, 707–710.

Milton JL, Horne RD and Goldstein GM (1980) Cross-pinning: a simple technique for treatment of certain metaphyseal and physeal fractures of the long bones. *Journal of the American Animal Hospital Association* **16**, 891–905

Newton CD and Nunamaker DM (1985) Paediatric fractures. In: *Textbook of Small Animal Orthopaedics*, eds CD Newton and DM Nunamaker, pp 461–466. Lippincott, Philadelphia, PA

Phillips IR (1979) A survey of bone fractures in the dog and cat. *Journal of Small Animal Practice* **20**, 661–674

Reynolds DA (1981) Growth changes in fractured long bones. A study of 126 children. *Journal of Bone and Joint Surgery*, **63B**, 83–88

Salter RB and Harris WR (1963) Injuries involving the epiphyseal plate. *Journal of Bone and Joint Surgery*, **45A**, 587

Sharrard WJW (1993) Fractures and joint injuries. In: *Pediatric Orthopaedics and Fractures*, 3rd edn, ed. WJW Sharrard, p. 1365. Blackwell Scientific Publications, Oxford

Wagner SD, Desch JP, Ferguson HR and Nassar RF (1987) Effect of distal femoral growth plate fusion on femoral-tibial length. *Veterinary Surgery* **16**, 435–439

PART THREE

Management of Specific Fractures

CHAPTER TWELVE

The Skull and Mandible

Harry W. Scott

INTRODUCTION

Trauma to the head may result in fractures of the calvarium, the maxillofacial region, the mandible, the dentition or any combination of these. Such injuries frequently produce severe disfigurement and pain, and are among the most distressing for patient and client alike. Many of these fractures pose special problems because they are open and involve concurrent trauma to soft tissue structures such as the oral mucosa, nasal passages and tongue. Treatment must not only address fracture fixation but also the soft tissues, the dentition and the maintenance of nutrition. Emergency treatment may be required in severely traumatized patients to maintain a patent airway and prevent further injury to soft tissue structures. Early reduction and stabilization are necessary when the fracture fragments obstruct the airway, impinge on the brain or eye, or prevent eating and drinking.

The location and nature of jaw fractures can frequently be visualized on physical examination; nevertheless, radiological examination should always be performed to assist in the identification of concomitant fractures, temporomandibular joint (TMJ) luxation and dental trauma. Evaluation of radiographs of this region is complicated by the great range of normal variation in skull shape and size between breeds of dog. Breed differences are less pronounced in the cat but the small size and the superimposition of structures complicates radiographic interpretation. With correct positioning distortion is eliminated and the bilateral symmetry of the skull can be used to advantage to facilitate assessment of unilateral abnormalities. Interpretation of radiographs obtained to assess fracture healing in the maxillofacial region and the calvarium is difficult because the thin cortical bone heals with less callus formation than that of long bone fractures. An external callus can be demonstrated radiologically during the healing of mandibular fractures but because the mandible is not a weight-bearing bone this is less extensive than that seen during the healing of most long bone fractures (Morgan and Leighton, 1995). Routine radiography includes the lateral and dorsoventral or ventrodorsal views and lateral oblique projections of both TMJs when fracture or luxation of either joint is suspected. Special projections and the use of intraoral non-screen film may be required to visualize individual structures, details of which may be found in standard texts.

PRINCIPLES OF JAW FRACTURE REPAIR

The basic principles of fracture repair are the same as those for fractures elsewhere, with the addition of factors that are unique to the jaw because of the presence of the teeth. Most of the dorsal two-thirds of the mandible is occupied by tooth roots; the ventral third includes the mandibular canal, which contains the mandibular alveolar artery and vein and the mandibular alveolar nerve. The mandibular canal has one caudomedial opening, the mandibular foramen, and two or three mental foramina on the rostrolateral aspect, the largest of which (the middle mental foramen) is located ventral to the septum between the first two premolars. The mandibular alveolar artery and its branches provide the sole blood supply to the alveolar bone, periodontal ligament and the teeth (Roush *et al.*, 1989). Disruption of the blood supply to the rostral fragment after osteotomy of the mandible is followed by the development of a transient extraosseous blood supply via the soft tissue attachments until the normal vascular pattern is re-established (Roush and Wilson, 1989). Thus the integrity of the rostral soft tissues is important for revascularization of bone and hence the prognosis for fracture union.

Considerations when undertaking fracture repair are the avoidance of iatrogenic trauma to the teeth and associated neurovascular structures, removal of diseased teeth within the fracture line, and – most important of all – restoration of correct dental occlusion. Implants should never be placed into or within the pulp or dentine of the root, including unerupted teeth in young animals, and the mandibular canal and its foramina should be avoided. Small malalignments that are well tolerated in diaphyseal fractures of the appendicular skeleton are usually unacceptable in the mandible. Caudal malalignment of only 2–3 mm may prevent closure of the mouth by up to 10 mm (Weigel,

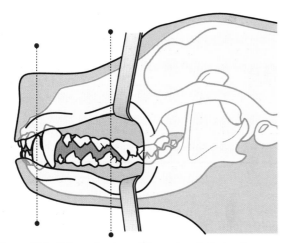

Figure 12.1: Schematic view of the canine skull showing normal dental occlusion.

1985). To achieve normal occlusion the mandibular canine tooth should be positioned in the middle of the space between the maxillary lateral incisor and canine tooth (Figure 12.1), and the cusp of the mandibular fourth premolar should be positioned between the maxillary third and fourth premolars (Ross, 1978). Malocclusion may result in complications such as impaired mastication, abnormal tooth wear, accumulation of plaque and tartar, periodontal disease, and degenerative disease of the TMJ (Chambers, 1981).

A number of methods of fracture repair have distinct advantages and are more readily adapted for use in the repair of jaw fractures in dogs. The surgical options in cats are limited by the small size of the fracture fragments, the irregular shape of the bones and the sparsity of the cortical bone. Almost all fractures of the mandible are open, due to the tight attachment of the gingiva to the underlying bone. The use of broad spectrum antibiotics has been associated with a reduced incidence of complications in open mandibular fractures in humans (Zallen and Curry, 1975) and dogs (Umphlet and Johnson, 1990). Cephalexin or potentiated amoxycillin are good empirical choices based on the type of micro-organisms composing the microbial flora of the mouth. Animals with concurrent severe periodontal disease may benefit from antibiotics directed at the type of micro-organisms associated with this disease, such as clindamycin, or metronidazole either alone or in combination with spiramycin.

The viability of the soft tissues should be assessed during fracture repair. Judicious debridement of devitalized soft tissue should be performed followed by primary closure of the resulting mucosal defect where possible. Primary repair of the gingiva is often limited by the lack of available purchase to secure the suture adjacent to the alveolar bone and the delicate nature of the tissues. Absorbable suture materials are preferred, such as small-diameter polyglactin (Vicryl; Ethicon) in a simple interrupted pattern. Soft tissue defects over intact bone will rapidly granulate and re-epithelialize;

defects at the fracture site, particularly in the presence of metal implants, should be avoided since they are associated with an increased incidence of osteomyelitis, delayed union and non-union (Ross and Goldstein, 1986). A large defect that cannot be closed by simple tissue apposition can be closed using a mucosal-submucosal advancement flap based on the lip margin. If necessary, alveolar bone can be removed beyond the mucosal margins to gain free tissue and facilitate flap advancement and suturing. Small fragments of bone devoid of soft tissue attachment should be discarded to prevent the development of sequestra; larger fragments should be retained even if they are avascular, provided they contribute to fracture stability.

Fractures frequently occur through dental alveoli either because of prior weakening caused by periodontal disease or because the alveolus serves as a stress riser. Some authorities have advocated the extraction of teeth on the fracture line based on the rationale that the presence of a tooth in the fracture line increases the incidence of osteomyelitis and non-union (Rossman *et al.*, 1985; Manfra Maretta and Tholen, 1990). Several studies in humans have shown that immediate extraction of the tooth does not prevent these complications (Neal *et al.*, 1978; Kahnberg and Ridell, 1979) and loss of teeth and associated alveolar bone increases the difficulty of achieving anatomical reduction. A recent study of mandibular fractures in the dog showed that there was an increased frequency of complications following removal of teeth (Umphlet and Johnson, 1990). Extraction of teeth should only be performed if there is severe periodontal disease, or if the tooth roots are fractured or loose and cannot be stabilized (Shields Henney *et al.*, 1992). If the dental fracture is coronal and the pulp cavity has not been invaded, the fragment should be removed and the tooth restored by enamel bonding. Fractured teeth with apical fragments can often be salvaged but usually require root canal therapy. Avulsed teeth may be re-implanted, provided the alveolar socket is intact, but will require root canal therapy once stable. Disruption of the blood supply to the teeth along the fracture line may cause inflammation of the pulpal tissues leading to periapical abscessation; such teeth should be monitored closely during the post-operative period and complications treated either by extraction or root canal therapy, as appropriate (Smith and Kern, 1995).

ANAESTHESIA

General anaesthesia is required for nearly all patients to allow a full physical and radiographic evaluation of the injury. The animal should be anaesthetized as soon as it is safe to do so following assessment and appropriate treatment of other injuries. Injectable agents may be used to allow examination of the oral cavity, the application of a muzzle, or for short procedures such as the wiring of a mandibular symphyseal fracture; for longer procedures inhalation agents should be administered through a cuffed endotracheal tube that will prevent the inhalation of blood and debris. A conventionally placed tube impedes oral manipulations and prevents closure of the mouth to check for correct reduction by alignment of the teeth; consequently pharyngostomy intubation should be used when undertaking repair of bilateral, comminuted or multiple fractures of the maxilla or mandible (Hartsfield *et al.*, 1977). After anaesthetic induction, intubation is performed in the usual way and the animal is positioned in lateral recumbency

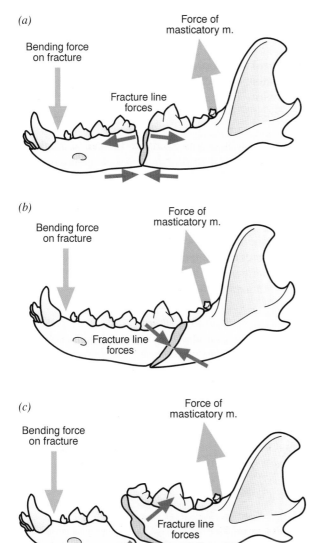

(a)

Force of masticatory m.

Bending force on fracture

Fracture line forces

(b)

Force of masticatory m.

Bending force on fracture

Fracture line forces

(c)

Force of masticatory m.

Bending force on fracture

Fracture line forces

Figure 12.2: *Biomechanics of mandibular fractures. (a) A fracture perpendicular to the long axis of the body of the mandible will tend to open at the dorsal end of the fracture line. (b) For oblique fractures, stability will depend on the angle and direction of the obliquity. A fracture line that runs from dorsocaudal to ventrorostral is favourable because muscle forces compress the fracture line and it will be inherently stable. (c) A fracture line that is orientated from dorsorostral to ventrocaudal is unfavourable because similar forces lead to distraction of the rostral fragment.*

with the neck extended (Egger, 1993). Using a finger inserted into the oropharynx, medial to lateral pressure is exerted in the piriform fossa, just caudal to the epihyoid bone. A skin incision is made approximately 1.5 times the diameter of the endotracheal tube and continued through the platysma muscle and sphincter colli muscle into the pharynx. Artery forceps inserted from the exterior are used first to grasp the cuff inflation tube and then the endotracheal tube itself, with the adapter removed, and pull it through the pharyngotomy incision. Following fracture repair the pharyngotomy wound is left unsutured and allowed to heal by second intention. For patients with concomitant upper airway obstruction, following routine endotracheal intubation, a tracheotomy should be performed for tracheostomy tube placement (Smith and Kern, 1995).

BIOMECHANICS OF JAW FRACTURES

The dominant muscle pull on the mandible is from the temporalis, masseter and the medial and lateral pterygoid muscles, whose combined effect is to close the jaw. In the dog these muscles are very strong and are capable of generating massive occlusal forces. The only muscle whose action is to open the jaw is the relatively weak digastricus muscle which attaches to the ventral aspect of the mandibular body. The primary force acting on the mandible during mastication is bending which induces maximum tensile stress at the oral or alveolar side of the mandible. Shear, rotational and compressive forces are of much less significance, particularly when fractures are unilateral due to the splinting effect of the hemimandible. The forces acting on the maxilla are similar but of smaller magnitude. To take advantage of the tension-band principle, all implants should be placed on the alveolar border unless this is likely to jeopardize the tooth roots and the neurovascular structures in the mandibular canal.

For simple mandibular fractures the direction of the fracture line will influence the inherent stability of the fracture and should be considered when choosing the method of fixation (Figure 12.2).

TECHNIQUES USED IN MANAGING HEAD FRACTURES

Long-term mouth closure
All of these techniques rely on interdigitation of the teeth of the upper and lower dental arcades to achieve fracture reduction through occlusal alignment. A 5–10 mm gap should be left between the upper and lower incisors to allow for the animal to lap a semi-liquid diet. If proper occlusion can only be maintained by closing the jaws then no gap is left and the animal is fed by gastrostomy or pharyngostomy, or by introducing

liquid food into the cheek pouch. The major disadvantage of all of these methods is that they interfere with normal masticatory function.

External coaptation

External coaptation may be indicated in the following circumstances:

- Stable fractures of the mandible and maxilla with minimal displacement
- Fractures in young animals, provided occlusion is good
- Unilateral or bilateral fissure or greenstick fractures
- Fractures of the ramus of the mandible including the condyloid process, provided displacement is not too severe
- Fractures secondary to periodontal disease where there is insufficient bone stock to accept implants
- As a temporary means of stabilization before definitive repair
- As an adjunct to other methods of stabilization

External support using a muzzle fashioned from adhesive tape (Withrow, 1981) (Figure 12.3) or a commercially available nylon muzzle (Mikki; MDC products) is a practical, cheap and non-invasive method of managing selected jaw fractures. Muzzle coaptation is probably the commonest definitive stabilization technique for mandibular fractures in dogs (Umphlet and Johnson, 1990). Despite its common usage, there are numerous disadvantages, some of which are similar to those for external coaptation of limb fractures:

- Less stability than a properly performed open reduction
- Reliance is made on the owner for daily maintenance of the muzzle
- Dermatitis may develop under the muzzle
- Immobilization may lead to soft tissue contraction.
- Some patients may not tolerate application of a muzzle
- Delay in return to normal eating and drinking
- Risk of heat stroke due to interference with panting
- Risk of inhalation pneumonia if the animal vomits
- Less suitable for cats and contraindicated in brachycephalic breeds because of interference with breathing. It is essential to check that an animal can breathe through its nose before application of a muzzle.

Intraoral techniques

Depending on the location of the fracture, dental occlusion is maintained by the placement of interarcade wires either around the incisor teeth (Merkley and Brinker, 1976), through drill holes in the alveolar ridge just caudal to the canine teeth, or between the tooth roots of the maxillary fourth premolar and the mandibular first molar (i.e. the carnassial teeth) bilaterally (Lantz, 1981). The endotracheal tube is removed following recovery from general anaesthesia and the wires are tightened to secure the jaw in the desired position. The technique may be used for comminuted fractures in which accurate bone fragment reconstruction is not possible, especially where the contralateral hemimandible is intact, and for combined fractures of the mandible and maxilla if they cannot be stabilized separately (Brinker *et al.*, 1990). A variation on this technique, applicable

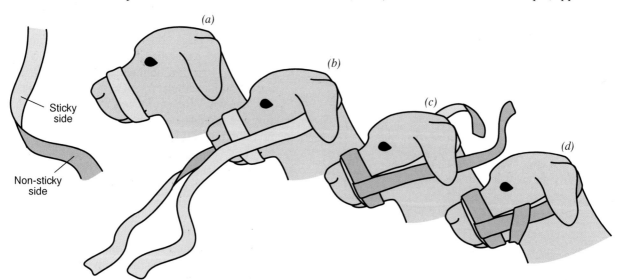

Figure 12.3: *The application of a tape muzzle. Three pieces of adhesive tape are used for the basic muzzle. (a) The first piece encircles the muzzle (sticky side out). (b) A second strip of tape is then placed around the back of the head with each end running alongside the muzzle (sticky side out). The ends should be of sufficient length to fold back behind the ears again after a third piece of tape has been applied. (c) A third strip of tape is placed around the muzzle (sticky side down) to bind in the second piece. The ends of the second piece are now folded back on themselves and anchored behind the head. (d) A fourth strip acting as a chin strap may be added.*

only to cats and small dogs, is the placement of screws in the mandible and maxilla caudal to the canine teeth; elastic bands are then placed over the screw heads which protrude into the buccal space to achieve alignment (Nibley, 1981). If the screws are placed unilaterally they should be positioned strategically to oppose any malalignment of the jaw. The client should be instructed how to remove the elastic bands in an emergency.

A technique that has been described more recently is the use of dental composite for the fixation of mandibular fractures and luxations in dogs and cats (Bennett *et al.*, 1994; Goeggerle *et al.*, 1996). The upper and lower canine teeth are bonded together to provide the same functional effect as a muzzle. This method of mouth closure is said to provide a better prognosis for restoration of occlusion compared with muzzling and eliminates the risk of iatrogenic damage to the teeth and periodontal structures that exists with interarcade wiring.

Advantages of intraoral methods over the use of muzzle fixation are as follows:

- No risk of dermatitis
- No risk of patient interference
- More applicable to the cat.

Disadvantages are as follows:

- Potential damage to teeth and periodontal tissues by the implants
- Tube feeding is necessary if the incisors are wired, or if the jaw is completely closed
- The appliance cannot be removed quickly in an emergency.

> **WARNING**
> Because of these drawbacks the use of alternative techniques is recommended whenever possible.

Interfragmentary and cerclage wire fixation

The most frequent application of wiring techniques is cerclage or circumferential wiring for the repair of fractures of the symphysis, and interfragmentary wiring, which involves the placement of wire directly across a fracture line. Interfragmentary wiring is a versatile and economical technique when properly performed and should be considered as the standard method of internal fixation of jaw fractures (Rudy and Boudrieau, 1992). However, it is an invasive procedure that requires a thorough knowledge of tooth root anatomy and is unforgiving of technical errors. The following are guidelines for correct placement of interfragmentary wires:

- Avoid tooth roots when drilling holes
- Drill all holes and place all wires before tightening
- Drill holes 5–10 mm from the fracture line and avoid weakened bone and soft alveolar bone

- Angle the drill holes towards the fracture site to facilitate the subsequent passage and tightening of the wire
- When drilling through the mandibular canal, use a Kirschner wire (K-wire) rather than a drill bit to reduce the risk of damaging the neurovascular structures
- Use the tension-band principle, i.e. place the first wire close to the alveolar border and tighten this wire first
- In all but the most stable fractures use two wires, preferably at an angle to one another. Place one wire perpendicular to the fracture line and the other parallel to the long axis of the mandibular body (Figure 12.4). A triangular configuration, with one hole in the rostral fragment and two holes in the caudal segment, is very effective for oblique fractures (Figure 12.5)
- When using a single wire, place the wire perpendicular to the fracture line to minimize iatrogenic shear forces
- Use wire of the correct size. Wire that is too thin will either break or cut through the bone; wire that is too thick will not be flexible enough to allow manipulation and tightening. Use 18–22 gauge wire, according to the size of the patient
- Avoid excessive soft tissue dissection and entrapment of soft tissue beneath the wire
- Tighten wires securely from caudal to rostral; symphyseal fractures should be wired last.

Interfragmentary wiring is not suitable for repair of fractures with comminution that cannot be reconstructed.

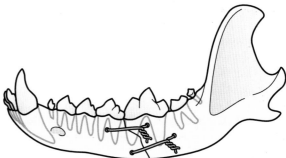

Figure 12.4: *Implant placement in the repair of a mandibular body fracture using interfragmentary wiring.*

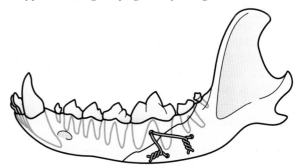

Figure 12.5: *Interfragmentary wiring of an oblique mandibular body fracture.*

Term	Definition
Interdental wiring	Fixation technique used in management of mandibular and maxillary fractures. Fragment alignment and stability are achieved by the placement of one or more wire loops that span the fractured region and are anchored around intact teeth on either side of the fracture.
Interdental splint	Uses the same principle as interdental wiring except that the wire is augmented with a dental acrylic splint which also spans the fractured region. In some circumstances the wire is omitted and the dental acrylic splint is bonded directly to tooth enamel.
Intraoral splint	Dental acrylic appliance placed against the hard palate and either wired or bonded to the teeth of the maxilla in order to maintain alignment and support of fracture fragments.
Interarcade wiring	Intraoral placement of wire between the mandible and maxilla to produce partial oral closure. Fracture fragment alignment is maintained as a result of interdigitation of teeth of the upper and lower dental arches.

Table 12.1: Wiring and splints used for fractures of the jaw.

Interdental wiring and splints

Interdental wiring is commonly used for the management of human jaw fractures and has been adapted for use in dogs, either as the sole method of repair for maxillary fractures and simple transverse mandibular body fractures, or as an adjunct to other techniques for the repair of more complex jaw fractures. Unfortunately, the dental anatomy of the dog and cat does not lend itself to this technique because of the large interdental spaces and the lack of a supragingival 'neck' to the teeth. Fractures often involve at least one of the roots of the adjacent teeth; therefore the wire should normally incorporate a minimum of two teeth on either side of the fracture line. The technique is only applicable to animals with an intact and healthy dentition. A number of configurations of wire have been described (Weigel, 1985) but a simple loop or figure-of-eight pattern works well. If interdental wire is to be used alone, the wire is passed through holes created in the gingiva at the neck of the tooth using a small K wire. Slipping of the wire can be prevented by creating a small notch in the teeth at the gingival margin, using a small round burr. Over-tightening of the wire must be avoided because this causes opening of the ventral side of the fracture line.

An alternative method of interdental fixation is the use of acrylic or dental composite to construct an interdental splint that is bonded directly to the enamel of the teeth after etching with phosphoric acid gel. Mandibular splints are created on the buccal and lingual surfaces of the first to third premolar teeth, and only the lingual surface of the fourth premolar and molars, to allow for the scissor bite of the carnassial teeth. The acrylic may be reinforced with interdental wiring or with a preformed metal splint. The combination of acrylic with metal reinforcement has been shown to be significantly stronger and stiffer than either metal or acrylic alone (Kern *et al.*, 1993). A recent study of this form of fixation showed that it is a viable alternative to bone plating and external skeletal fixation for the repair of mandibular fractures (Kern *et al.*, 1995). The technique is quick, economical, simple to perform and avoids the risk of iatrogenic damage to the tooth roots and neurovascular structures of the mandibular canal.

Intraoral splints

The most effective type of intraoral splint is fabricated from acrylic and is wired or bonded directly to the coronal surfaces of the teeth. The surfaces of the teeth for attachment of the splint are acid-etched and a thin layer of lubricating jelly is applied to protect the soft tissues. Polymerization is an exothermic reaction and there is a risk of thermal necrosis of oral tissue. This can be avoided by applying the acrylic powder in multiple thin layers in an alternating pattern with liquid monomer to build up the splint, or more simply by the use of cold-cure acrylics. The wire may be interdental or may be placed around the maxilla or through holes drilled in the maxilla. Disadvantages with this technique include interference with the management of soft tissue injuries and development of stomatitis and gingivitis secondary to entrapment of food between the appliance and the gingiva. Care must be exercised to prevent entry of acrylic into the fracture site during construction of the splint, since this increases the risk of delayed healing.

External skeletal fixation

The standard Kirschner–Ehmer splint with connecting bars and clamps can be used for the fixation of mandibular and maxillary fractures. Such splints are heavy and cumbersome, and difficult to apply, but these problems can be overcome by the use of dental acrylic for pin stabilization (Tomlinson and Constantinescu, 1991; Davidson and Bauer, 1992). The general principles are similar but the use of acrylic permits the placement of numerous pins of differing sizes and at variable angles, and the splint can be curved around the jaw rostrally to incorporate bilateral pins. Standard intramedullary pins, threaded pins or K-wires, can be used as transfixation pins and may be inserted either as half-pins or full pins. At least two and preferably three pins of the correct diameter should be used in each main fragment to provide rigid fixation. Threaded pins are recommended because they can be placed perpendicular to the long axis of the bone, they grip more securely, and they prolong the stability of the pin–bone interface (Aron *et al.*, 1986; Bennett *et al.*, 1987). Threaded pins with an outer thread diameter greater than the shaft diameter may be used but are more expensive and probably confer little advantage when used for jaw fractures. Pin breakage is much less of a problem following repair of jaw fractures than with fractures of the weight-bearing bones of the appendicular skeleton, because the forces on the jaw are smaller and can be more easily controlled by appropriate post-operative care. The pins may be bent over to lie parallel to the skin to increase the strength of the pin–acrylic interface. The acrylic can either be injected into flexible tubing or a penrose drain, using a catheter syringe, or be allowed to become doughy before being moulded over the bent fixation pins by hand. A 20 mm diameter acrylic rod is stiffer and stronger than a medium Kirschner–Ehmer connecting bar (Willer *et al.*, 1991) and is strong enough for the largest of dogs. Advantages of the technique are: that it is easy to apply to a wide variety of fracture configurations; it is minimally invasive; the fracture fragments and associated soft tissue and blood supply are not disturbed; and there are no implants at the fracture site to potentiate infection. Indications include fractures where there is comminution and those where there is gross soft tissue damage. Furthermore, stable fixation can be achieved in fractures where there are deficits due to loss of bone or teeth.

Intramedullary pinning

This technique has been advocated for the repair of mandibular fractures (Brinker *et al.*, 1990) but has little to commend it. The pin inevitably causes disruption of the neurovascular structures in the mandibular canal and damages the tooth root apices and associated soft tissues (Weigel, 1985; Roush and Wilson, 1989). Umphlet and Johnson (1990) reported that intramedullary pinning of mandibular fractures was associated with more complications than other methods of fixation. The mandibular canal is relatively straight from the root of the canine to the first molar but it then curves upwards until it opens on the medial aspect of the ramus as the mandibular foramen. A large pin tends to cause malocclusion as the bone accommodates to the shape of the pin, whereas a smaller pin provides insufficient stability. The pin is usually inserted retro-

grade, starting with the shorter segment. Fractures in the segment of the mandible between the second premolar and the first molar are the most amenable to pin fixation but alternative methods of fixation are recommended because of the aforementioned disadvantages.

Bone plating

Although bone plating provides an opportunity for rigid fixation, rapid return to pain-free normal function and primary bone healing, the technique has numerous disadvantages when used for the repair of jaw fractures. Application involves considerable disruption of soft tissues and fracture fragment vascular supply, which may compromise healing (Roush *et al.*, 1989). Furthermore, damage to the tooth roots or neurovascular structures during screw placement is almost inevitable and may result in endodontic disease. Precise contouring of the plate is required if malocclusion is to be avoided when the screws are tightened. Application of the plate on the tension side of the bone near the alveolar border provides the best fixation but is not recommended, because of the likelihood of interference with the tooth roots and the risk of complications due to gingival erosion over the implants (Verstraete and Lighthelm, 1987). Some of these problems can be overcome by using ASIF-style plates that enable the surgeon to angle the screws away from the tooth roots; reconstruction plates have the added advantage of allowing more precise three-dimensional contouring. To avoid some of these complications, the screws may be inserted in monocortical fashion so that they only engage the cortex in contact with the plate. In two recent experimental studies six-hole ASIF plates were applied in compression mode with the screws penetrating the cortex on only the ventrobuccal aspect of the mandible (Roush and Wilson, 1989; Kern *et al.*, 1995). Stable fixation was achieved as indicated by primary bone healing and most of the recognized complications were avoided. Conventional bone plating is most useful for large or giant breed dogs with unstable unilateral or bilateral mandibular body

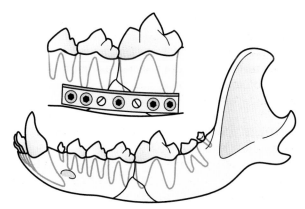

Figure 12.6: Plating of a mandibular body fracture (see text for details).

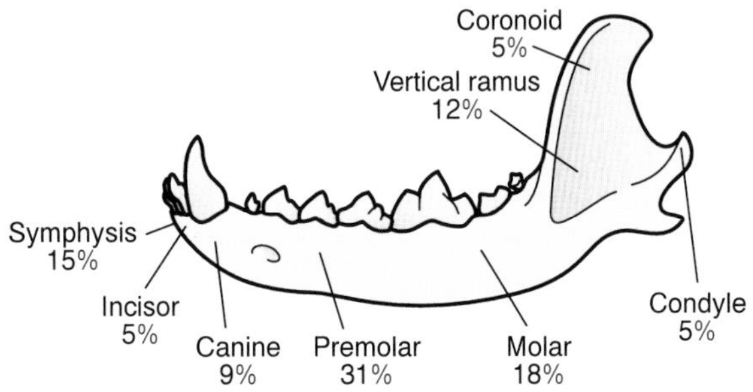

Figure 12.7: The distribution of mandibular fractures in the dog.

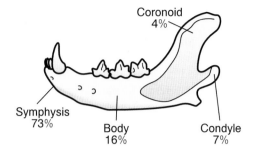

Figure 12.8: The distribution of mandibular fractures in the cat.

fractures (Harvey and Emily, 1993). The plate is placed on the ventral third of the lateral surface of the mandible and may be combined with interdental fixation or the use of a muzzle for 3–4 weeks postoperatively (Figure 12.6).

Recently the use of miniplates and screws designed specifically for the treatment of humans with maxillofacial trauma has been described for the repair of mandibular and maxillofacial fractures in dogs and cats (Boudrieau and Kudisch, 1996). The ability to perform precise three-dimensional contouring of the miniplates, combined with their small size, makes them applicable for fractures where conventional plates would be unsuitable or difficult to apply. The authors concluded that maxillofacial miniplates are particularly indicated in the management of selected comminuted fractures or fractures in which gaps are present, thus precluding the use of interfragmentary wire. Currently available miniplate systems are expensive and their use is therefore likely to be confined to referral institutions with a particular interest in these types of injury.

Partial mandibulectomy/maxillectomy

These techniques are widely used for the management of oral neoplasia and are well tolerated in dogs and cats. Hemimandibular instability and TMJ degeneration are inevitable sequels of mandibulectomy (Umphlet *et al.*, 1988). Mandibulectomy has been recommended for the management of fractures where primary repair is likely to fail because of the presence of extensive trauma or infection, or in cases where primary repair has already failed and resulted in an inability to eat or drink (Lantz and Salisbury, 1987). The technique should be regarded as a salvage procedure and, with rare exceptions, should not be used for primary repair unless there are financial constraints that preclude the use of other methods.

APPLICATION OF FIXATION TECHNIQUES TO SPECIFIC FRACTURES

Fractures of the mandible

Fractures of the mandible are the third most common fracture in the cat, accounting for between 11% and

23% of all fractures in cats and 1.5% and 2.5% in dogs (Hill, 1977; Phillips, 1979). In two recent retrospective studies of mandibular fractures, in cats (Umphlet and Johnson, 1988) and in dogs (Umphlet and Johnson, 1990), the commonest method of treatment for cats was cerclage wiring of symphyseal fractures, whereas for dogs the commonest technique was the use of a tape muzzle for fractures caudal to the second premolar teeth. The distribution of mandibular fractures in these studies is shown in Figures 12.7 and 12.8. The predominance of symphyseal fractures in the cat was largely responsible for the high incidence of mandibular fractures in this species. Road traffic accidents were the most frequent cause, followed by fights, falls and iatrogenic effects as a result of dental extractions.

Decision making in mandibular fracture repair

The choice of technique will be based on the size, age and use of the animal, the location and stability of the fracture, concurrent injuries and economic considerations. It will also be influenced by the personal preferences and expertise of the surgeon and the equipment available. The number and diversity of techniques that have been described for mandibular fracture repair are matched only by the variety and unpredictability of fracture configurations. Before embarking on treatment it is important to formulate a fracture plan tailored to the individual patient. A lack of available expertise or equipment for optimum repair should prompt consideration of referral. Table 12.2 gives a summary of the commonly used techniques and their suitability for fracture repair based on the anatomical location and stability of the fracture.

Fractures of the mandibular symphysis

The symphysis of the mandible is a fibrocartilaginous joint or synchondrosis uniting the right and left mandibular bodies. The joint is flexible and permits a moderate amount of independent movement of the two hemimandibles. The simplest method of repair is the use of a circumferential wire (Figure 12.9). The wire (18–20 gauge for dogs, 20–22 gauge for cats) is placed using a large-bore needle which is inserted through the skin of the ventral midline chin along the lateral aspect of the mandible to exit the gingiva just caudal to the canine tooth. The wire is then threaded through the needle,

Fracture location	Fracture type	Procedures
Symphysis	Simple separation Comminuted fractures	**Circumferential wiring** Tape muzzle **Dental composite and wire** Partial mandibulectomy Dental composite bonding of canines/interarcade wiring
Rostral body	Stable Unstable	**Tape muzzle** Interfragmentary wire Interdental acrylic splint **External fixator** **Interfragmentary wire +/– interdental wire** Interdental acrylic splint Partial mandibulectomy Dental composite bonding of canines/interarcade wiring
Caudal body	Stable Unstable	**Tape muzzle** Interfragmentary wiring +/– interdental wiring Interdental acrylic splint **Plate** **External fixator** **Interfragmentary wiring +/– interdental wiring** Interdental acrylic splint Dental composite bonding of canines/interarcade wiring
Ramus	Stable Unstable	**Tape muzzle** **Tape muzzle** **Plate** **Interfragmentary wiring +/– K-wire** Dental composite bonding of canines/ interarcade wiring
Coronoid process	Stable Unstable	**Tape muzzle** **Tape muzzle** Dental composite bonding of canines/interarcade wiring
Condyloid process	Stable Unstable	**Tape muzzle** **Tape muzzle** Interfragmentary wiring +/– K-wire Mandibular condylectomy

Table 12.2: Decision making in the management of mandibular fractures. Bold type indicates the author's preferred methods.

which is withdrawn and the procedure is repeated on the contralateral side using the same hole in the skin. The wire is tightened by twisting the ends together until stability is achieved. After 6 weeks the wire is removed under a general anaesthetic. Clinical union usually occurs within this period, although in some animals stability may occur in the absence of bone healing, owing to the formation of a fibrous union.

For comminuted or oblique symphyseal fractures the addition of a figure-of-eight wire or a wire brace (Kitto, 1972) around the base of the canine teeth may be necessary to avoid collapse of the teeth medially. Alternatively, an intraoral acrylic splint can be used to achieve normal occlusion, either incorporating the wire or bonded to the canine teeth (Harvey and Emily, 1993) (Figure 12.9).

Fractures of the body of the mandible
The body of the mandible is the tooth-bearing portion of the bone. The premolar region is the commonest site of jaw fractures in the dog (Umphlet and Johnson, 1990). If the fracture is inherently stable almost all repair techniques are applicable and the simplest method

that will provide adequate stability with the least potential for complications should be chosen. Muzzle fixation can be used for fractures where there is innate stability, especially in young animals where healing is expected to be rapid, provided the canine teeth are able to occlude normally when the mouth is gently closed. The stability of the fracture will depend on the location and direction of the fracture line, as previously stated. Healing times for mandibular fractures may be longer than the previously reported period of 3–5 weeks (Brinker *et al.*, 1990). Umphlet and Johnson (1990) found that clinical union for canine mandibular fractures in the premolar region occurred in an average time of 9 weeks (range 4–16 weeks). Overall it was found that the more caudally placed the fracture, the longer was the time required for healing.

The ventral surgical approach is preferred for access to most mandibular fractures (Piermattei, 1993) (Operative Technique 12.1).

Bilateral fractures immediately caudal to the canine teeth or in the rostral premolar region can be managed using either external skeletal fixation (Figure 12.10) or tension-band wiring of the dorsal surface.

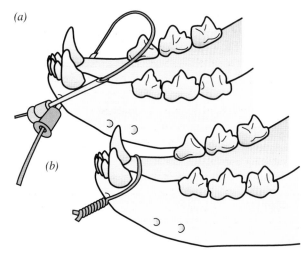

(a)

(b)

Figure 12.9: *Circumferential wiring of a mandibular symphyseal fracture in a cat. (a) A small, midline skin incision is made on the ventral aspect of the jaw below the canine teeth. A large bore hypodermic needle (see text) is inserted through the skin incision to emerge intraorally between the mandibular mucosa and the skin, just caudal to a lower canine tooth. One end of the wire is passed through the centre of the needle to emerge ventrally. The needle is withdrawn leaving the wire in position and the procedure is repeated on the other side. (b) The wire ends are then twisted to stabilize the reduced fracture. The twisted ends can then be bent over or left protruding.*

For tension-band wiring a ventral approach is used first to reduce the fracture and place the interfragmentary wires; intraoral tension-band wires are then placed through holes drilled in the alveolar bone of the two fragments. The drill holes must be placed carefully to avoid the root of the mandibular canine tooth, which occupies a large portion of the rostral fragment. The rostral hole is drilled between the canine teeth and the lateral incisors, and the caudal hole between the second and third premolars. To provide secure fixation, the holes are placed well below the dorsal margin of the alveolar bone.

External skeletal fixation has two distinct advantages over tension-band wiring. Firstly, the implants are not placed immediately adjacent to the fracture site in an area where there may be little bone stock; and secondly, stability can be achieved where there is loss of bone fragments or even of an entire canine tooth. For comminuted fractures where the canine teeth are intact and stable, the canine teeth can be bonded together, as previously described, to maintain normal occlusion during the healing process. Where there are multiple small fragments of bone and broken teeth, an alternative approach for comminuted fractures is a partial mandibulectomy.

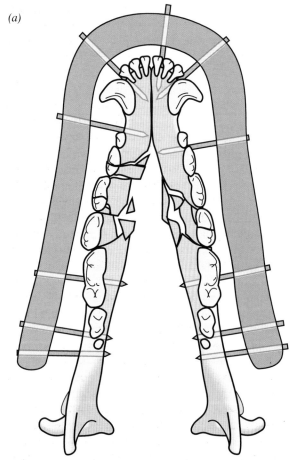

(a)

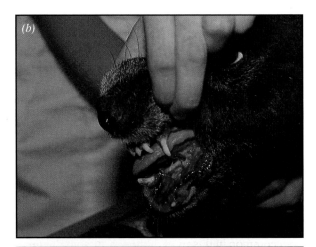

(b)

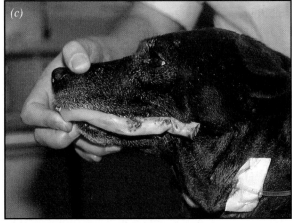

(c)

Figure 12.10: *External skeletal fixation of mandibular fractures. (a) Schematic view of a bilateral comminuted mandibular body fracture repaired with pins and a dental acrylic connecting bar (see text for details of application). (b) Bilateral open fractures of the rostral mandibular body in a dog following a road traffic accident. (c) The same dog 24 hours after repair of the fractures using an acrylic fixator.*

Interfragmentary wiring, combined with interdental wiring if necessary, is adequate for most other unstable fractures.

Where fractures are bilateral or there is comminution, gross soft tissue trauma, or loss of bone stock, external skeletal fixation is a more appropriate method of repair. If the fracture is bilateral it is best to place the fixation pins as half-pins. An alternative technique for bilateral or comminuted fractures is bone plating, especially for caudal body fractures, where it is easier to avoid the mandibular canal and the tooth roots. However, plating is not a good choice for cats or for young dogs with growing teeth.

Fractures of the ramus of the mandible

The (vertical) ramus is the caudal non-tooth-bearing vertical part of the bone. It has three processes: the coronoid process, the condyloid or articular process and the angular process. The mandibular notch is located between the coronoid and the condyloid processes; the angle of the mandible is its caudoventral portion. Because of its protected location, fractures of the ramus are less common than fractures of the body of the mandible. The ramus differs from the rest of the mandible in that the bone is thinner and weaker and, because of its shape, it is more difficult to hold in alignment using internal fixation. However, the bone is surrounded by broad muscular insertions over its entire surface, the coronoid process in particular being well protected by the overlying zygomatic arch and masseter muscle. Fractures in this region are usually closed, stable and minimally displaced. If significant malocclusion is present, concomitant TMJ luxation or fracture/luxation should be suspected.

Muzzle fixation is the preferred technique for most fractures of the ramus. The options for grossly displaced or unstable fractures, especially in larger dogs, include Kirschner wires, interfragmentary wires or mini-plates (Sumner-Smith and Dingwall, 1973). Dental malocclusion as a complication of fracture repair is less common in this region of the mandible (Umphlet and Johnson, 1990). For surgical approach, see Operative Technique 12.2.

Fractures of the condyloid process

Condylar fractures are uncommon and when they do occur are often associated with fractures of the rostral mandibular body or mandibular symphysis. The condylar fracture is easily overlooked even when radiographic examination is performed. As with other articular fractures, rigid internal fixation and an early return to function have been recommended. However, most fractures are minimally displaced and internal fixation is difficult because of the small size of the fragments and the inaccessibility of the joint. In most cases good results can be obtained with conservative management, and post-operative periarticular fibrosis is avoided (Salisbury and Cantwell, 1989). A muzzle is

applied for 2–4 weeks and the animal is fed a semi-liquid diet. Clinical union takes an average of 11 weeks (range 10–13 weeks) (Umphlet & Johnson, 1990). In some cases a fibrous union may develop because of motion at the fracture site but good mandibular function may still result (Chambers, 1981). Open reduction and internal fixation may be indicated for severely displaced condylar fractures, using interfragmentary wire, small intramedullary pins or K-wires.

Mandibular condylectomy and meniscectomy are well tolerated in normal dogs (Tomlinson and Presnell, 1983) and this is the preferred method of managing painful non-union fractures, DJD, and ankylosis attributable to periarticular fibrosis (Lantz et al., 1982; Lantz, 1991). The surgical approach to the TMJ is described in Operative Technique 12.3.

Fractures of the maxillofacial region

Fractures of this region account for approximately 1–2% of all fractures in the dog and cat (Leonard, 1971; Phillips, 1979). In addition to the maxilla, the other bones rostral to the orbital region are frequently involved. These are the incisive, nasal and palatine bones which constitute the hard palate, the upper dental arcades and the muzzle. Fractures of the face near the orbit may involve the frontal, zygomatic, temporal and ethmoid bones. There is often epistaxis due to concurrent trauma to the nasal turbinates but haemorrhage tends to be self-limiting and these injuries are not of primary concern, provided reduction of the fractured bones is achieved. The extent of the fracture may be determined by physical and radiographic examination. As with fractures of the mandible, restoration of normal dental occlusion and masticatory function is paramount.

The majority of fractures are stable and minimally displaced and can be treated using external coaptation. Because the muscular forces on the maxilla are much less than those on the mandible, less rigid fixation is required and a fibrous union may produce a satisfactory functional result, provided dental occlusion has not been compromised. Fractures that communicate with the nasal cavity or the sinuses are likely to be contaminated and the patient should be treated with antibiotics, as in any other open fracture. Frontal bone fractures may develop subcutaneous emphysema if fracture fragments penetrate the frontal sinus. These rarely require surgical intervention unless they impinge on the eye, in which case small fragments should be removed and larger fragments should be stabilized. Conservative treatment may require aspiration of the emphysema, if extensive, followed by application of a compressive dressing to prevent recurrence. Fractures of the zygomatic arch are relatively common and may require surgery if they interfere with mastication or compress ocular structures. An occasional complication of healing of fractures of the zygomatic arch or the ramus of the mandible is the production of excessive bony callus that interferes with normal jaw movement (Bennett and Campbell, 1976; Van Ee and Pechman, 1987). The condition is treated by resection of a portion of the zygomatic arch and fibrous tissue adhesions as necessary. The surgical approach is made through the skin and platysma muscle directly over the bone.

Most of the standard internal fixation techniques are applicable for comminuted or displaced fractures in this region, particularly interfragmentary and interdental wiring. Draping of the maxilla is similar to that of the mandible. The surgical approach should be made directly over the site of the fracture, although for multiple fractures (especially along the nose) a dorsal midline approach with retraction of soft tissues laterally may be best to avoid neurovascular structures. Care should be taken to avoid the infraorbital artery and nerve exiting through the large infraorbital foramen of the maxilla which lies dorsal to the septum between the third and fourth maxillary premolars. The osseous lacrimal canal should be avoided when drilling holes for orthopaedic wire in the small lacrimal bone in the rostral margin of the orbit.

Intraoral approaches are used for fractures of the hard palate or along the dental arcade. Longitudinal fractures of the hard palate or nasal bones are not uncommon in the cat and may be seen as one component of the specific triad of injuries (thoracic injury, facial trauma and extremity fractures), first termed the 'high-rise syndrome' by Robinson (1976), that occurs when an animal jumps or falls from a height and lands on its forelimbs and chin. Traumatic clefts of the hard palate can be repaired using wire fixation perpendicular to the fracture line, anchored between the teeth on either side of the buccal cavity – usually the fourth premolars in the cat, and additionally the canine teeth in the dog. Where more support is required the wire is anchored over the ends of a small pin or K-wire passed just dorsal to the hard palate. The mucoperiosteum along the fracture line may sometimes require suturing to prevent the development of an oronasal fistula.

External skeletal fixation is particularly suited to bilateral or severely comminuted maxillary fracture repair since the presence of multiple small fragments makes these fractures difficult to stabilize by any other means (Stambaugh and Nunamaker, 1982). The only requirement is that there must be sufficient bone stock caudal to the fracture line to allow placement of the fixation pins. A type 2 fixator is most commonly employed and the pins are driven as either half-pins or full pins, depending on the configuration of the fracture. If the fracture is bilateral they are driven as full pins across the nasal cavity, taking care to avoid the tooth roots and the infraorbital foramen. Fixation pins are always inserted parallel to the hard palate, with the teeth held in the correct alignment, using at least two pins for each major fragment. Once inserted, the pins may be used to manipulate the bone fragments to achieve dental occlusion before they are embedded in acrylic.

POST-OPERATIVE MANAGEMENT OF JAW FRACTURES

Post-operative care for all animals with jaw fractures includes the feeding of a liquid diet for the first 4–7 days after surgery, followed by avoidance of hard foods until the fracture has healed. Animals that are anorexic may require tube feeding. Nasopharyngeal tube placement can be performed in the conscious patient and is particularly useful for cats, where insertion is very easy. In cases where long-term nutritional support is anticipated (more than 7 days) a gastrostomy tube should be placed at the time of fracture repair. A technique of blind percutaneous placement of the tube has been described (Fulton and Dennis, 1992). In animals with oral wounds or where an intraoral appliance has been used for fracture repair, the mouth should be rinsed daily with warm water or an antiseptic mouthwash. Intraoral appliances may cause trauma to soft tissues and will inevitably cause a degree of stomatitis and gingivitis secondary to food entrapment between the appliance and the gingiva. This problem generally resolves spontaneously within 7 days of removal of the appliance.

PROBLEMS ENCOUNTERED IN REPAIRING JAW FRACTURES

There are two situations where an increase in the frequency of complications of fracture repair can be predicted:

- Fractures where there is severe comminution or bone loss
- Fractures where there is advanced periodontal disease.

The critical size of a bone defect that will not heal is probably about 20–40 mm (Schmitz and Hollinger, 1986). External skeletal fixators and bone plates are the best techniques for bridging deficits. A cancellous bone graft should be used for all fractures where a problem is anticipated if an open approach is performed. Substantial defects may be managed as partial mandibulectomies requiring no further treatment (Lantz and Salisbury, 1987); alternatively, plate fixation and cortical bone grafting may be performed (Boudrieau et al., 1994).

Approximately 85% of all dogs and cats older than 6 years have periodontal disease (Tholen and Hoyt, 1983). If an animal has clinically significant periodontal disease a complete dental prophylaxis should be performed, with dental extractions as appropriate, at the same time as fracture fixation. Pathological fracture may occur in animals with severe periodontal disease as a result of minimal trauma through an alveolus already weakened by osteolysis. These animals are also at risk of iatrogenic fracture as a result of attempted extraction of teeth where there has been extensive bone loss but the teeth are still securely maintained in their sockets. Management of iatrogenic fractures is frequently complicated by the bone loss and the presence of poor quality osteoporotic bone, with limited osteogenic potential, and infected bone secondary to the periodontal disease. Typically these patients are geriatric small-breed dogs with incomplete dentition caused by previous extractions or shedding of teeth. Internal fixation is generally not a good option because of the poor bone quality. Judicious extraction of diseased teeth is indicated where there is periapical abscess formation, though this may result in further weakening of the bone. Options for fracture management are limited to long-term mouth closure techniques or mandibulectomy, the choice of technique depending on the type of fracture. A functional result is to be expected for fractures that are unilateral and stable even in cases where the bone fails to heal and a fibrous union develops. For unstable fractures, especially when bilateral, it may be preferable to perform a primary mandibulectomy rather than risk a prolonged and potentially unsuccessful attempt at fracture repair.

POST-OPERATIVE COMPLICATIONS OF JAW FRACTURE REPAIR

Complications of jaw fracture repair and their associated management are essentially the same as those described for fractures of the appendicular skeleton but with the addition of problems relating to the dentition. These include osteomyelitis, delayed union, non-union, malunion and malocclusion, bone sequestration, facial deformity, oronasal fistula and dental abnormality. Complications were reported in 34% of mandibular fractures in 105 dogs (Umphlet and Johnson, 1990) and 24.5% of mandibular fractures in 62 cats (Umphlet and Johnson, 1988) – figures which are higher than those for long bone fractures. The most frequent complication in dogs and cats was dental malocclusion, which, besides adversely affecting function, increases the risk of delayed union and non-union by increasing the forces of leverage against the fixation device. Treatment for this complication is determined by the severity of the associated clinical signs. Options include immediate removal of the fixation device followed by correct reduction and fixation, and extraction or orthodontic movement of the maloccluded teeth (Manfra Maretta et al., 1990). Malocclusion secondary to segmental defects may be corrected by bone grafting and plate fixation (Boudrieau et al., 1994).

FRACTURES OF THE CALVARIUM

Fractures of the calvarium are uncommon and this may be due in part to the fact that most animals are either killed outright or die soon after injury as a result of severe brain trauma (Hill, 1977; Phillips, 1979). These fractures are invariably associated with injury to the underlying neurological structures. Brain trauma can be classified as concussion, contusion and laceration, in increasing order of severity. All three types of injury may occur in association with fractures of the skull but laceration is the commonest (Dewey et al., 1992).

All animals with head trauma constitute a medical emergency and in a small proportion of cases rapid surgical intervention may also be indicated. Details of medical therapy for head injury are not within the scope of this book. The level of consciousness and brainstem reflexes are important in the initial assessment and in the monitoring of animals with head trauma. Transient loss of consciousness followed by a rapid recovery may occur when the brain is concussed and this is associated with a good prognosis.

Most skull fractures can be managed conservatively (Newton, 1985; Egger, 1993). The benefits of surgical intervention must be weighed against the complications of administering a general anaesthetic to a neurologically compromised patient. In the absence of neurological deterioration, surgery may be delayed for 24–48 hours if time is needed for patient stabilization. Surgical intervention may be indicated in the following circumstances (Dewey et al., 1993):

- Open fractures
- Fractures where there is depression of the fragments more than the width of the calvarium in the fracture area
- Retrieval of contaminated bone fragments or foreign material
- Persistent leakage of cerebrospinal fluid
- For decompression where there is a deteriorating neurological status despite medical therapy.

Fractures of the base of the skull are rarely treated because of the severity of the injury and their inaccessibility for surgical intervention.

The surgical approach to the calvarium is made with the patient positioned in ventral recumbency with the head supported and stabilized. A midline skin incision is made extending from the external occipital protuberance to the level of the eyes (Piermattei, 1993) (Figure 12.11). Alternatively a lateral curved incision may be made, depending on the location of the fracture. The superficial temporal fascia is incised and the temporalis muscle elevated subperiosteally and retracted laterally to expose the area of the fracture. Multiple holes are drilled in the calvarium around the periphery of the fracture, enabling the insertion of small instruments to elevate the fragments (Oliver,

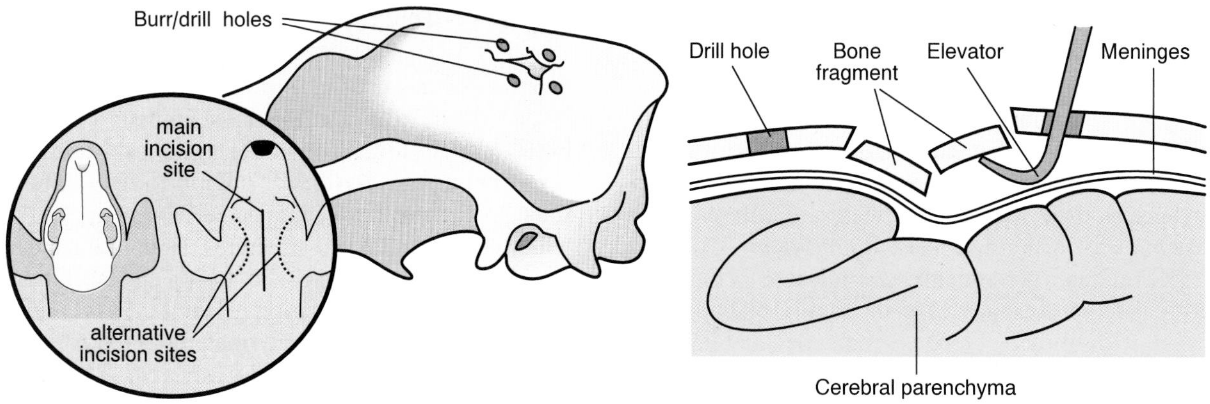

Figure 12.11: *Exposure and reduction of fractures of the calvarium.*

1975). Unstable fragments can be removed even if large since the temporalis muscle provides adequate protection of the brain parenchyma.

REFERENCES

Aron DN, Toombs JP and Hollingsworth SC (1986) Primary treatment of severe fractures by external skeletal fixation: threaded pins compared with smooth pins. *Journal of the American Animal Hospital Association* **22**, 659.

Bennett D and Campbell JR (1976) Mechanical interference with lower jaw movement as a complication of skull fractures. *Journal of Small Animal Practice* **17**, 747.

Bennett JW, Kapatkin AS and Manfra Maretta S (1994) Dental composite for the fixation of mandibular fractures and luxations in 11 cats and 6 dogs. *Veterinary Surgery* **23**, 190.

Bennett RA, Egger EL, Histand M and Ellis AB (1987) Comparison of the strength and holding power of 4 pin designs for use with half pin (type 1) external skeletal fixation. *Veterinary Surgery* **16**, 207.

Boudrieau RJ and Kudisch M (1996) Miniplate fixation of mandibular and maxillary fractures in 15 dogs and 3 cats. *Veterinary Surgery* **25**, 277.

Boudrieau RJ, Tidwell AS, Ullman SL and Gores BR (1994) Correction of mandibular nonunion and malocclusion by plate fixation and autogenous cortical bone grafts in two dogs. *Journal of the American Veterinary Medical Association* **204**, 744.

Brinker WO, Piermattei DL and Flo GL (1990) Fractures and dislocations of the upper and lower jaw. In: *Handbook of Small Animal Orthopaedics and Fracture Treatment*, 2nd edn. WB Saunders, Philadelphia.

Chambers JN (1981) Principles of management of mandibular fractures in the dog and cat. *Journal of Veterinary Orthopaedics* **2**, 26.

Davidson JR and Bauer MS (1992) Fractures of the mandible and maxilla. *Veterinary Clinics of North America Small Animal Practice* **22**, 109.

Dewey CW, Budsberg SC and Oliver JE (1992) Principles of head trauma management in dogs and cats – Part 1. *Compendium on Continuing Education for the Practising Veterinarian* **14**, 199.

Dewey CW, Budsberg SC and Oliver JE (1993) Principles of head trauma management in dogs and cats – Part 2. *Compendium on Continuing Education for the Practising Veterinarian* **15**, 177.

Egger EL (1993) Skull and mandibular fractures. In: *Textbook of Small Animal Surgery*, 2nd edn (ed. D Slatter). WB Saunders, Philadelphia.

Fulton RB and Dennis JS (1992) Blind percutaneous placement of a gastrostomy tube for nutritional support in dogs and cats. *Journal of the American Veterinary Medical Association* **201**, 697.

Goeggerle UA, Inskeep GA and Toombs JP (1996) Managing mandibular fractures in dogs. *Compendium on Continuing Education for the Practising Veterinarian* **18**, 511.

Hartsfield SM, Gendreau CL, Smith CW *et al.*, (1977) Endotracheal intubation by pharyngotomy. *Journal of the American Animal Hospital Association* **13**, 71.

Harvey CE and Emily PP (1993) Oral surgery. In: *Small Animal Dentistry*. Mosby, St Louis, MO.

Hill FWG (1977) A survey of bone fractures in the cat. *Journal of Small Animal Practice* **18**, 457.

Kahnberg KE and Ridell A (1979) Prognosis of teeth involved in the line of mandibular fractures. *International Journal of Oral Surgery* **8**, 163.

Kern DA, Smith MM, Grant JW and Rockhill AD (1993) Evaluation of bending strength of five interdental fixation apparatuses applied to canine mandibles. *American Journal of Veterinary Research* **54**, 1177.

Kern DA, Smith MM, Stevenson S. *et al.* (1995) Evaluation of three fixation techniques for repair of mandibular fractures in dogs. *Journal of the American Veterinary Medical Association* **206**, 1883.

Kitto HW (1972) A technique of mandibular fixation in cat symphyseal fractures. *The Veterinary Record* **91**, 591.

Lantz GC (1981) Interarcade wiring as a method of fixation for selected mandibular fractures. *Journal of the American Animal Hospital Association*, **17**, 599.

Lantz GC (1991) Surgical correction of unusual temporomandibular joint conditions. *Compendium on Continuing Education for the Practising Veterinarian* **13**, 1570.

Lantz GC and Salisbury SK (1987) Partial mandibulectomy for treatment of mandibular fractures in dogs: eight cases (1981–1984). *Journal of the American Veterinary Medical Association* **191**, 243.

Lantz GC, Cantwell HD, Vanvleet JF and Cechner PE (1982) Unilateral mandibular condylectomy: experimental and clinical results. *Journal of the American Animal Hospital Association* **18**, 883.

Leonard EP (1971) In: *Orthopaedic Surgery of the Dog and Cat*. WB Saunders, Philadelphia.

Manfra Maretta S and Tholen MA (1990) Extraction techniques and management of associated complications. In: *Small Animal Oral Medicine and Surgery* (eds. MJ Bojrab and MA Tholen). Lea & Febiger, Philadelphia.

Manfra Maretta S, Schrader SC and Matthiesen DT (1990) Problems associated with the management and treatment of jaw fractures. *Problems in Veterinary Medicine* **2**, 220.

Merkley DF and Brinker WO (1976) Facial reconstruction following massive bilateral maxillary fracture in the dog. *Journal of the American Animal Hospital Association* **12**, 831.

Morgan JP and Leighton RL (1995) Axial skeletal trauma. In: *Radiology of Small Animal Fracture Management*. WB Saunders, Philadelphia.

Neal DC, Wagner WF and Albert B (1978) Morbidity associated with teeth in the line of mandibular fractures. *Journal of Oral Surgery* **36**, 859.

Newton CD (1985) Fractures of the skull. In: *Textbook of Small Animal Orthopaedics*. JB Lippincott, Philadelphia.

Nibley W (1981) Treatment of caudal mandibular fractures: a preliminary report. *Journal of the American Animal Hospital Association* **17**, 555.

Oliver JE (1975) Craniotomy, craniectomy, and skull fractures. In: *Current Techniques in Small Animal Surgery* (ed. MJ Bojrab). Lea & Febiger, Philadelphia.

Phillips IR (1979) A survey of bone fractures in the dog and cat. *Journal of Small Animal Practice*, **20**, 661.

Piermattei DL (1993) The head. In: *An Atlas of Surgical Approaches to the Bones and Joints of the Dog and Cat*, 3rd edn. WB Saunders, Philadelphia.

Robinson GW (1976) The high rise trauma syndrome in cats. *Feline Practice* **6**, 40.

Ross DL (1978) Evaluation of oral abnormalities. In: *Proceedings American Animal Hospital Association, 45th Annual Meeting, Salt*

Lake City, UT, 79.

Ross DL and Goldstein GS (1986) Oral surgery basic techniques. *Veterinary Clinics of North America Small Animal Practice* **16**, 967.

Rossman LE, Garber DA and Harvey CE (1985) Disorders of teeth. In: *Veterinary Dentistry* (ed. C.E. Harvey). WB Saunders, Philadelphia.

Roush JK and Wilson JW (1989) Healing of mandibular body osteotomies after plate and intramedullary pin fixation. *Veterinary Surgery* **18**, 190.

Roush JK, Howard PE and Wilson JW (1989) Normal blood supply to the canine mandible and mandibular teeth. *American Journal of Veterinary Research* **50**, 904.

Rudy RL and Boudrieau RJ (1992) Maxillofacial and mandibular fractures. *Seminars in Veterinary Medicine and Surgery (Small Animal)* **7**, 3.

Salisbury SK and Cantwell HD (1989) Conservative management of fractures of the mandibular condyloid process in three cats and one dog. *Journal of the American Veterinary Medical Association* **194**, 85.

Schmitz JP and Hollinger JO (1986) The critical size defect as an experimental model for craniomandibulofacial nonunions. *Clinical Orthopaedics,* **205**, 299.

Shields Henney LH, Galburt RB and Boudrieau RJ (1992) Treatment of dental injuries following craniofacial trauma. *Seminars in Veterinary Medicine and Surgery (Small Animal)* **7**, 21.

Smith MM and Kern DA (1995) Skull trauma and mandibular fractures. *Veterinary Clinics of North America Small Animal Practice* **25**, 1127.

Stambaugh JE and Nunamaker DM (1982) External skeletal fixation of comminuted maxillary fractures in dogs. *Veterinary Surgery* **11**, 72.

Sumner-Smith G and Dingwall JS (1973) The plating of mandibular fractures in giant dogs. *The Veterinary Record* **92**, 39.

Tholen MA and Hoyt RF (1983) Oral pathology. In: *Concepts in Veterinary Dentistry* (ed. MA Tholen). Veterinary Medicine Publishing, Edwardsville, Kansas.

Tomlinson JL and Constantinescu GM (1991) Acrylic external skeletal fixation of fractures. *Compendium on Continuing Education for the Practising Veterinarian* **13**, 235.

Tomlinson J and Presnell KR (1983) Mandibular condylectomy effects in normal dogs. *Veterinary Surgery* **12**, 148.

Umphlet RC and Johnson AL (1988) Mandibular fractures in the cat. A retrospective study. *Veterinary Surgery* **17**, 333.

Umphlet RC and Johnson AL (1990) Mandibular fractures in the dog. A retrospective study of 157 cases. *Veterinary Surgery* **19**, 272.

Umphlet RC, Johnson AL, Eurell JC and Losonsky J (1988) The effect of partial rostral hemimandibulectomy on mandibular mobility and temporomandibular joint morphology in the dog. *Veterinary Surgery* **17**, 186.

van Ee RT and Pechman RD (1987) False ankylosis of the temporomandibular joint in a cat. *Journal of the American Veterinary Medical Association* **191**, 979.

Verstraete FJM and Lighthelm AJ (1987) Dental trauma caused by screws used in internal fixation of mandibular osteotomies in the canine. *Journal of Veterinary Dentistry* **4**, 5.

Weigel JP (1985) Trauma to oral structures. In: *Veterinary Dentistry* (ed. CE Harvey). WB Saunders, Philadelphia.

Willer RL, Egger EL and Histand MB (1991). A comparison of stainless steel versus acrylic for the connecting bar of external skeletal fixators. *Journal of the American Animal Hospital Association* **27**, 541.

Withrow SJ (1981) Taping of the mandible in treatment of mandibular fractures. *Journal of the American Animal Hospital Association* **17**, 27.

Zallen RD and Curry JT (1975) A study of antibiotic usage in compound mandibular fractures. *Journal of Oral Surgery* **33**, 431.

OPERATIVE TECHNIQUE 12.1
Surgical exposure of the mandibular body

Positioning
The animal is placed in dorsal recumbency and routine aseptic preparation of the surgical field is performed. In those cases where access to the oral cavity is required the mouth is repeatedly irrigated with dilute povidone iodine solution and the tongue is reflected back on itself into the pharynx so that it does not interfere with assessment of dental occlusion. An intraoral drape fastened to the skin at the level of the oral commissures is used to cover the anaesthetic apparatus in those animals intubated conventionally. The drape may be reflected rostrally to allow observation of the oral cavity following pharyngostomy endotracheal tube placement. In either case the anaesthetic machine is placed to the side of the patient to allow unimpeded access to the surgical field.

Assistant
Optional.

Tray Extras
Pointed reduction forceps; Gelpi and Hohmann retractors; selected implants and hardware for insertion.

Surgical Approach
Exposure of the mandible is achieved by incising the thin sheet-like platysma muscle, which is then retracted laterally with the fascia and skin (Figure 12.12). Exposure of the medial aspect of the bone can be increased by separating the mylohyoideus muscle from the medial edge of the mandible and retracting it medially. Although subperiosteal elevation of the digastricus muscle from the ventral aspect of the mandible may be performed for access to caudal body fractures, it is preferable to preserve the attachment by retraction of the muscle to either side as necessary. It is important to avoid the facial vein and accompanying nerve trunks laterally.

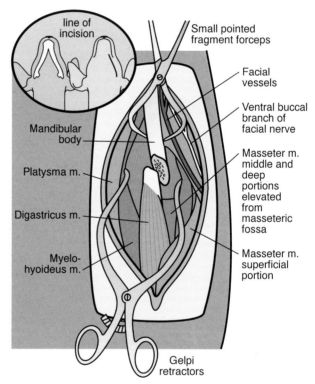

Figure 12.12: Ventral exposure of a mandibular body fracture (see text for details).

Wound Closure
The intermuscular septum between the digastricus and masseter muscles is sutured using absorbable material of the surgeon's choice. The rest of the closure is routine.

OPERATIVE TECHNIQUE 12.2

Surgical exposure of the mandibular ramus

Positioning
Lateral recumbency with the head supported. Intubation as described in main text.

Assistant
Optional.

Tray Extras
Pointed reduction forceps; Gelpi and Hohmannn retractors; selected implants and hardware for insertion.

Surgical Approach
The surgical approach to the angle of the mandible is hampered by the heavy musculature, the parotid gland and the neurovascular structures in this region (Figure 12.13). After incising the platysma muscle, the dorsal and ventral buccal branches of the facial nerve, and the parotid gland and its duct should be identified (Piermattei, 1993). Exposure of the fracture is achieved by incising across the superficial layers of the masseter muscle parallel with the caudal border of the mandible. The middle and deep layers of the muscle are elevated subperiosteally from their insertion on the masseteric fossa and retracted dorsally, allowing exposure of the ramus to the level of the TMJ.

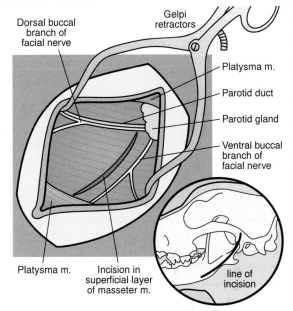

Figure 12.13: Surgical approach to the mandibular ramus (see text for details).

Wound Closure
The aponeurosis covering the superficial layer of the masseter muscle is sutured. The rest of the closure is routine.

OPERATIVE TECHNIQUE 12.3
Surgical exposure of the temporomandibular joint

Positioning
Lateral recumbency with the head supported. Intubation as described in text.

Assistant
Optional.

Tray Extras
Pointed reduction forceps; Gelpi and Hohmannnn retractors.

Surgical Approach
The skin incision is made along the ventral border of the zygomatic arch and crosses the TMJ caudally (Piermattei, 1993) (Figure 12.14). The platysma muscle and fascia are incised and retracted with the skin; the attachment of the origin of the masseter muscle on the zygomatic arch is incised and subperiosteal elevation of the muscle is performed. The palpebral nerve and the transverse facial vessels and dorsal branch of the facial nerve should be avoided. Reflection of the tissue ventrally exposes the lateral surface of the joint and the upper portion of the condyloid process. This approach may be combined with the approach to the ramus of the mandible when greater exposure of this region is required.

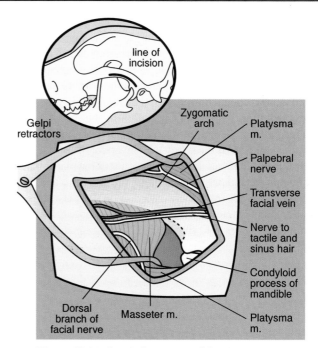

Figure 12.14: Surgical exposure of the temporomandibular joint (see text for details).

Wound Closure
The aponeurosis covering the superficial layer of the masseter muscle is sutured. The rest of the closure is routine.

CHAPTER THIRTEEN

The Spine

W. Malcolm McKee

INTRODUCTION

Traumatic spinal injuries are relatively common in small animal practice. They generally result from road traffic accidents. Other forms of trauma include falls from heights, gunshot injuries and collision with stationary objects. Of key importance is the potential for concomitant injury to the spinal cord or cauda equina. This may result in various degrees of neurological dysfunction.

Cases with acute spinal cord injury should be considered as emergencies. The use of the neuroprotective drug methylprednisolone sodium succinate may be beneficial in animals presented within a few hours of injury. Open reduction and internal fixation of caudal thoracic and lumbar fractures and luxations is often indicated in order to decompress the spinal cord and reduce pain; surgery can be challenging and thus referral to a specialist should be considered. However, other injuries, such as cervical fractures, can often be managed non-surgically with external splinting, or cage confinement. The prognosis in patients that retain pain sensation is generally favourable.

Vertebral fractures and luxations are the most common types of injury. Although this chapter deals primarily with vertebral fractures, many of the principles of assessment and management are applicable to vertebral luxations and fracture/luxations. It is therefore considered appropriate that the management of spinal luxations should also be considered here.

EVALUATION OF THE PATIENT

Physical examination

Dogs and cats with traumatic spinal injuries should be handled with care as they are often distressed and in significant pain. The use of a muzzle is advisable. Avoidance of further spinal cord injury is of paramount importance. A temporary splint may be applied, or alternatively the animal may be strapped to a rigid board or stretcher, especially when being transported.

A thorough clinical examination is essential since trauma that is sufficient to cause a vertebral fracture or luxation may result in significant concomitant injuries. Particular reference should be made to the cardiopulmonary system and the patient should be monitored for evidence of pneumothorax, cardiac dysrhythmia and shock. In one study of 67 dogs with lumbar fractures and luxations, 24 dogs had cardiopulmonary trauma, 13 had pelvic fractures and five had urogenital injuries (Turner, 1987). Concurrent pelvic trauma may be difficult to detect in non-ambulatory patients. Rectal examination and careful assessment of pelvic symmetry may be helpful. Failure to detect pelvic fractures and sacroiliac separations may result in an overestimation of the severity of spinal cord injury.

Neurological examination

A detailed neurological examination should enable the level of vertebral column injury to be identified (Wheeler and Sharp, 1994) and the severity of spinal cord damage to be graded (Table 13.1). Malalignment of the spine may be palpable, or indeed visible, and there may be external evidence of trauma. Certain postural reaction tests (for example, hemi-walking and wheelbarrowing) should be avoided due to the possibility of instability and further spinal cord trauma. The

Grade	Neurological dysfunction
1	Spinal pain (no neurological deficits)
2	Ambulatory paraparesis/tetraparesis
3a	Non-ambulatory paraparesis/tetraparesis
3b	Paraplegia/tetraplegia
4	Paraplegia/tetraplegia; urinary incontinence
5a	Paraplegia/tetraplegia; urinary incontinence; loss of superficial (digital pressure) pain perception
5b	Paraplegia/tetraplegia; urinary incontinence; loss of deep pain perception
5c	Grade 5b and evidence of ascending-descending myelomalacia

Table 13.1: Grading spinal cord injury. The combination of tetraplegia and loss of deep pain perception is rare; cervical spinal cord injuries of this severity tend to be fatal.

severity of cord injury is primarily determined on the presence or absence of motor function (purposeful limb movement) and conscious pain perception caudal to the lesion. The presence or absence of deep pain perception (as assessed with pump plier stimulation of periosteum, e.g. metatarsals, tibia, tail) is a key prognostic factor.

> **WARNING**
> **It is essential to remember that the reflex withdrawal of a limb is not evidence of pain perception. The patient must show a behavioural response, such as turning of the head.**

The possibility of injury at more than one area of the vertebral column should be considered and also the potential for concomitant peripheral nerve damage, e.g. brachial plexus avulsion.

> **WARNING**
> **Serial neurological examinations are important to detect changes in neurological status.**

DIFFERENTIAL DIAGNOSIS

Diagnosis is generally straightforward from the history and neurological findings; however, on occasions the owner may be unaware of trauma. Other causes of acute onset neurological dysfunction must be considered in these cases.

Common causes of acute onset neurological dysfunction:

- Degenerative intervertebral disc extrusion
- Ischaemic myelopathy (e.g. fibrocartilaginous embolism)
- Cervical spondylopathy (wobbler syndrome)
- Atlantoaxial subluxation (developmental).

Uncommon causes of acute onset neurological dysfunction:

- Pathological vertebral fracture
  - neoplasia (e.g. osteosarcoma)
  - osteoporosis (e.g. nutritional secondary hyperparathyroidism)
  - infection (e.g. osteomyelitis, discospondylitis)
- Spontaneous spinal haemorrhage (+/– coagulopathy)
- Non-osseous spinal neoplasia (possible haemorrhage)
- Acute inflammatory central nervous system disorders.

RADIOGRAPHIC EXAMINATION

Radiographs of the chest are mandatory in all spinal trauma cases to detect potentially life-threatening problems, such as pulmonary contusion and pneumothorax. Rupture of the diaphragm and rib fractures are less common. Radiographs of the pelvis should be obtained if there is any doubt regarding possible injury (Figure 13.1).

General anaesthesia is generally mandatory when performing spinal radiography in order to obtain diagnostic images. However, light sedation is preferable initially in trauma patients so that the protective role of the paraspinal and abdominal musculature is preserved. More detailed films may be obtained under general anaesthesia when the nature of the injury and degree of vertebral instability have been determined, and a potential therapeutic plan may be discussed with the owner.

Survey radiography
Lateral and ventrodorsal projections of the spine should be obtained (Brawner *et al.*, 1990). Horizontal beam techniques should be employed in cases with vertebral instability in order to avoid further cord injury. Oblique views may be useful for detecting articular facet fractures. The entire spine should be radiographed in animals where there is a clinical suspicion of more than one lesion. Multiple fractures or luxations are uncommon: 3 of 51 cases in one study (McKee, 1990) and 2 out of 112 cases in another series (Selcer *et al.*, 1991).

It is important to remember that radiographs do not necessarily represent the position of the vertebrae at the time of trauma. This is one explanation for the poor correlation that often exists between the degree of vertebral displacement and the severity of the neurological dysfunction (McKee, 1990). Conversely, many dogs with significant displacement of vertebral fractures and luxations, especially in the cervical and caudal lumbar spine, retain pain perception and variable motor function. This is primarily due to the large ratio of vertebral canal to spinal cord and cauda equina diameter respectively.

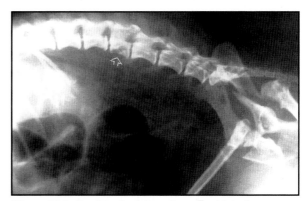

Figure 13.1: *Combined pelvic and vertebral injuries resulting from a road traffic accident in a terrier. Note the compression fracture L4 (shortened vertebral body) (arrowed), ilial fractures and coxofemoral luxations.*

Stress radiography

Stress view radiographs are seldom necessary; however, on occasions they can provide valuable information, especially about vertebral stability. For example, vertebral subluxations with minimal displacement and traumatic disc extrusions may be difficult to differentiate on survey radiographs, especially in the thoracic spine where there is superimposition of rib heads. Stressed views may aid differentiation and this information can be critical for management (e.g. stabilization versus decompressive surgery). Traction views are preferable to flexion–extension views, but the latter are often more informative. The risk of further spinal cord injury is significant and thus these techniques should be performed with great care and using fluoroscopy where possible.

Myelography

Myelography is not routinely performed in all spinal trauma cases. It is indicated in the following situations:

- Survey films are normal or inconclusive (e.g. spinal haemorrhage, spinal cord concussion, subtle intervertebral disc extrusion)
- Survey radiographic findings are inconsistent with neurological findings (e.g. thoracolumbar luxation in a patient with absent patellar reflexes)
- Decompressive surgery is contemplated (e.g. to remove disc material, bone fragments or blood clots)
- Exploratory surgery is considered in cases with no deep pain perception (grade 5b) (Figure 13.5) (transection of the spinal cord may on occasions be identified).

Myelography should be performed with care since flexion of the spine may exacerbate spinal cord compression where vertebral instability exists; consideration should be given to cisternal versus lumbar puncture.

Myelography enables space-occupying lesions to be localized:

- Extradural (e.g. fracture, luxation, disc material, bone fragments, haemorrhage)
- Intradural-extramedullary (e.g. haematoma)
- Intramedullary (e.g. haematoma, spinal cord oedema).

The vast majority of spinal trauma lesions are extradural.

MANAGEMENT OF THE SPINAL TRAUMA PATIENT

The appropriate management of traumatic spinal injuries necessitates an understanding of:

- Pathophysiology of acute spinal cord injury
- Spinal biomechanics
- Types of spinal injury
- Assessment of vertebral stability.

Pathophysiology of acute spinal cord injury

Vertebral trauma may result in varying degrees of spinal cord concussion and compression. The magnitude and relative contribution of these features is important with regard to the potential for reversible (or irreversible) cord injury and the most appropriate method of management.

Pathological changes within the spinal cord may be considered as primary and secondary. The primary changes are associated with the initial concussive injury and include axonal disruption, vascular damage, grey matter haemorrhage and necrosis, and oedema. Cord compression may result in nerve conduction blockage, interruption of neuronal axoplasmic flow, demyelination and additional vascular compromise. Secondary metabolic and vascular mechanisms may subsequently cause additional neuronal and supporting tissue damage. These processes may result in vicious cycles of autodestruction.

Metabolic mechanisms of secondary spinal cord injury

Spinal cord trauma and resultant ischaemia result in increased production of oxygen free-radicals which may overwhelm natural scavenging systems. Cell membrane phospholipids are particularly prone to free-radical attack, with resultant membrane disruption and the production of lipid peroxides – a process referred to as lipid peroxidation (Brown and Hall, 1992). Further free-radicals are released, thus perpetuating the process, which may ascend and descend the spinal cord (ascending–descending myelomalacia). Arachidonic acid production will contribute to the lipoxygenase and cyclooxygenase pathways to form leucotrienes and prostaglandins. Free-radicals may damage the microvasculature and contribute to ischaemia. Acute spinal cord injury may also result in elevated intraneuronal calcium levels and cell death.

Vascular mechanisms of secondary spinal cord injury

Following acute spinal cord injury, there is an immediate marked fall in grey matter blood flow. There is also a loss of autoregulation of spinal cord blood flow, and endogenous opioids may be released and cause

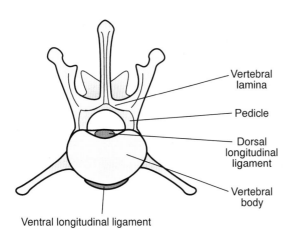

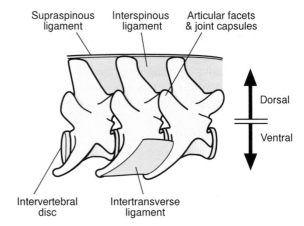

Figure 13.2: Dorsal and ventral compartment structures of the vertebral column.

systemic hypotension. These two factors may result in an additional fall in spinal blood flow (Tator and Fehlings, 1991). Vasoconstrictive substances (e.g. thromboxane A2, serotonin) and free-radical induced lipid peroxidation may also adversely affect the microcirculation.

For further discussion of the mechanisms of acute cord injury, refer to reviews in Brown and Hall (1992) and Coughlan (1993).

Spinal biomechanics

Structures that provide strength in the normal vertebral column may be divided into dorsal and ventral compartments (Figure 13.2).

Dorsal compartment structures:

- Articular facets/joint capsules
- Vertebral lamina/pedicles
- Supraspinous ligament
- Interspinous ligament.

Ventral compartment structures:

- Vertebral body
- Intervertebral disc
- Dorsal longitudinal ligament
- Ventral longitudinal ligament
- Intertransverse ligament.

The vertebral bodies and (to a lesser degree) the articular facets resist compressive forces, whereas the ligamentous structures and the facet joint capsules provide tensile strength. Rotational stability is derived from the intervertebral disc and articular facets (Shires *et al.*, 1991). The effect on strength and stability of removing various of these support structures, thus mimicking various traumatic injuries, has been studied (Smith and Walter, 1988; Shires *et al.*, 1991). A combination of discectomy and bilateral facetectomy markedly weakens and destabilizes the rotational integrity of the spine, compared with either of these procedures in isolation.

Traumatic vertebral column instability may be caused by bending (e.g. dorsoventral and lateral), rotational, compressive or shear forces. Naturally occurring injuries tend to result from a combination of these forces.

Types of spinal injury

Injuries tend to occur between stable and more mobile parts of the vertebral column, such as the thoracolumbar and lumbosacral junctions, although any vertebra(e) may be affected. The various types of injury are listed in Table 13.2.

Fractures of the vertebral body are the most common and may be oblique, transverse, physeal, compressive or comminuted (Figure 13.3). Concomitant luxation of the vertebral facets is not uncommon. Vertebral luxation and subluxation involve tearing of the annulus fibrosus of the intervertebral disc, with

Common	Uncommon
Vertebral fracture	Haemorrhage/ haematoma
Vertebral (sub)luxation	Spinal cord concussion
Vertebral fracture–luxation Intervertebral disc extrusion	

Table 13.2: Types of traumatic spinal injury.

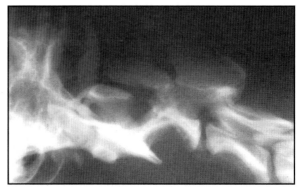

Figure 13.3: Fracture of the axis in a Staffordshire Bull Terrier.

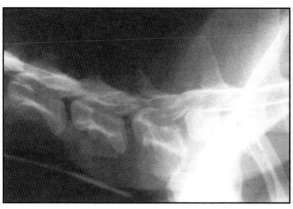

Figure 13.4: C6-C7 luxation in a Skye Terrier.

damage to the facet joints and supporting ligaments (Figure 13.4). This is in contrast to intervertebral disc extrusion where the nucleus pulposus is rapidly extruded through a previously healthy annulus. A specific syndrome caused by dorsolateral explosion of cervical discs has been described (Griffiths, 1970). Spinal cord concussion, and indeed necrosis, may occur in the absence of vertebral column injury (Griffiths, 1978).

Traumatic spinal injuries may be divided into three groups on the basis of which structures are affected:

- Dorsal compartment injury (e.g. articular facet fracture)
- Ventral compartment injury (e.g. intervertebral disc extrusion)
- Combined compartment injury (e.g. vertebral body fracture/articular facet luxation).

Combined compartment injuries are the most common. Dorsal compartment injury in combination with vertebral body fracture is the most serious, allowing bending, rotational and translational displacement, as well as vertebral collapse. In contrast, injury to the dorsal compartment structures in combination with vertebral luxation is less serious since a ventral buttress remains. Disc extrusions are inherently stable, because of an intact ventral buttress and articular facets. Isolated dorsal compartment injuries are uncommon and are often not of clinical significance, although cicatricial scar formation may on occasions result in delayed spinal cord compression (Waters *et al.*, 1994).

Assessment of vertebral stability

Assessing the degree of stability at the site of injury is an important factor in spinal trauma management. Although somewhat subjective, certain clinical and radiographic features may provide an index of suspicion.

Clinical features of spinal instability:

- Detection of crepitus when palpating the spine, or as the patient moves
- Progressive neurological dysfunction (14% of cases in one study; McKee, 1990)

The possibility of secondary mechanisms of spinal cord injury and ascending–descending myelomalacia should also be considered.

Radiographic features of spinal instability:

- Significant displacement of vertebrae
- Combined dorsal and ventral compartment injury
- Change in alignment on subsequent radiographs
- Change in alignment with stress radiography (take care!).

GENERAL PRINCIPLES OF MANAGEMENT

It is essential that vertebral fractures with concomitant neurological dysfunction are treated promptly. Medical management of acute spinal cord injury is aimed at reducing the secondary mechanism of lipid peroxidation and maintaining spinal cord blood flow. The need for surgery should be considered according to individual status. Decompression of the spinal cord and/or stabilization of the vertebral column are frequently indicated. These techniques are often technically demanding and thus referral of the patient to a surgical specialist should be considered. A temporary splint should be applied, or alternatively the patient may be strapped to a rigid board, in order to reduce the possibility of further spinal cord injury during transport.

Medical management of acute spinal cord injury

The judicious use of intravenous fluids is indicated to aid maintenance of spinal cord blood flow, especially when the patient is anaesthetized, since the injured spinal cord is unable to regulate its own perfusion. Monitoring of mean systemic arterial pressure is advisable in order to avoid hypertension and increased cord oedema.

The neuroprotective drug methylprednisolone sodium succinate may inhibit lipid peroxidation and thus reduce secondary spinal cord injury (Hall, 1992). The following protocol is currently recommended (Coughlan, 1993):

- Use within 8 hours of injury
- 30 mg/kg initially
- 15 mg/kg 4 and 8 hours after the initial dose
- Slowly administer intravenously over a few minutes to avoid hypotension and vomiting.

Other corticosteroids (for example, dexamethasone) and non-steroidal anti-inflammatory drugs should not be administered, as no beneficial effects have been demonstrated. In addition, they may result in potentially serious and even lethal gastrointestinal complications, especially when used in combination.

> **WARNING**
> **The use of non-steroidal anti-inflammatory drugs in combination with corticosteroids is contraindicated.**

Tirilazad mesylate, a 21-amino steroid which lacks glucocorticoid activity and thus side-effects, is a potent inhibitor of lipid peroxidation and may be the drug of choice in the future (Meintjes *et al.*, 1996).

Analgesia

Spinal fractures and luxations often cause significant pain. It is thus important that analgesics are administered as soon as possible following neurological assessment.

Narcotic analgesics – for example, morphine (cat 0.1 mg/kg IM, dog 0.25–1.0 mg/kg IM q 4 hours) and buprenorphine (0.006–0.01 mg/kg IV or IM q 6–8 hours) – are more effective than non-steroidal anti-inflammatory drugs. However, combination therapy is often the preferred therapy, provided corticosteroids have not been used. Pre-operative administration of opioids reduces the requirement for post-operative

analgesics, but they cause respiratory depression and thus should be avoided in patients with cranial, cervical and chest injuries.

Non-steroidal anti-inflammatory drugs should be used with care as spinal surgery patients have a tendency for intestinal ulceration. Carprofen (2 mg/kg IV or SC q 24 hours) does not appear to inhibit prostaglandin E levels in the gut (McKellar *et al.*, 1991) and thus is the author's drug of choice. It has not been determined whether carprofen and methylprednisolone sodium succinate may be used in combination safely in spinal injury patients.

Methocarbamol (20 mg/kg PO q 8 hours), a centrally acting skeletal muscle relaxant, and diazepam (2–15 mg PO q 8 hours) may reduce the pain associated with muscle spasm. They are often helpful in combination with analgesics.

SURGICAL VERSUS NON-SURGICAL MANAGEMENT

The choice of treatment for animals with spinal trauma is a subject of controversy. Many authors adopt a

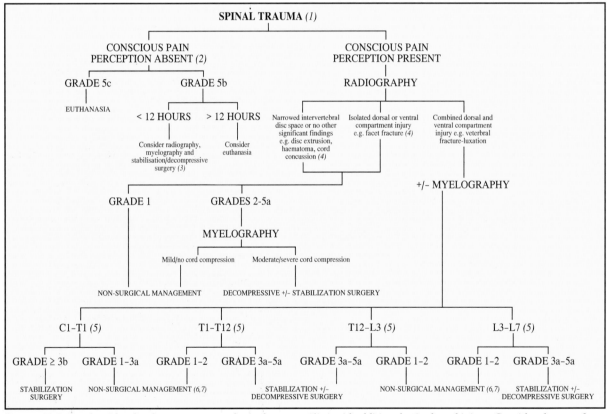

Figure 13.5: *An algorithm for the management of spinal trauma. (1) Avoid additional spinal cord injury. Consider the use of methylprednisolone sodium succinate. (2) Refer to text for grading of spinal cord injury. (3) These animals have a very guarded prognosis. Surgery should be reserved for cases where vertebral displacement on radiographs is not severe. Spinal cord integrity should be assessed prior to consideration of vertebral stabilization. Application of a pedicle of intact omentum to the injured cord may be useful to reduce oedema and aid neovascularization (Goldsmith et al., 1985). (4) Consider possibility of non-displaced vertebral subluxation and use of stress view radiography to demonstrate instability. Surgery is seldom indicated in the management of traumatic disc extrusions and cord concussion, since neither a mass effect nor instability is a significant feature (Griffiths, 1970; Griffiths, 1978). (5) Consider 'other factors' listed above. (6) Consider further investigation and surgery if there is progressive neurological dysfunction or where there is no neurological improvement within 10 days, also if relentless pain is a feature. (7) The use of an external splint should be strongly considered.*

conservative approach while others favour vertebral stabilization and/or decompressive procedures (Carberry *et al.*, 1989). A number of neurological and other factors should be considered (Figure 13.5).

Neurological factors:

- Nature of spinal lesion
- Evidence of vertebral instability
- Grade of spinal cord injury
- Degree of spinal pain
- Myelographic evidence of spinal cord compression
- Anatomical location of injury
- Interval between injury and presentation.

Other factors:

- Size of the patient
- Concurrent orthopaedic injuries
- Concurrent non-orthopaedic injuries
- Disposition and function of the patient
- Available equipment and expertise
- Financial restrictions and owner compliance.

Vertebral stabilization allows early pain-free ambulation and unimpeded physiotherapy, including hydrotherapy, compared with non-surgical management. This is particularly important in large dogs, where the standard of nursing care should not be underestimated. In addition, internal fixation generally reduces the hospitalization and recovery times and thus the incidence of decubital ulcers and other complications of prolonged recumbency. However, one of the key disadvantages of surgery is the potential for iatrogenic spinal cord injury.

NON-SURGICAL MANAGEMENT

External splinting and/or cage rest are advocated in the majority of non-surgical patients with vertebral fractures and luxations. Cage rest alone is not recommended for combined or ventral compartment injuries in the thoracolumbar region of the spine, where the cord occupies the majority of the vertebral canal, unless the fracture or luxation is inherently stable. In contrast, the majority of cervical fractures and luxations can successfully be managed non-surgically since the spinal cord occupies less of the vertebral canal. It is essential, however, that the patient is monitored for evidence of neurological deterioration.

External splinting

External splints are most applicable to thoracolumbar fractures and luxations in animals with an intact ventral buttress or intact facets. They are not recom-

mended for combined compartment injuries since their ability to counteract major disruptive forces is limited. Back splints may be used as the sole means of providing stability or as an adjunct to internal fixation techniques. The following advantages and disadvantages are worthy of consideration.

Advantages of back splints:

- Inexpensive
- Unlikely to cause harm during application
- Can move patient safely when applied
- Myelography not necessary
- Less expertise/equipment required.

Disadvantages of back splints:

- Require intact ventral or dorsal buttress
- Significant risk of decubital ulcers
- Hindrance of manual bladder expression
- Necessity for fluoroscopy when reducing fracture/luxation and applying splint
- Inability to manage concurrent traumatic chest and abdominal wounds
- Necessity to monitor/adjust splint on a weekly basis
- Inability to institute hydrotherapy.

> **WARNING**
> **Significant complications may result from pressure sores and urine scalding if a high level of nursing care is not practised with back splints.**

Back splints may be constructed from aluminium sheeting or thermoplastic materials. Mason metasplints are an alternative in small dogs and cats (Figure 13.6). They are secured to the patient with Velcro straps or sticking plaster. The former may allow the splint to be changed, or adjusted, more readily. Refer to Patterson and Smith (1992) for further details.

Cage confinement

Animals with cervical and (to a lesser degree) lumbosacral fractures and luxations may respond favourably to strict cage confinement (Denny, 1983; Turner, 1987) (Figure 13.7). Closed reduction of these injuries is extremely difficult and provision of adequate stability with external splints is practically impossible. The two key disadvantages of cage confinement are the possibility of prolonged pain and the risk of vertebral instability increasing spinal cord compression and neurological dysfunction.

SURGICAL MANAGEMENT

The surgical management of spinal fractures has three major aims:

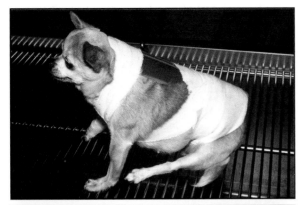

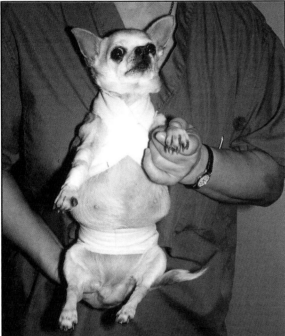

Figure 13.6: A Mason metasplint provided temporary vertebral stabilization in this Chihuahua with a mid thoracic fracture–luxation.

- Fracture/luxation reduction
- Fracture stabilization
- Spinal cord/cauda equina decompression.

Ideally the technique employed should be sufficiently rigid to encourage fracture or luxation healing and strong enough to withstand the intrinsic and extrinsic forces exerted on the vertebral column during this period.

Biomechanics of spinal fixation techniques
The potential post-operative bending (especially flexion), rotational, shear and compressive forces which may disrupt vertebral fracture or luxation fixation techniques must be carefully considered. The possibility of inadvertent injury when nursing paretic and ataxic patients is significant. Walter *et al.* (1986) estimated the bending moment at the thoracolumbar junction in a 45 kg dog, supported by the chest with the hindlimbs hanging free, to be greater than three times the strength provided by vertebral body plating.

The following biomechanical properties of fixation techniques should be considered when planning surgery and post-operative management:

- When subjected to bending, vertebral body plating is the most strong and most rigid single technique (strength = load at failure; rigidity = load-related deformation). However, the strength at failure is only one-third the strength of the normal intact spine (Walter *et al.*, 1986)
- When subjected to rotational deformation, vertebral body pins and bone cement provided the greatest stability and strength compared with other techniques (Waldron *et al.*, 1991)
- The resistance to bending of pins and screws depends on their area moment of inertia and for these implants a small increase in core diameter dramatically increases their bending strength (Muir *et al.*, 1995). When interconnected with bone cement, 3.2 mm vertebral body pins are significantly stronger than 3.5 mm vertebral body screws (Garcia *et al.*, 1994)
- Vertebral body four-pin fixation techniques appear to be strongest when the implants converge towards the fracture/luxation. In contrast, eight-pin techniques appear to be strongest when the implants angle away from the site of injury (Garcia *et al.*, 1994).

Choice of fixation technique
Many spinal fixation techniques have been described.

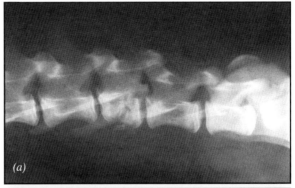

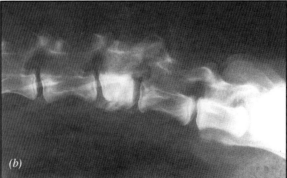

Figure 13.7: (a) Lumbar fracture–luxation in an immature Labrador Retriever with mild paraparesis which was managed by cage confinement. (b) Ten weeks post-trauma the fracture had healed and the neurological deficits had resolved.

Location of injury*	Technique of choice	Alternative technique(s)†
C1–C2	Articular facet screws *(Operative Technique 13.1)*	Ventral pins or screws and bone cement Ventral plating (Stead *et al.*, 1993) Dorsal cross pinning (Jeffery, 1996)
C2–T1	Vertebral body pins or screws and bone cement (+/– screwing of luxated articular facets in large dogs) *(Operative Technique 13.2)*	Transvertebral screw(s) +/– intervertebral spacer (McKee, 1990)
T1–T11	Dorsal spinous process plating# *(Operative Technique 13.3)*	Spinal stapling#
T11–T12	Vertebral body pins or screws and bone cement# *(Operative Techniques 13.4 & 13.5)*	Dorsal spinous process plating Spinal stapling
T12–L3	Vertebral body (+/– ilial) pins or screws and bone cement# *(Operative Technique 13.5)*	Dorsal spinous process plating and transilial pin(s)# Spinal stapling#
L7	Transilial pin(s)# *(Operative Technique 13.6)*	Vertebral body and ilial screws and bone cement# (Beaver *et al.*, 1996)
Sacrum and coccygeal vertebrae	See *Operative Technique 13.7* for discussion of management	

Table 13.3: *Fixation techniques at various levels of the vertebral column.*

* = Although rare, traumatic atlanto-occipital subluxation has been reported (DeCamp et al., 1991)
† = Refer to Shores et al. (1989) and Phillips and Blackmore (1991) for techniques employing external skeletal fixation
# = Luxated (non-fractured) facet joints may be screwed, preferably with washers, or stabilized with K-wires.

The choice of technique depends on characteristics of the vertebral injury and biomechanical factors.

Fracture/luxation characteristics:

- Location of the injury
- Potential for accurate reduction
- Necessity for laminectomy/hemilaminectomy.

Biomechanical factors:

- Inherent fracture/luxation stability
- Ability of technique to counteract disruptive forces
- Size and activity of the patient
- Concurrent orthopaedic injuries.

Techniques that utilize the vertebral bodies (ventral compartment) are generally preferred since the dorsal compartment structures are inherently weak and implant failure is common. However, the technique of choice is often dictated by the location of the fracture or luxation. The author's spinal fixation technique of choice applicable at various levels of the vertebral column and the advantages and disadvantages of the more common techniques are listed in Tables 13.3 and 13.4, respectively.

In view of the potential for iatrogenic spinal cord injury during reduction and stabilization of vertebral fractures and luxations, it is strongly recommended that frequent reference is made to a cadaver spine for anatomical details.

The value of decompressive surgery

Myelography plays an important role in selecting patients for decompressive surgery. The technique of choice is primarily governed by the method of spinal fixation, since this dictates the surgical approach to the affected area. Hemilaminectomy is generally preferable to dorsal laminectomy, because the former results in less instability (Smith and Walter, 1988; Shires *et al.*, 1991). Such procedures enable the removal of extruded disc material, bone fragments and blood clots from within the vertebral canal. Their importance following reduction and stabilization of a fracture or luxation is debatable. Following decompressive surgery it is essential that fractured or luxated vertebrae are stabilized by internal fixation.

GENERAL COMMENTS ON POST-OPERATIVE MANAGEMENT

Post-operative management is an extremely important

Technique	Advantages	Disadvantages
Vertebral body pins or screws and bone cement	Excellent flexibility in terms of number and position of pins/screws Accurate reduction of fracture/luxation not essential Strong since utilizes vertebral bodies Good resistance to rotational forces Avoids important spinal nerve roots Applicable at most levels of the vertebral column Not necessary to resect rib heads Minimal instrumentation/implants Can apply bilaterally	Poor resistance to bending forces Can only span one intervertebral space Potential soft tissue complications, e.g. oesophageal obstruction, hindrance of wound closure Possible thermal injury to spinal cord Potential for pin migration Risk of infection
Vertebral body plating	Strong since utilizes vertebral bodies Resists flexion–extension bending forces Readily combined with hemilaminectomy Can apply bilaterally in large dogs	Only applicable in caudal thoracic and cranial lumbar spine (T12–L3) Poor resistance to rotational forces Accurate reduction necessary Screw positioning determined by size and design of plate Potential pneumothorax if rib head resection necessary
Atlantoaxial facet screwing	Reduced risk of iatrogenic cord injury Permanent fixation/fusion	Utilizing compression rather than tension side of spine Technical difficulty in placing screws in small dogs Retraction injuries to soft tissues
Transilial pinning	Avoids important spinal nerve roots Minimal instrumentation required	Does not provide rigid fixation Pin migration if not bent or clamped
Dorsal spinous process plating	Avoids important spinal nerve roots Easy exposure and application of plates Minimal instrumentation required	Poor resistance to bending and rotational forces Immobilizes large segment of vertebral column Processes weak and prone to fracture Implant loosening Avascular necrosis of processes
Spinal stapling	Avoids important spinal nerve roots Effective when ventral buttress intact Minimal instrumentation required	Poor strength where ventral compartment injury Immobilizes large segment of vertebral column Articular and dorsal spinous processes prone to fracture Injures articular facets (osteoarthritis/ankylosis)

Table 13.4: Advantages and disadvantages of internal fixation techniques used in the spine.

aspect of care of neurosurgical patients. Analgesics (narcotics and non-steroidal anti-inflammatory drugs) should be used routinely. Antimicrobial agents, if considered necessary, should be used peri-operatively. Routine post-operative use should be avoided. If an infection develops (for example, urinary or wound), the choice of antimicrobial agent should be based on aerobic and anaerobic culture and sensitivity. Faeces should be monitored for evidence of melaena since gastrointestinal ulceration is not uncommon in spinal injury patients treated with anti-prostaglandin drugs, especially corticosteroids.

WARNING
Corticosteroids have no role in the post-operative management of spinal trauma patients.

A high standard of nursing care is essential in order to prevent urinary tract infections, faecal and urine scalding, decubital ulcers and pneumonia. The bladders of incontinent animals must be emptied at least three times daily. Pharmacological drugs may be necessary – for example, bethanechol and phenoxybenzamine. Patients must be kept clean and dry on non-retentive, well padded bedding. Recumbent animals should be turned regularly. Both active (whirlpool bath or bathtub) and passive physiotherapy (flexion and extension exercises) are invaluable. Medium and large dogs should be assisted with belly band or other support since internal fixation techniques have a limited ability to resist bending and rotational forces.

PROGNOSIS

The prognosis depends on a number of factors, the most important of which is the severity of the neurological dysfunction. Cases that retain some degree of voluntary motor function generally have a good prognosis. Patients with no voluntary motor function and with urinary incontinence have a guarded prognosis and cases with loss of conscious pain perception rarely recover (McKee, 1990; Selcer *et al.*, 1991). Serial neurological examinations are an important factor in assessing the prognosis more accurately. A functional recovery is only likely if there is at least one grade of improvement within 2-4 weeks of the initial injury.

REFERENCES

Anderson A and Coughlan AR (1997) Sacral fractures in dogs and cats: a classification scheme and review of 51 cases. *Journal of Small Animal Practice* **38**, 404-409

Beaver DP, MacPherson GC, Muir P and Johnson K A (1996) Methylmethacrylate and bone screw repair of seventh lumbar vertebral fracture-luxations in dogs. *Journal of Small Animal Practice* **37**, 381-386

Blass CE and Seim HB (1984) Spinal fixation in dogs using Steinmann pins and methylmethacrylate. *Veterinary Surgery* **13**, 203-210

Brawner WR, Braund KG and Shores A (1990) Radiographic evaluation of dogs and cats with acute spinal cord trauma. *Veterinary Medicine* **85**, 703-723

Brown SA and Hall ED (1992) Role for oxygen-derived free radicals in the pathogenesis of shock and trauma, with focus on central nervous system injuries. *Journal of the American Veterinary Medical Association* **200**, 1849-1859

Carberry CA, Flanders JA, Dietze AE, Gilmore DR and Trotter EJ (1989) Nonsurgical management of thoracic and lumbar spinal fractures and fracture/luxations in the dog and cat: a review of 17 cases. *Journal of the American Animal Hospital Association* **25**, 43-54

Clary EM and Roe SC (1996) *In vitro* biomechanical and histological assessment of pilot hole diameter for positive-profile external skeletal fixation pins in canine tibiae. *Veterinary Surgery* **25**, 453-462

Coughlan AR (1993) Secondary injury mechanisms in acute spinal cord trauma. *Journal of Small Animal Practice* **34**, 117-122

DeCamp CE, Schirmer RG and Stickle RL (1991) Traumatic atlanto-occipital subluxation in a dog. *Journal of the American Animal Hospital Association* **27**, 415-418

Denny HR (1983) Fractures of the cervical vertebrae in the dog. *Veterinary Annual* **23**, 236-240

Denny HR, Gibbs C and Waterman A (1988) Atlantoaxial subluxation in the dog; a review of 30 cases and an evaluation of treatment by lag screw fixation. *Journal of Small Animal Practice* **29**, 37-47

Garcia J, Milthorpe BK, Russell D and Johnson KA (1994) Biomechanical study of canine spinal fracture fixation using pins or bone screws with polymethylmethacrylate. *Veterinary Surgery* **23**, 322-329

Goldsmith HS, Steward E and Duckett S (1985) Early application of pedicled omentum to the acutely traumatised spinal cord. *Paraplegia* **23**, 100-112

Griffiths IR (1970) A syndrome produced by dorsolateral 'explosions' of the cervical intervertebral discs. *Veterinary Record* **87**, 737-741

Griffiths IR (1978) Spinal cord injuries: a pathological study of naturally occurring lesions in the dog and cat. *Journal of Comparative Pathology* **88**, 303-315

Hall ED (1992) The neuroprotective pharmacology of methylprednisolone. *Journal of Neurosurgery* **76**, 13-22

Jeffery ND (1996) Dorsal cross pinning of the atlantoaxial joint: New surgical technique for atlantoaxial subluxation. *Journal of Small Animal Practice* **37**, 26-29

Kuntz CA, Waldron D, Martin RA, Shires PK, Moon M and Shell L (1995) Sacral fractures in dogs: a review of 32 cases. *Journal of the American Animal Hospital Association* **31**, 142-150

Lewis DD, Stampley A, Bellah JR, Donner GS and Ellison GW (1989) Repair of sixth lumbar vertebral fracture-luxations using transilial pins and plastic spinous-process plates in six dogs. *Journal of the American Veterinary Medical Association* **194**, 538-542

Lumb WV and Brasmer TH (1970) Improved spinal plates and hypothermia as adjuncts to spinal surgery. *Journal of the American Veterinary Medical Association* **157**, 338-342

McAnulty JF, Lenehan TM and Maletz LM (1986) Modified segmental spinal instrumentation in repair of spinal fractures and luxations in dogs. *Veterinary Surgery* **15**, 143-149

McKee WM (1990) Spinal trauma in dogs and cats: a review of 51 cases. *Veterinary Record* **126**, 285-289

McKellar QA, Lees P, Ludwig B and Tiberghien MP (1991) Pharmacokinetics, tolerance and serum thromboxane inhibition of carprofen. *Journal of Small Animal Practice* **31**, 443-448

Meintjes E, Hosgood G and Daniloff J (1996) Pharmaceutic treatment of acute spinal cord trauma. *Compendium of Continuing Education for the Practising Veterinarian* **18**, 625-635

Muir P, Johnson KA and Markel MD (1995) Area moment of inertia for comparison of implant cross-sectional geometry and bending stiffness. *Veterinary and Comparative Orthopaedics and Traumatology* **8**, 146-152

Patterson RH and Smith GK (1992) Backsplinting for treatment of thoracic and lumbar fracture/luxation in the dog: principles of application and case series. *Veterinary and Comparative Orthopaedics and Traumatology* **5**, 179-187

Phillips L and Blackmore J (1991) Kirschner-Ehmer device alone to stabilise caudal lumbar fractures in small dogs. *Veterinary and Comparative Orthopaedics and Traumatology* **4**, 112-115

Selcer RR, Bubb WJ and Walker TL (1991) Management of vertebral column fractures in dogs and cats; 211 cases (1977-1985). *Journal of the American Veterinary Medical Association* **198**, 1965-1968

Shires PK, Waldron DR, Hedlund CS, Blass CE and Massoudi L (1991) A biomechanical study of rotational instability in unaltered and surgically altered canine thoracolumbar vertebral motion units. *Progress in Veterinary Neurology* **2**, 6-14

Shores A, Nichols C, Rochat M, Fox SM and Burt GJ (1989) Combined Kirschner-Ehmer device and dorsal spinal plate fixation technique for caudal lumbar vertebral fractures in dogs. *Journal of the American Veterinary Medical Association* **195**, 335-339

Shores A, Haut R and Bonner JA (1991) An *in-vitro* study of plastic spinal plates and Luque segmental fixation of the canine thoracic spine. *Progress in Veterinary Neurology* **2**, 279-285

Slocum B and Rudy RL (1975) Fractures of the seventh lumbar vertebra in the dog. *Journal of the American Animal Hospital Association* **11**, 167-174

Smeak DD and Olmstead ML (1985) Fracture/luxations of the sacrococcygeal area in the cat. A retrospective study of 51 cases. *Veterinary Surgery* **14**, 319-324

Smith GK and Walter MC (1988) Spinal decompressive procedures and dorsal compartment injuries: comparative biomechanical study in canine cadavers. *American Journal of Veterinary Research* **49**, 266-273

Sorjonen DC and Shires PK (1981) Atlantoaxial instability: A ventral surgical technique for decompression, fixation and fusion. *Veterinary Surgery* **10**, 22-29

Stead AC, Anderson AA and Coughlan A (1993) Bone plating to stabilise atlantoaxial subluxation in four dogs. *Journal of Small Animal Practice* **34**, 462-465

Stone EA, Betts CW and Chambers JN (1979) Cervical fractures in the dog: a literature and case review. *Journal of the American Animal Hospital Association* **15**, 463-471

Swaim SF (1971) Vertebral body plating for spinal immobilisation. *Journal of the American Veterinary Medical Association* **158**, 1683-1695

Tator CH and Fehlings MG (1991) Review of the secondary injury theory of acute spinal cord trauma with emphasis on vascular mechanisms. *Journal of Neurosurgery* **75**, 15-26

Turner WD (1987) Fractures and fracture-luxations of the lumbar spine: a retrospective study in the dog. *Journal of the American Animal Hospital Association* **23**, 459-464

Ullman SL and Boudrieau RJ (1993) Internal skeletal fixation using a Kirschner apparatus for stabilisation of fracture/luxations of the lumbosacral joint in six dogs. *Veterinary Surgery* **22**, 11-17

Waldron DR, Shires PK, McCain W, Hedlund C. and Blass CE (1991) The rotational stabilising effect of spinal fixation techniques in an unstable vertebral model. *Progress in Veterinary Neurology* **2**, 105-110

Walter MC, Smith GK and Newton CD (1986) Canine lumbar spinal internal fixation techniques: a comparative biomechanical study. *Veterinary Surgery* **15**, 191-198

Waters DJ, Wallace LJ and Roy RG (1994) Myelopathy in a dog secondary to scar tissue (cicatrix) formation: a complication of vertebral articular facet fracture. *Progress in Veterinary Neurology* **5**, 105-108

Wheeler SJ and Sharp NJH (1994) Patient examination. In: *Small Animal Spinal Disorders: Diagnosis and Surgery*. Mosby-Wolfe, London

OPERATIVE TECHNIQUE 13.1
Atlantoaxial (C1–C2) (sub)luxation

Background
Atlantoaxial (sub)luxation is most commonly a developmental disorder; however, trauma (for example, collision with a patio door) may occasionally disrupt a previously normal articulation (Figure 13.8). Fixation of the articular facets using screws via a ventral approach is the treatment of choice (Sorjonen and Shires, 1981).

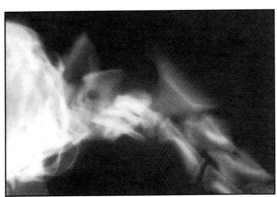

Figure 13.8: Radiograph showing atlantoaxial subluxation.

Positioning
Dorsal recumbency with the cranial cervical spine extended over a sand bag; initially gentle traction (Figure 13.9a).

PRACTICAL TIP
Symmetrical positioning of patient is critical.

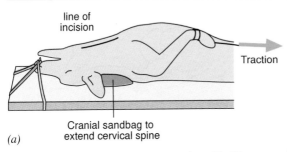

(a)

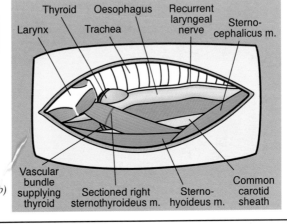

(b)

Figure 13.9: Ventral surgical approach to C1–C2.

Assistant
Useful.

Tray Extras
Gosset and Gelpi retractors; periosteal elevator; small curette or pneumatic burr; drill; cortical screws (1.5, 2.0, 2.7 or 3.5 mm) and corresponding instrumentation for insertion; drill bit (or gouge and mallet) for making bone graft hole; dental tartar scraper.

Surgical Approach
A midline incision is made from cranial to the larynx to the manubrium. The sternohyoideus muscles are separated and the right sternothyroideus muscle is sectioned near the thyroid cartilage (Figure 13.9b). The trachea, oesophagus and left common carotid sheath are retracted to the left.

PRACTICAL TIP
An oesophageal stethoscope aids identification of oesophagus.

The prominent ventral process of the atlas is palpated and the tendons of the longus colli muscles are dissected from this structure and retracted laterally. The atlantoaxial synovial joints are opened and the articular cartilage is removed with a small burr or curette.

→

OPERATIVE TECHNIQUE 13.1 (CONTINUED)
Atlantoaxial (C1–C2) (sub)luxation

Reduction and Fixation

Release aforementioned traction; maintain extension of spine. Drill one set of facets and leave drill bit *in situ* as the other set are drilled, measured, tapped and screwed. Screws are positioned at an angle of 30° away from the midline and 20° dorsally (Figure 13.10). Lag screws are preferable to positional.

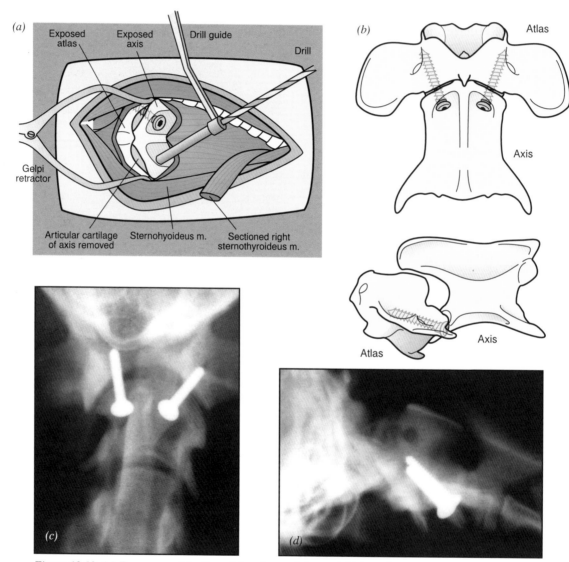

Figure 13.10: *(a) Exposure and fixation of the atlantoaxial synovial joints. (b) Schematic views of the atlas and axis to show the ideal positions of atlantoaxial fixation screws. (c) A ventral post-operative radiograph showing screw position in the case of atlantoaxial subluxation shown in Figure 13.8. (d) Lateral radiograph of the case shown in (c).*

→

OPERATIVE TECHNIQUE 13.1 (CONTINUED)

Atlantoaxial (C1–C2) (sub)luxation

PRACTICAL TIP
Prevent dorsal displacement of axis when drilling by levering it ventrally with small dental tartar scraper.

In most small dogs 2.0 mm screws are appropriate; 1.5 mm screws may be used in miniature dogs (positional rather than lag) and 3.5 mm screws in large breeds. Cancellous bone is obtained from the proximal aspect of a humerus and packed in and around the joint spaces to promote fusion.

WARNING
It is technically difficult to position the implants sufficiently ventral in the atlas and this may result in fixation failure. Avoid injury to recurrent laryngeal nerves and prolonged retraction of trachea.

Closure
Routine, including repair of right sternothyroideus muscle.

Post-operative Care
Light support dressing to extend head/neck for 4 weeks. Strict rest for 6 weeks. Harness preferable to collar.

WARNING
Dorsal wiring techniques are to be avoided because of the significant incidence of iatrogenic cord injury (Denny *et al.*, 1988) and fixation failure.

OPERATIVE TECHNIQUE 13.2
Cervical fractures and luxations (C2–T1)

Background

The axis is the most frequently fractured cervical vertebra, due to concentration of force in this area which is a transition point between the atlanto-occipital unit and the caudal cervical spine (Stone *et al.*, 1979). When deemed necessary, fractures and luxations of the cervical spine are most appropriately stabilized with vertebral body pins or screws and bone cement (Blass and Seim, 1984).

Positioning

Dorsal recumbency, with the affected region of the spine supported with sand bags.

(a)
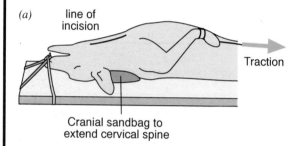

> **PRACTICAL TIP**
> Symmetrical positioning of patient is critical and this is aided with gentle cervical traction (Figure 13.11a). Traction also aids reduction of fracture/luxation.

(b)
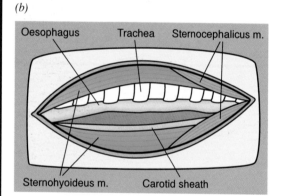

(c)
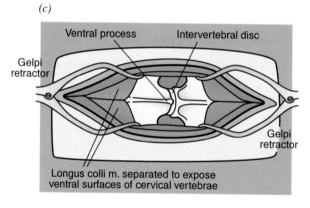

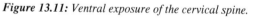

Figure 13.11: Ventral exposure of the cervical spine.

Assistant

Yes.

Tray Extras

Gosset, Hohmann and Gelpi retractors; periosteal elevator; end-threaded positive profile pins (2, 3, 4 mm); variable speed battery drill (+/- shroud); drill bits; bone cement; pin cutters.

Surgical Approach

A midline incision is made from the larynx to the manubrium. The sternocephalicus and sternohyoideus muscles are separated and branches of the caudal thyroid vein are cauterized (Figure 13.11b). The trachea, oesophagus and left common carotid sheath are retracted to the left. The prominent ventrally directed transverse processes of C6 are a useful landmark. The longus colli muscles are elevated from the affected vertebrae and retracted laterally (Figure 13.11c).

> **PRACTICAL TIP**
> An oesophageal stethoscope aids identification of oesophagus.

OPERATIVE TECHNIQUE 13.2 (CONTINUED)
Cervical fractures and luxations (C2–T2)

Reduction and Fixation

The caudal segment is generally displaced dorsally. Reduction is achieved by leverage with a Hohmann retractor and gentle traction/counter-traction. Reduction can be maintained using carefully positioned vertebral body/transvertebral K-wire(s).

Ideally, positive profile threaded pins are then placed into the vertebral bodies, directed away from the vertebral canal (Figure 13.12). It is important to ensure that the transcortices are penetrated. A minimum of two pins should be placed in pre-drilled holes both cranial and caudal to the fracture or luxation. Polymethylmethacrylate bone cement is placed around the pins and lavaged with saline, preferably cooled, to dissipate heat during hardening. Aseptic technique is of utmost importance.

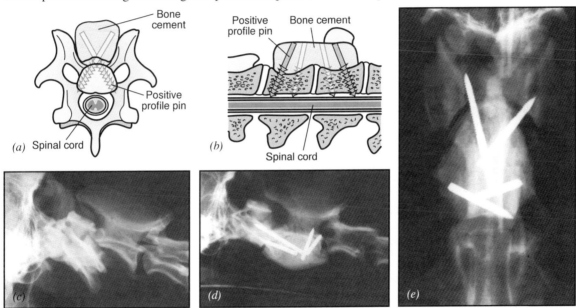

Figure 13.12: (a), (b) Schematic views of the cervical vertebrae to show the ideal positioning of vertebral body pins and bone cement. (c) C2 fracture in a dog. (d), (e) Lateral and ventrodorsal post-operative radiographs of the case shown in (c). Fixation was achieved using ventral pins and bone cement.

> **WARNING**
> **Excessive cement is to be avoided in order to reduce the possibility of tracheal or oesophageal injury.**

> **WARNING**
> **Avoid penetrating the vertebral canal!**

> **WARNING**
> **Monitor closely for potential bradycardia.**

Closure

Routine, including apposition of longus colli muscles where possible. Penrose or closed suction drain should be employed for a short period if haemostasis is suboptimal.

Post-operative Care

Strict rest for 6 weeks. Harness preferable to collar. Dressing generally not helpful.

Alternative Technique

Application of a bone plate is difficult because of the irregular shape of the vertebral bodies.

→

OPERATIVE TECHNIQUE 13.2 (CONTINUED)
Cervical fractures and luxations (C2–T1)

Additional Comments

When using bone cement techniques the surgeon has a choice of vertebral body pins or screws. The advantages of screws compared with non-threaded pins are that they have greater pull-out resistance, are less likely to migrate, are interchangeable if length is inappropriate, and do not need to be bent or cut. However, screws are debatably more difficult to insert than pins. The author's preference is to use positive profile threaded pins (negative profile have a tendency to break), which combines the advantages of screws and non-threaded pins. Although accurate insertion is aided by their self-tapping nature, it is beneficial to pre-drill a pilot hole whose diameter approximates to but does not exceed the inner diameter of the pin. This improves pin stability and reduces microstructural damage that may lead to excessive bone resorption and premature pin loosening (Clary and Roe, 1996). Pre-drilling also enables the depth of the vertebral body to be measured accurately prior to pin insertion.

OPERATIVE TECHNIQUE 13.3
Thoracic vertebral fractures and luxations (T1–T11)

Background
Injuries in this area of the spine are fortunately uncommon. They tend to be inherently stable because of the epaxial musculature. Utilization of the vertebral bodies is extremely difficult because of their triangular cross-section and the relative lack of bone stock in the centre of the vertebrae. Dorsal spinous processes plating is the most applicable technique (Lumb and Brasmer, 1970; Shores *et al.*1991).

Positioning
Ventral recumbency (symmetrical).

Assistant
Yes.

Tray Extras
Gelpi and Hohmann retractors; periosteal elevator; plastic or metal spinal plates; bolts and nuts; spanners; drill and drill bit for metal plates.

Surgical Approach
Dorsal midline with elevation and retraction of the epaxial muscles from the dorsal spinous processes and dorsal laminae (Figure 13.13).

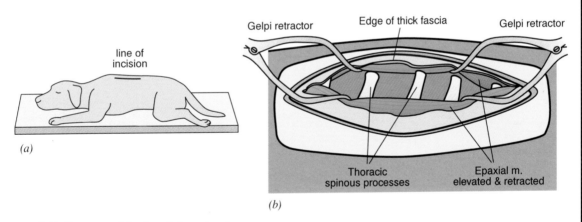

Figure 13.13: Exposure of the dorsal thoracic spine.

Reduction and Fixation
Towel clamps or artery forceps attached to the dorsal spinous processes cranial and caudal to the fracture/luxation may be distracted with a Gelpi retractor. Alternatively, an assistant may apply traction and counter-traction. The tip of a small Hohmann retractor can be placed under the lamina of the ventrally displaced vertebra and levered on the lamina of the dorsal vertebra to aid final reduction. Reduction is maintained using traction and counter-traction by assistant. In addition, non-fractured facet joints may be stabilized with K-wires.

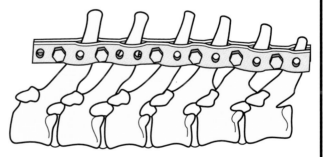

Figure 13.14: Schematic view of the thoracic spine to show the ideal position of plastic spinal plates.

→

OPERATIVE TECHNIQUE 13.3 (CONTINUED)
Thoracic vertebral fractures and luxations (T1–T11)

Fixation is achieved using paired metal or plastic plates secured to the dorsal spinous processes by bolts placed either through (metal) or between (plastic) the processes (Figure 13.14).

PRACTICAL TIP
Position plates as ventral as possible on processes.

WARNING
The processes are inherently weak and failures due to implant slippage, fracture or avascular necrosis are common complications.

Closure
Routine, including the midline tendinous raphe.

Post-operative Care
Strict confinement for 6 weeks. Consider use of external splint in large dogs with mid to caudal thoracic injuries since the fixation technique is inherently weak. Belly band support.

OPERATIVE TECHNIQUE 13.4
Thoracolumbar fractures and luxations (T12–L3)

Background
Vertebral body plates (Swaim, 1971) can be readily applied in this region of the spine and bilateral plating may be performed in large dogs.

Positioning
Lateral recumbency – preferably right lateral for right-handed surgeon. Apply gentle traction by securing fore limbs cranially and hind limbs caudally (Figure 13.15a).

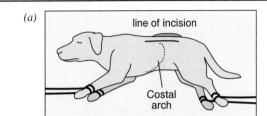

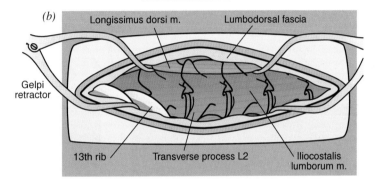

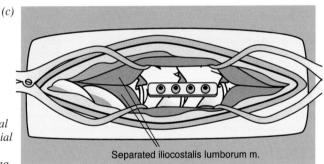

Figure 13.15: Lateral exposure of the cranial lumbar spine for vertebral body plating.

Assistant
Useful.

Tray Extras
Gelpi and Hohmann retractors; periosteal elevator; drill; bone plates/cortical screws and corresponding instrumentation for insertion.

Surgical Approach
Lateral approach with elevation and retraction of the epaxial muscle mass. In the thoracic region, resection (or disarticulation) of rib heads is required and removal of the short transverse processes (Figure 13.15 b, c).

Reduction and Fixation
Reduction is achieved by traction/counter-traction and leverage with a Hohmann retractor.

Intact articular facet processes may be used to assess accuracy of reduction.

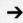

OPERATIVE TECHNIQUE 13.4 (CONTINUED)
Thoracolumbar fractures and luxations (T12–L3)

Articular facets may be luxated and require careful reduction. There is inherent stability if facet processes are intact (may secure with K-wire). Increasing traction/counter-traction on limbs may aid maintenance of vertebral body fractures in cases with no ventral buttress. The bone plate is positioned on transverse process ostectomy sites in the thoracic region and at the junction of the transverse processes and vertebral bodies in the lumbar region. Screws should engage a minimum of four cortices cranial and caudal to the fracture or luxation. It is essential that they are directed ventral to the vertebral canal (Figure 13.16).

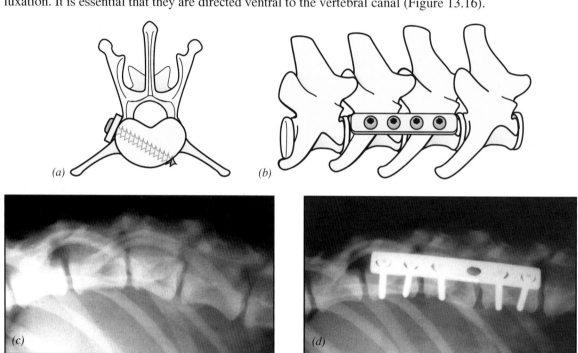

Figure 13.16: (a), (b) Schematic views of the lumbar spine to show the ideal position of a vertebral body plate and screws. (c) Lateral radiograph of a German Shepherd Dog with a cranial lumbar fracture–luxation. (d) Lateral post-operative radiograph of the case shown in (c). Fixation was achieved using vertebral body plating.

PRACTICAL TIP
Ascertain appropriate plate size from pre-operative radiographs; consider a custom-made plate if standard plates inappropriate. In order to avoid inappropriate screw placement, identify intervertebral disc spaces with a hypodermic needle. Converge screws in vertebral body to increase pull-out resistance.

WARNING
Inappropriate plate positioning or angle of drilling may result in catastrophic iatrogenic spinal cord injury, or implant loosening.

Closure
Routine, including repair of the lumbodorsal fascia.

Post-operative Care
Strict rest for 6 weeks. Belly band support.

OPERATIVE TECHNIQUE 13.5
Caudal thoracic fractures and luxations (T11–T12)
Lumbar fractures and luxations (L3–L7)

Background
Vertebral body pins, or screws, and bone cement are less likely to interfere with important hind limb spinal nerves compared with plates in the L3–L7 region of the spine.

Positioning
Ventral recumbency with hind limbs positioned alongside the abdomen (Figure 13.17a).

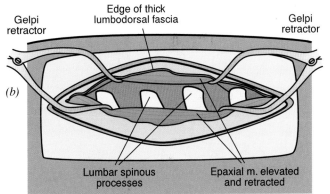

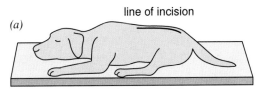

(a)   line of incision

(b)

Gelpi retractor · Edge of thick lumbodorsal fascia · Gelpi retractor · Lumbar spinous processes · Epaxial m. elevated and retracted

Figure 13.17: *Dorsal exposure of the lumbar spine.*

Assistant
Yes.

Tray Extras
Gelpi and Hohmann retractors; periosteal elevator; end threaded positive profile pins (2, 3, 4 mm); drill bits; variable speed battery drill (+/– shroud) (e.g. Makita); bone cement; pin cutters.

Surgical Approach
The affected vertebrae are exposed via a dorsal midline approach with elevation and retraction of the epaxial musculature (Figure 13.17b).

Reduction and Fixation
Towel clamps or artery forceps attached to the dorsal spinous processes cranial and caudal to the fracture/ luxation may be distracted with a Gelpi retractor. Alternatively, an assistant may apply traction and counter-traction. The tip of a small Hohmann retractor can be placed under the lamina of the ventrally displaced (usually caudal) vertebra and levered on the lamina of the dorsal (usually cranial) vertebra to aid final reduction. Reduction may often be maintained with screws or K-wires, placed across intact articular processes. Manual reduction by the assistant surgeon is occasionally necessary. Threaded pins (pre-drilled) or screws are placed bilaterally in the vertebral bodies where the transverse processes originate. A minimum of two pins or screws, and preferably three, should be placed both cranial and caudal to the fracture or luxation. Bone cement is placed around the implants and lavaged with saline to dissipate heat during hardening (Figure 13.18 a–e).

> ### PRACTICAL TIP
> **Placement of pins/screws in L7 vertebral body leaving sufficient implant available for incorporation in cement is technically difficult because of the proximity of the ilial wings. Placing screws in the ilial wings is an alternative (Figure 13.18).**

> ### WARNING
> **Protect vital hindlimb spinal nerves. Excessive cement may make wound closure difficult. Ensure pins do not unduly penetrate the abdominal (or thoracic) cavity, since they may result in vascular injury (immediate or delayed) i.e. measure, rather than eye-ball, their depth.**

→

OPERATIVE TECHNIQUE 13.5 (CONTINUED)
Caudal thoracic fractures and luxations (T11–T12)
Lumbar fractures and luxations (L3–L7)

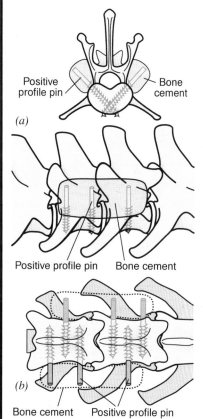

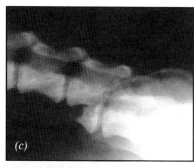

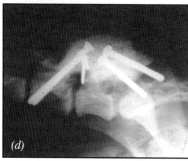

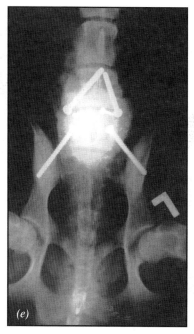

Figure 13.18: (a), (b) Schematic views of the lumbar spine to show the ideal position of a vertebral body, pins and bone cement. (c) A sixth lumbar vertebral fracture in a dog. (d), (e) Lateral and ventrodorsdal post-operative radiographs of the case shown in (c). The fracture was stabilized using screws and bone cement, with the caudal screws placed through the wings of the ilia. The luxated articular facets were screwed together after reduction.

Closure
Routine; including, where possible, repair of the lumbodorsal fascia.

Post-operative Care
Strict rest for 6 weeks. Belly band support.

Alternative Techniques
Dorsal spinous process plating in combination with transilial pins (Figure 13.19) (Lewis *et al.*, 1989) and spinal stapling (McAnulty *et al.*, 1986) are alternative methods of fixation. In the latter technique, several pins are wired to the articular and/or dorsal spinous processes. Additional fixation may be obtained in the lumbosacral region by bending the pins and anchoring them in the wings of the ilia (Figure 13.20).

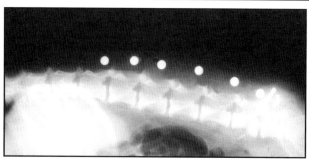

Figure 13.19: Dorsal spinous process plating in combination with transilial pins for the management of a sixth lumbar vertebral fracture.

Courtesy of Dr DD Lewis.

→

OPERATIVE TECHNIQUE 13.5 (CONTINUED)

Caudal thoracic fractures and luxations (T11–T12)
Lumbar fractures and luxations (L3–L7)

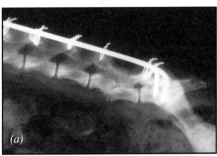

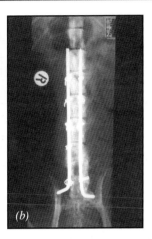

Figure 13.20: Lateral and ventrodorsal post-operative radiographs illustrating the use of pins wired to the articular facets and anchored through the wings of the ilia to manage a caudal lumbar fracture in a dog.

Additional Comments

When using bone cement techniques the surgeon has a choice of vertebral body pins or screws. The advantages of screws compared with non-threaded pins are that they have greater pull-out resistance, are less likely to migrate, are interchangeable if length is inappropriate, and do not need to be bent or cut. However, screws are debatably more difficult to insert than pins. The author's preference is to use positive profile threaded pins (negative profile have a tendency to break), which combine the advantages of screws and non-threaded pins. Although accurate insertion is aided by their self-tapping nature it is beneficial to pre-drill a pilot hole whose diameter approximates to but does not exceed the inner diameter of the pin. This improves pin stability and reduces microstructural damage that may lead to excessive bone resorption and premature pin loosening (Clary and Roe 1996). Pre-drilling also enables the depth of the vertebral body to be measured accurately prior to pin insertion.

OPERATIVE TECHNIQUE 13.6
Seventh lumbar vertebra fractures (L7)

Background
Injury to L7 typically involves luxation of the articular facets and an oblique fracture of the vertebral body with cranioventral displacement of the caudal segment. Transilial pin(s) may be employed to maintain reduction (Slocum and Rudy, 1975; Ullman and Boudrieau, 1993). Since this technique does not provide rigid fixation, shortening of the vertebral body during healing is to be expected.

Positioning
Ventral recumbency with hindlimbs positioned alongside the abdomen (Figure 13.21a).

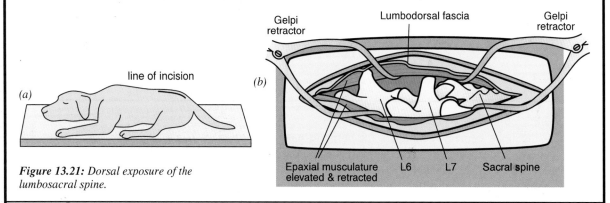

Figure 13.21: Dorsal exposure of the lumbosacral spine.

Assistant
Useful.

Tray Extras
Gelpi and Hohmann retractors; periosteal elevator; drill; cortical screws (generally 2.0 or 2.7 mm) and corresponding instrumentation for insertion; spiked washers; external skeletal fixation clamps and connecting bars (generally small or medium); Jacob's chuck; pin cutters.

Surgical Approach
The lumbosacral spine is exposed via a dorsal midline approach with elevation and retraction of the epaxial musculature. Articular facets L7–S1 are identified. The middle gluteal musculature is elevated from the lateral aspect of the wings of the ilia (Figure 13.21b).

Reduction and Fixation
Towel clamps attached to the dorsal spinous processes of L7 and the sacrum may be distracted with a Gelpi retractor. Alternatively, an assistant may apply traction and counter-traction. The tip of a small Hohmann retractor can be placed under the lamina of L7 vertebra and levered on the dorsal lamina of L6 to aid final reduction. Reduction may be maintained with screws (+/– washers) placed across luxated articular facet processes (Figure 13.22). One or two pins are placed through one ilial wing, projected just dorsal to the caudal lamina of L7 (or facet screws/washers), and through the contralateral ilial wing. External skeletal fixation clamps are attached to the ends of the pins to prevent migration (Figure 13.22).

> **PRACTICAL TIP**
> Drilling one set of articular facet processes and leaving the drill bit *in situ* as the other set are drilled, measured, tapped and screwed aids the unassisted surgeon.

→

OPERATIVE TECHNIQUE 13.6 (CONTINUED)

Seventh lumbar vertebra fractures (L7)

WARNING
Bending the ends of transilial pins may result in bowing with subsequent rotation and loss of fracture reduction. Prevention of pin migration with clamps is preferable.

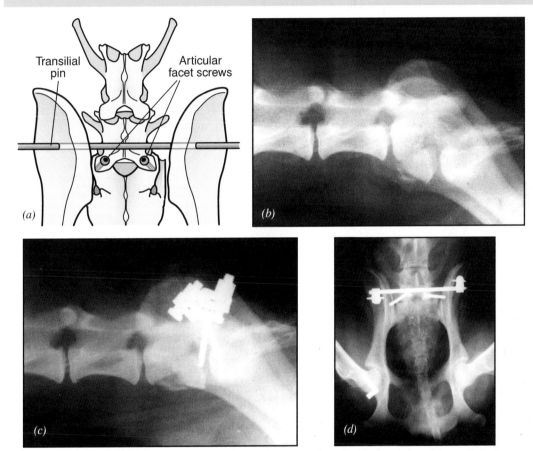

Figure 13.22: *(a) Schematic view of the lumbosacral spine to show the ideal position of a transilial pin for maintaining reduction of L7 vertebral body fractures. The L7-S1 articular facets are shown screwed together. (b) L7 fracture in a dog. (c), (d) Lateral and ventrodorsal post-operative radiographs of the case shown in (c) illustrating the use of a transilial pin and articular facet screws in the management of L7 fractures. External skeletal fixation clamps prevented migration of the transilial pin.*

Closure
Routine, including repair of the lumbodorsal fascia.

Post-operative Care
Strict rest for 6 weeks. Belly band support.

OPERATIVE TECHNIQUE 13.7

Sacral fractures and caudal vertebral fractures and luxations

Sacral fractures

Sacral fractures commonly have concomitant pelvic injuries; for example, ilial fracture or sacroiliac separation (Anderson and Coughlan, 1997). Pain is often a feature and neurological deficits can be significant (e.g. urinary and faecal incontinence), especially when fractures traverse the sacral canal or sacral foraminae. Fractures lateral to the sacral foraminae and those involving the spinous processes are of less clinical significance (Kuntz *et al.*, 1995). A classification for sacral fractures has recently been proposed (Figure 13.23).

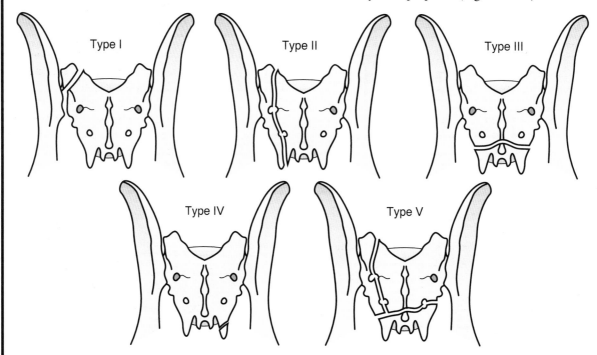

Figure 13.23: *Classification of sacral fractures (redrawn from Anderson and Coughlan, 1997).*

Many sacral fractures can be managed non-surgically, e.g. avulsion of the sacrotuberous ligament. Others may benefit from surgical reduction and stabilization, e.g. a sagittal foraminal (Type II fracture). The options for stabilizing foraminal fractures after open reduction are lag screwing, transilial pin(s) or bolt(s) (Figures 13.22 and 17.6) or a combination of the two techniques (Figure 13.24). Reduction and fixation of sagittal fractures can be challenging. Refer to Operative Technique 17.1 (managing sacroiliac luxations) for guidance on exposure and fixation of sagittal foraminal fractures of the sacrum.

Caudal vertebral fractures and luxations

These are most commonly seen in cats, and on occasion the tail may be avulsed. Caudal spinal nerve injury is often severe. In addition, traction on the tail may affect sacral nerves cranial to the vertebral lesion, causing urinary incontinence.

Fractures and luxations of the caudal vertebrae are usually treated non-surgically or by tail amputation. Reduction and fixation may be contemplated on occasions, especially in larger dogs. Possible fixation techniques would include wiring, screwing and plating. The prognosis for return of bladder function is good in animals with good anal tone and perineal skin sensation. Failure to regain continence within 4 weeks indicates a poorer prognosis (Smeak and Olmstead, 1985).

CHAPTER FOURTEEN

The Scapula

Andy Torrington

INTRODUCTION

Scapular fractures are uncommon. When they do occur they are mainly confined to fractures of the neck or the acromial process, or involve the articular surface. Fractures of the body are less common.

The scapula is the point of insertion of the trapezius, omotransversarius and the serratus ventralis thoracis muscles. Medial to the scapula the major structures include the brachial plexus from which the nerves supplying the forelimb originate and the axillary artery from which the major arteries supplying the forelimb arborize.

Fracture of the scapula may be associated with rib and/or cervical fractures. Thoracic trauma, including pulmonary contusion, pneumothorax and traumatic myocarditis, may also be found in association with these fractures (see Chapter 6). The presence or absence of these concomitant injuries must be thoroughly investigated before other injuries are considered.

Because of the proximity to neurovascular structures whose integrity is paramount for continued function of the forelimb following fracture repair, these must be assessed prior to surgical intervention.

Both caudocranial and mediolateral radiographic views of the scapula are necessary in order to assess the fracture adequately. Rotating the body of the patient 30 degrees away from the affected limb facilitates the caudocranial view. This reduces interpretational difficulties associated with overlying bony densities.

Fractures of the scapula can be divided into five types:

- Fractures of the scapular body and spine
- Fractures of the scapular neck
- Fractures involving the glenoid cavity
- Fractures of the supraglenoid tubercle
- Fractures of the acromial process.

FRACTURES OF THE SCAPULAR BODY

The majority of scapular body fractures are not severely displaced, because of the splinting effect of the surrounding musculature. These types of fractures may be treated conservatively (Chapter 7). Confinement, with or without a support dressing, should be continued for 4-6 weeks. When displacement does occur, the distal fragment usually overrides medially and proximally, with the fracture site of the proximal fragment overlying the shoulder joint area (Figure 14.1). Failure to repair these fractures adequately may result in degenerative joint disease of the shoulder, resulting from non-physiological loading. Surgical management is described in Operative Technique 14.1.

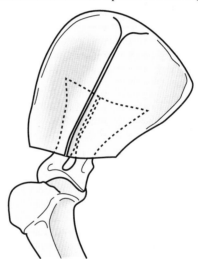

Figure 14.1: *Relative displacement of proximal and distal fragments in a transverse scapular fracture.*

FRACTURES OF THE SCAPULAR NECK

The glenoid cavity is most commonly displaced medially and proximally (Figure 14.2a). The presence of displacement is an indication for open reduction and rigid internal fixation (Operative Technique 14.2).

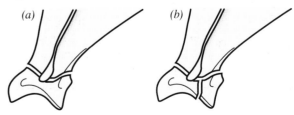

Figure 14.2: *(a) Transverse scapular neck fracture. (b) T-fracture of scapular neck with involvement of glenoid cavity.*

FRACTURES INVOLVING THE GLENOID CAVITY

These are usually T-fractures (Figure 14.2b). They are articular fractures and should be managed by open reduction and rigid internal fixation (Operative Technique 14.3).

> **WARNING**
> **Successful surgical treatment of T-fractures requires a substantial degree of orthopaedic experience.**

FRACTURES OF THE SUPRAGLENOID TUBEROSITY

Supraglenoid fractures are most commonly seen in skeletally immature dogs less than 7 months of age, but they are occasionally seen in the adult.

The supraglenoid tuberosity is the point of origin of the biceps brachii; thus these fractures are avulsion injuries (Figure 14.3). As such they are more commonly associated with low-grade trauma, during exercise. Because these injuries are often not associated with overtly traumatic incidents, many cases do not present until some time after the injury – often up to 3 weeks or more. On occasion they will be seen in association with scapular body fractures following road traffic accidents (Figure 14.4).

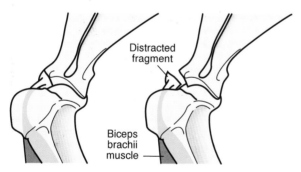

Figure 14.3: Avulsion fracture of supraglenoid tuberosity.

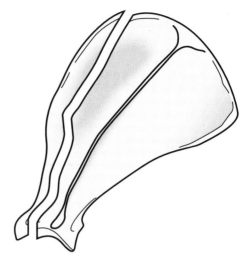

Figure 14.4: Fracture of supraglenoid tuberosity associated with longitudinal scapular body fracture.

Diagnosis requires radiography. The lateral view is usually more helpful than other projections. Radiographs will show the displaced supraglenoid tuberosity.

Placing the shoulder joint in flexion during radiography may help in identifying the injury. The condition is managed surgically (Operative Technique 14.4).

FRACTURES OF THE ACROMIAL PROCESS

See Operative Technique 14.2 for fixation techniques.

REFERENCES

Caywood D, Wallace LJ and Johnson GR (1977) The use of a plastic plate for repair of a comminuted scapular body fracture in a dog. *Journal of American Animal Hospital Association* **13**, 176.

Cheli R (1976) Surgical treatment of fractures of the scapula in the dog and cat. *Folia Vet. Lat.* **6**, 189.

Holt PE (1978) Longitudinal fracture of the scapula in a dog. *Veterinary Record* **102**, 311.

Piermattei DL (1993) *An Atlas of Surgical Approaches to the Bones of the Dog and Cat. 3rd edn.* WB Saunders, Philadelphia.

Ticer JW (1975) *Radiographic Techniques in Small Animal Practice.* WB Saunders, Philadelphia.

OPERATIVE TECHNIQUE 14.1
Fractures of the scapular body

Positioning
Lateral recumbency with affected limb uppermost.

Assistant
Optional.

Tray Extras
Gelpi self-retaining retractors (2 pairs); appropriate size screw and plate set; drill and bits.

Surgical Approach
The scapular body is approached through a lateral incision over the scapular spine. Incising through the deep fascia over the spine permits caudal retraction of the spinous head of the deltoideus muscle and cranial retraction of the trapezius and omotransversarius muscles. The supraspinatus and infraspinatus muscles are elevated from the body of the scapula and held in retraction using two pairs of Gelpi self-retaining retractors, one positioned proximally and the other distally (Figure 14.5).

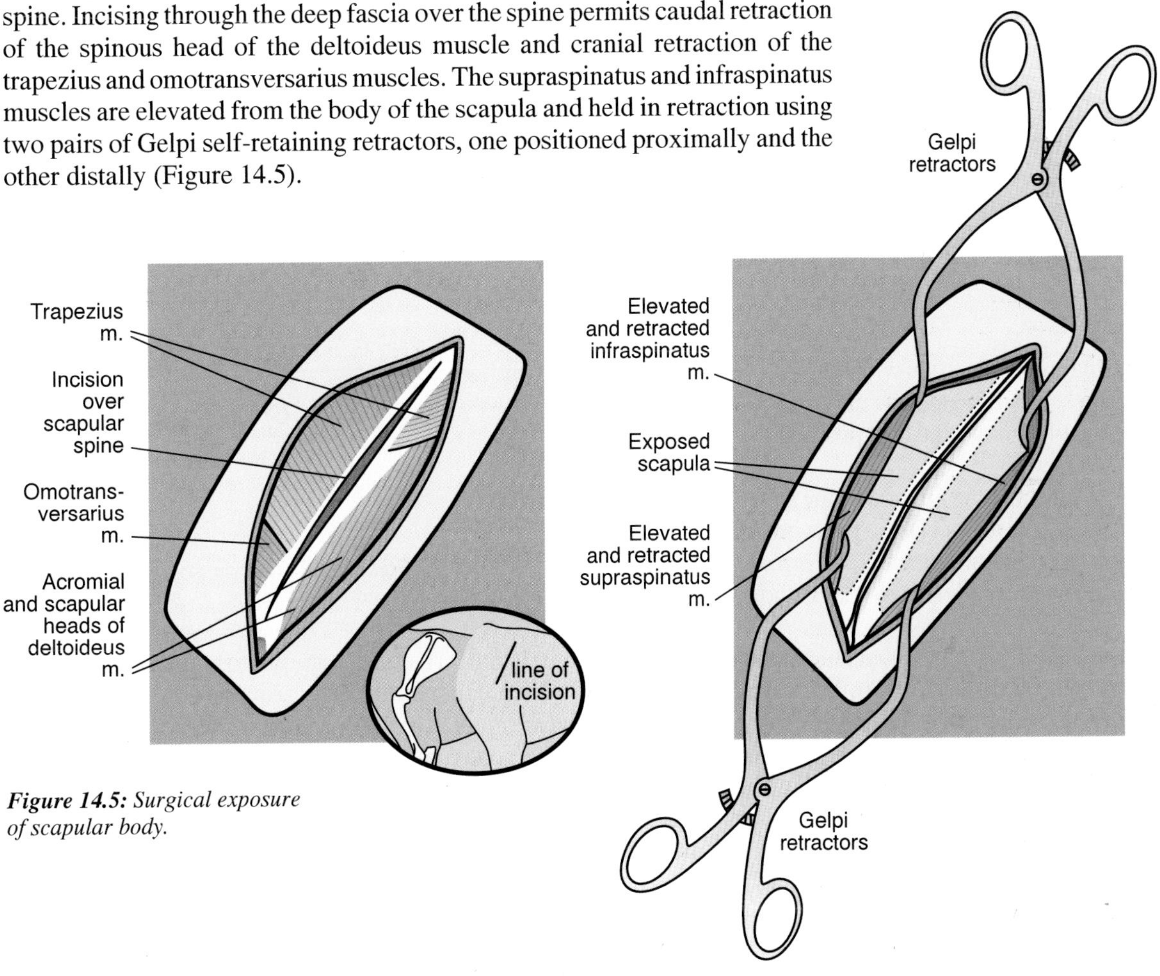

Figure 14.5: Surgical exposure of scapular body.

Reduction and Fixation
Reduction of the fracture is achieved by a combination of linear traction on the limb and gentle leverage applied to the distal fragment. It is often helpful to over-reduce the fracture initially by bringing the medially displaced distal fragment into a position that is lateral to the proximal fragment.

→

OPERATIVE TECHNIQUE 14.1 (CONTINUED)
Fractures of the scapular body

In general, scapular body fractures that require open reduction are best repaired using plates and screws. In smaller patients (under 15 kg) the use of wire sutures, 18 to 22 gauge, has been described. The plate should be secured to the distal fragment first whilst the fracture is over-reduced. The fracture is then reduced and the screws are inserted in the proximal fragment (Figure 14.6).

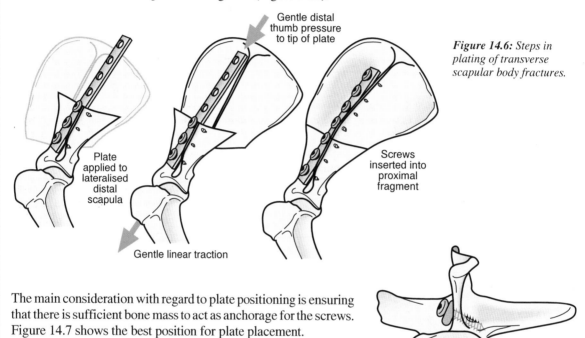

Gentle distal thumb pressure to tip of plate

Plate applied to lateralised distal scapula

Gentle linear traction

Screws inserted into proximal fragment

Figure 14.6: Steps in plating of transverse scapular body fractures.

The main consideration with regard to plate positioning is ensuring that there is sufficient bone mass to act as anchorage for the screws. Figure 14.7 shows the best position for plate placement.

Plates may also be applied to the spine to stabilize scapular body fractures. The use of plastic (polyvinylidine fluoride) plates has also been described, where their conformability to the scapular surface was deemed an advantage (Caywood *et al.*, 1977).

Figure 14.7: Transverse view of scapula to show plate and screw positioning

The main role of the implant in scapular body fractures is, as in other fracture locations, to maintain anatomical alignment until the fracture has gained sufficient physiological stability. The scapula differs from other appendicular bones in that it is not subject to the loads that are applied to the more distal bones of the forelimb. Because of the scapula's excellent blood supply, scapular fractures generally heal extremely well and more rapidly than fractures of the cortical bone of the lower limb. These two factors permit the use of plates that are mechanically weaker than those that would be applied in lower limb fractures. In general, 2.0 mm and 2.7 mm plates (Synthes) are adequate for most scapular body fractures in most patients.

> **WARNING**
> **Care must be taken to avoid iatrogenic damage to structures medial to the scapula: brachial plexus, axillary artery and thorax. It is also important to be aware of the suprascapular nerve running under the acromial process (see Figure 14.8c), when positioning the plate on the distal fragment.**

Post-operative Care
Depending on the stability achieved surgically, a Velpeau sling or scapular support bandage may be applied for 4–6 weeks. The patient should be restricted to short lead exercise during this period.

Implant removal is usually only undertaken if there are problems associated with its continued presence, such as screw loosening or infection.

OPERATIVE TECHNIQUE 14.2
Fractures of the scapular neck

Positioning
Lateral recumbency with affected limb uppermost.

Assistant
Optional.

Tray Extras
Gelpi self-retaining retractors (2 pairs); appropriate size screw and plate set; drill and bits; K-wire set (if pinning); chuck (if pinning); pin/wire cutters.

Surgical Approach
A lateral incision is made commencing at the midpoint of the scapular spine curving caudally over the proximal third of the humerus (Figure 14.8a). The deep fascia over the spine is incised and retracted cranially and caudally (Figure 14.8b). The acromion is osteotomized and retracted with the acromial head of the deltoideus muscle distally (Figure 14.8c). The osteotomy should leave sufficient bone attached to the deltoids to permit later reattachment. The supraspinatus and infraspinatus muscles are either retracted or they are freed from their humeral attachment in order to permit greater visualization of the fracture site. Exposure of the lateral and caudal aspects of the scapular neck is gained by tenotomy of the infraspinatus or teres minor muscle. Proximal retraction of the supraspinatus muscle requires osteotomy of the greater tubercle of the humerus.

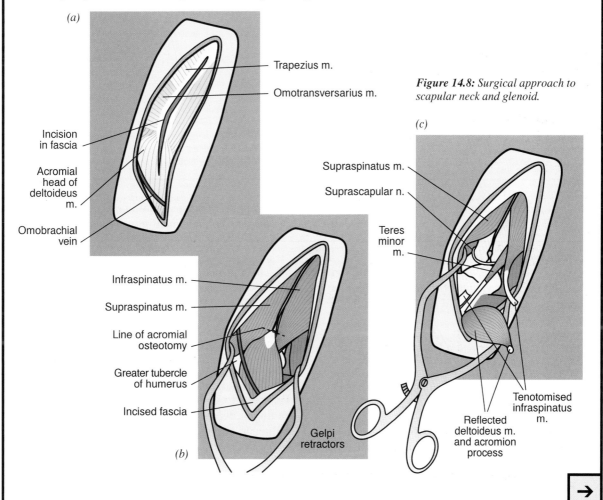

Figure 14.8: Surgical approach to scapular neck and glenoid.

(a) Trapezius m. — Omotransversarius m. — Incision in fascia — Acromial head of deltoideus m. — Omobrachial vein

(b) Infraspinatus m. — Supraspinatus m. — Line of acromial osteotomy — Greater tubercle of humerus — Incised fascia — Gelpi retractors

(c) Supraspinatus m. — Suprascapular n. — Teres minor m. — Reflected deltoideus m. and acromion process — Tenotomised infraspinatus m.

OPERATIVE TECHNIQUE 14.2 (CONTINUED)
Fractures of the scapular neck

Reduction and Fixation
Reduction of the fracture is achieved by a combination of linear traction on the limb and gentle leverage applied to the distal fragment.

Plating is superior to cross-pinning in providing rigid fixation. In general, because of the small size of the distal fragment, a T-plate is required in order to fulfil the orthopaedic principle of a minimum of two screws in each fragment (Figure 14.9).

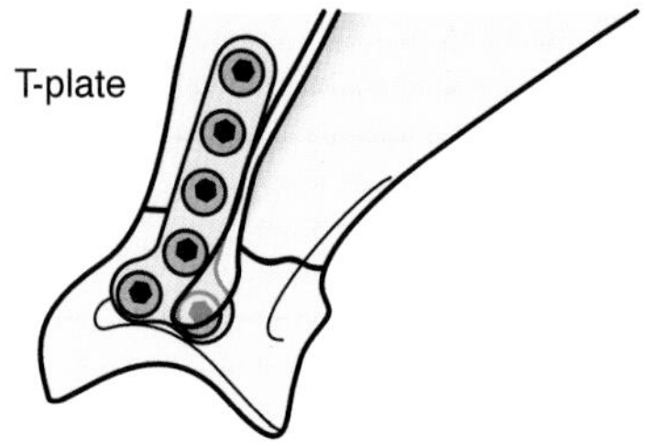

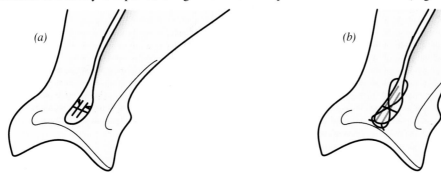

Figure 14.9: *T-plate fixation of a simple (non-articular) fracture of the scapular neck.*

> ### WARNING
> **The suprascapular nerve should be identified and avoided.**

Closure
The surgical site should be closed in layers. The greater tubercle, if osteotomized, should be reattached with pins and tension-band wire. The infraspinatus and teres minor tenotomies are repaired with a Bunnell–Mayer or horizontal mattress suture pattern of polydioxanone (PDS-Ethicon) or non-absorbable suture material. The acromial osteotomy is repaired using wire sutures or pins and a tension band (Figure 14.10).

(a)

(b)

Figure 14.10: *Acromial process osteotomy repair: (a) wire suture; (b) pin and tension-band wire.*

Post-operative Care
If cross-pinning alone has been used (see below), a scapular support bandage should be applied for 10–14 days. Plating techniques may permit early weight bearing and passive movement physiotherapy.

Alternative Technique
Cross-pinning alone, using K-wires or small Steinmann pins, may provide sufficient stability in simple non-articular fractures (Figure 14.11). This technique is complicated because the scapula tapers proximally and care must be taken to avoid penetration of the medial cortex.

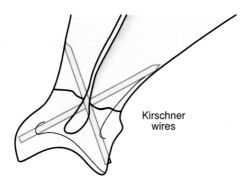

Kirschner wires

Figure 14.11: *Cross-pin fixation of simple (non-articular) fracture of scapular neck.*

> ### PRACTICAL TIP
> **Well positioned post-operative craniocaudal radiographs should be checked thoroughly for failure to engage the proximal fragment.**

OPERATIVE TECHNIQUE 14.3
Fractures involving the glenoid cavity

Positioning
Lateral recumbency with affected limb uppermost.

Assistant
Helpful during fracture reduction but not essential.

Tray Extras
Gelpi self-retaining retractors (2 pairs); appropriate size screw and plate set; drill and bits; K-wire set (if pinning); chuck (if pinning); pin/wire cutters.

Surgical Approach
See Operating Technique 14.2.

Reduction and Fixation
In the case of articular fractures, it is important to achieve accurate reconstruction of the articular surface. This can be achieved using a lag screw, which is generally introduced caudocranially. This reduces the fracture to a simple scapular neck fracture and thus it can be dealt with by using either of the techniques described in Operative Technique 14.2). The accuracy of screw placement is simplified by pre-drilling the glide hole in the caudal fragment from the fracture surface (Figure 14.12).

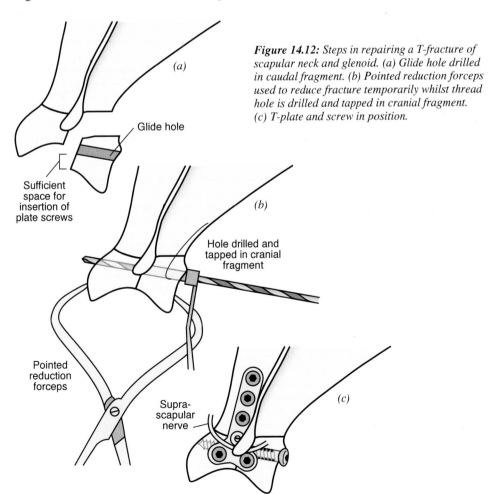

Figure 14.12: Steps in repairing a T-fracture of scapular neck and glenoid. (a) Glide hole drilled in caudal fragment. (b) Pointed reduction forceps used to reduce fracture temporarily whilst thread hole is drilled and tapped in cranial fragment. (c) T-plate and screw in position.

OPERATIVE TECHNIQUE 14.3 (CONTINUED)
Fractures involving the glenoid cavity

The following points should be considered when placing the interfragmentary screw:

- The glenoid cavity is concave; thus too distal a position may result in penetration of the articular surface.
- Placing the screw in a position that will interfere with plate screw positioning may compromise the application of a plate.

The fracture is reduced and pointed reduction forceps are used to maintain reduction. It is wise at this point to inspect the articular surface for accuracy of reduction and make any adjustments in order to ensure preservation of the anatomy of the articular surface. Gentle countersinking of the pilot hole should be performed. An insert sleeve with inner diameter equal to the core diameter of the selected screw is inserted in the pre-drilled hole. The hole in the cranial fragment is then drilled. The joint surface should now be inspected again. Following tapping, the screw can be inserted and tightened, thus reducing the articular fracture. The articular surface should finally be checked for accuracy of reconstruction.

If a T-plate is used to reduce the resultant transverse fracture, the horizontal bar should be positioned distal to the lag screw, such that the interfragmentary screw does not interfere with placement of the plate screws (Figure 14.12).

WARNING
The suprascapular nerve should be identified and avoided.

Closure
See Operating Technique 14.2.

Post-operative Care
See Operating Technique 14.2.

OPERATIVE TECHNIQUE 14.4
Fractures of the supraglenoid tuberosity

Positioning
Lateral recumbency with affected limb uppermost.

Assistant
Optional.

Tray Extras
Gelpi self-retaining retractors (2 pairs); appropriate size screw set (if lag screw fixation); drill and bits; K-wire set (if pinning); chuck (if pinning); pin/wire cutters.

Surgical Approach
See Operating Technique 14.2. Surgical approach is made by reflecting the brachiocephalicus muscle cranially. It may be necessary to osteotomize the greater tuberosity of the humerus to facilitate adequate exposure (Piermattei, 1993).

Reduction and Fixation
Two small K-wires (generally 1–1.5 mm diameter) are inserted in caudoproximal direction. A tension-band wire is anchored proximally (Figure 14.13a).

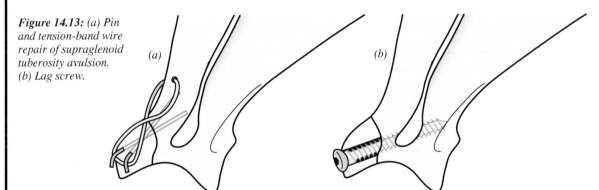

Figure 14.13: *(a) Pin and tension-band wire repair of supraglenoid tuberosity avulsion. (b) Lag screw.*

A single screw may be used in lag fashion, inserted in a caudoproximal direction. This procedure is facilitated by pre-drilling and tapping the screw hole in the scapular body, prior to reduction of the fracture. The glide hole is then drilled in the avulsed fragment, and the screw inserted (Figure 14.13b).

Chronic injuries may not permit anatomical reduction and fixation using the above techniques. In such instances, or where the avulsed fragment is too small to accommodate implants, it may be secured to the craniomedial surface of the humerus. This can be accomplished using a screw and washer, or using a ligament staple.

Closure
The surgical site should be closed in layers. The greater tubercle, if osteotomized, should be reattached with pins and tension-band wire.

Post-operative Care
Post-operative exercise should be restricted to short lead walks for four weeks.

CHAPTER FIFTEEN

The Humerus

Hamish R. Denny

INTRODUCTION

With the exception of condylar fractures, the majority of humeral fractures result from road traffic accidents. In a recent survey, fractures of the humerus accounted for 10% of all appendicular fractures (Johnson *et al.*, 1994). Most humeral fractures are treated by internal fixation because it is difficult to satisfy the main criteria for using external support.

Chest injuries, particularly pneumothorax, are common complications of humeral fractures. Other possibilities include intrapulmonary haemorrhage, diaphragmatic rupture, rib fractures and occasionally chylothorax. A careful clinical and radiological examination should be done to check for chest injuries. The patient's condition should be stabilized before embarking on fracture fixation.

> **WARNING**
> **Humeral fractures are frequently accompanied by chest injuries.**

Fractures of the humerus can be broadly classified into three groups (Braden, 1975):

- Fractures involving the proximal epiphysis and metaphysis
- Fractures of the diaphysis
- Distal humeral fractures (supracondylar, condylar and intercondylar fractures).

The approximate distribution of fractures between these three groups has been quoted as 8%, 40% and 52%, respectively (Braden, 1975).

Humeral fractures in the cat

There are important anatomical differences between the humerus of the cat and dog. The humeral diaphysis in the cat is straighter and the medullary cavity has a more uniform diameter than that of the dog. Consequently, intramedullary fixation provides a satisfactory method of treatment for many feline diaphyseal fractures. Another important anatomical difference between the dog and cat is the position of the median nerve; in the dog the nerve lies just cranial to the medial epicondyle, while in the cat

the medial epicondyle is pierced by an epicondyloid fossa which contains the median nerve. The supratrochlear fossa is not completely penetrated in the cat.

PROXIMAL HUMERUS

Approximately 8% of humeral fractures involve the proximal third. These can be divided into :

- Fractures involving the proximal growth plate
- Fractures of the humeral head
- Fractures of the proximal metaphyseal region.

Fractures involving the proximal growth plate

Salter-Harris I and II (Figure 15.1)

- Uncommon
- Usually severe caudo-medial overriding of the fragments occurs
- Open reduction is essential (Operative Technique 15.1).

Salter-Harris III (Figure 15.2)

- Rare (Dejardin *et al.*, 1995)
- May be fracture of the lesser tubercle
- Greater tubercle tends to remain close to the glenoid but there is marked caudal displacement of the humeral head
- Articular fracture, therefore open reduction is essential to allow accurate anatomical reduction of the fragments (Operative Technique 15.2).

Fractures of the humeral head

This is a very rare injury: one reported case occurred in a 3-year-old Miniature Dachshund (Holt, 1990). The fracture was stabilized using two K-wires (Figure 15.3). An alternative would have been the use of a K-wire in combination with a lag screw. For surgical approach see Operative Technique 15.2. Implants are inserted from the craniolateral aspect of the greater tuberosity and are directed caudally into the humeral head.

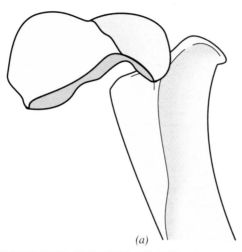

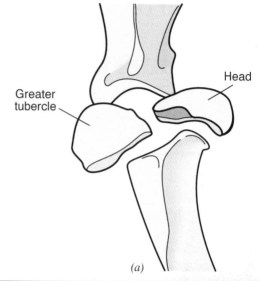

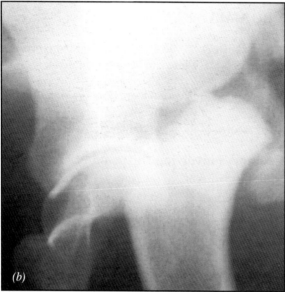

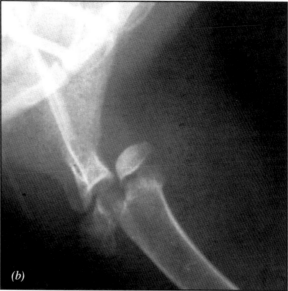

Figure 15.1: *(a) Salter-Harris Type I separation of proximal humeral epiphysis. (b) Radiograph of Salter-Harris Type I separation of proximal humeral epiphysis in a Golden Retriever.*

Figure 15.2: *(a) Salter-Harris Type III fracture of the proximal humeral epiphyses. (b) Salter-Harris Type III fracture of the proximal humeral epiphyses in a 9-month-old Domestic Shorthaired cat.*

Fractures of the proximal metaphyseal region

- Uncommon
- Usually transverse and impacted
- Nutritional secondary hyperparathyroidism in pups or osteosarcoma formation in adults are predisposing factors.

In puppies or kittens, because of the inherent stability of the fracture, cage rest may be sufficient to allow healing to occur. However, if there is displacement then an intramedullary pin is used for fixation.

Positioning, instrumentation and surgical approach are as described in Operative Technique 15.1. After fracture reduction, a Steinmann pin is inserted through the skin and bone just lateral to the ridge of the greater tuberosity and driven well down into the distal shaft of the humerus.

Post-operatively, check diet and restrict exercise for 4 weeks. Remove pin once healing is complete (4–6 weeks).

HUMERAL DIAPHYSIS

In the dog the medullary cavity of the humerus is wide proximally and gradually decreases in size towards the supratrochlear foramen. Consequently, although fractures do occur in the proximal shaft, the majority involve the distal two-thirds and in particular the distal third. Fractures of the proximal and mid-shaft regions tend to be transverse while the more distal fractures follow the curvature of the musculospiral groove and are spiral or oblique. Many are also comminuted.

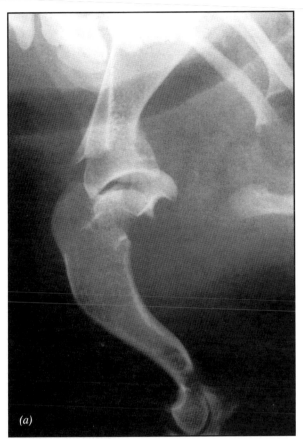 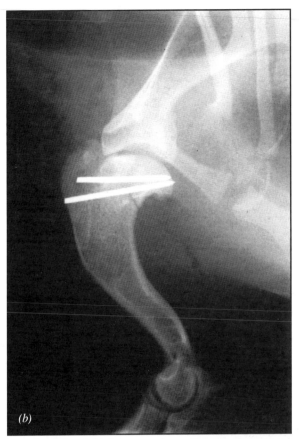

Figure 15.3: *(a) Fracture of the humeral head in a 3-year-old Miniature Dachshund. (b) Post-operative radiograph showing K-wire fixation.*

Courtesy of PE Holt.

Bone plating* (*Operative Techniques 15.3 and 15.4*)	Plate fixation is the preferred method of treatment for most humeral diaphyseal fractures in dogs.
Intramedullary pinning (*Operative Technique 15.5*)	This method should be reserved for transverse or blunt oblique fractures in small dogs and cats but can also be used in longer oblique fractures in cats.
External fixation (*Operative Technique 15.6*)	The external fixator can be used to stabilize most types of diaphyseal fracture of the humerus. However, it is used most often for comminuted fractures and open fractures.

Table 15.1: *Decision making in the surgical management of humeral diaphyseal fractures.*
* *Ideally the plate should be placed on the cranial surface of the bone; this is the tension side. However the plate may also be placed on the lateral or the medial side of the bone. Careful pre-operative planning is essential and the prognosis following plate fixation is generally good.*

The radial nerve lies close to the fracture site (see Figure 15.16b) and radial paresis is a common complication. In the author's experience, this is invariably transient and resolves within 2–3 weeks of fracture repair. The nerve should be inspected during open reduction and carefully protected during the insertion of implants.

The method of fixation will depend on age, size of animal and nature of the fracture (Table 15.1).

Choice of aspect for plating
This depends on:

- Location of the fracture

- Position of lag screws in relation to a neutralization plate.

Fractures in the mid-section of the humerus are generally plated laterally or cranially. Lag screws are used for initial fixation of oblique or comminuted fractures and the position of these screws in relation to the neutralization plate must be considered. This is illustrated in case studies A and B below.

The medial approach is used in preference to the lateral for dealing with fractures of the distal third of the humeral shaft (case study C).

Case Study A: (Fig 15.4) Labrador with comminuted mid-shaft humeral fracture

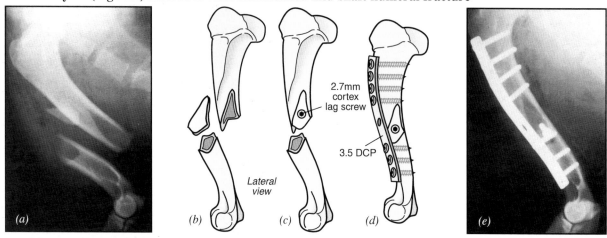

Figure 15.4: (a) Pre-operative radiograph; (b) tracing from pre-operative radiograph; (c) craniolateral approach – fragment reduced, lag screw fixation (2.7 mm cortex screw); (d) cranial application of plate (8-hole 3.5 DCP); (e) post-operative radiograph.

Case Study B: (Fig 15.5) Newfoundland with comminuted fracture involving the distal third of the humeral shaft

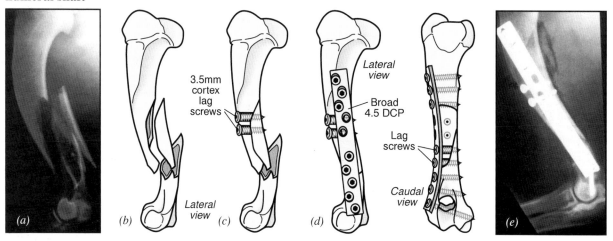

Figure 15.5: (a) Pre-operative radiograph; (b) tracing from pre-operative radiograph; (c) craniolateral approach – reconstruction of shaft using two lag screws (3.5 cortex screws); (d) lateral and caudal view of humerus showing application of a plate to the lateral side of the humerus (broad 4.5 DCP) – screws 4 and 5 cross a fracture line and are placed as lag screws; (e) post-operative lateral radiograph.

Case Study C: (Fig 15.6) Chow with oblique fracture involving distal third of the humeral shaft

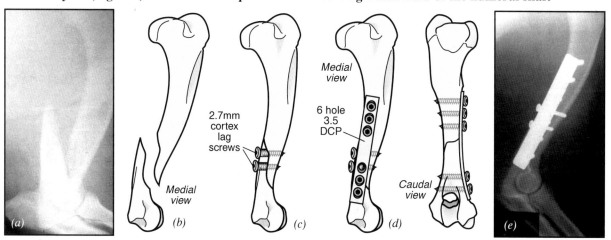

Figure 15.6: (a) Pre-operative lateral radiograph; (b) tracing from pre-operative lateral radiograph; (c) medial approach – reconstruction of shaft using two lag screws (2.7 screws); (d) lateral and caudal view of humerus showing application of a plate to the medial surface of the humerus (6-hole 3.5 DCP); (e) post-operative lateral radiograph.

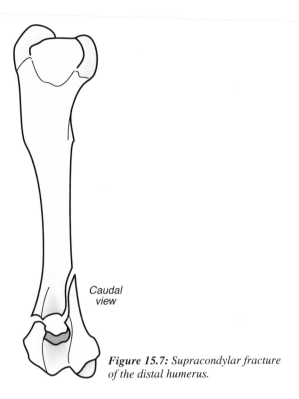

Figure 15.7: *Supracondylar fracture of the distal humerus.*

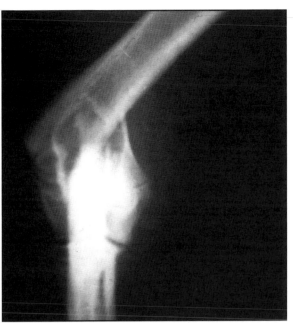

Figure 15.8: *Six-month-old German Shepherd Dog with a supracondylar fracture involving the growth plate (Salter-Harris Type II injury).*

DISTAL HUMERUS

Supracondylar fractures

Adult

The fracture line passes through the supratrochlear foramen. Fractures are usually transverse or oblique. Supracondylar fractures (Figures 15.7 and 15.8) should be accurately reduced and rigidly stabilized because of their close proximity to the elbow (Operative Technique 15.7). An intramedullary pin used in conjunction with a K-wire to prevent rotation is the simplest method of fixation (Brinker, 1974). Alternatively, in large dogs, a plate can be applied to the medial supracondylar ridge of the humerus (Braden, 1975).

Skeletally immature animals

Supracondylar fractures which involve the growth plate are generally Salter-Harris type II injuries (Figure 15.8). The medial cortex is usually fractured obliquely and this area can be readily stabilized with a K-wire or a lag screw placed transversely from medial to lateral, proximal to the growth plate. After this initial fixation, K-wires are driven up from the medial and the lateral condyle across the fracture site in a cruciate pattern (see Figure 15.23).

Condylar fractures

Condylar fractures (Figure 15.9) (Denny, 1983) usually result from a violent upward stress transmitted through the head of the radius to the humeral trochlea. Falls, jumping and sudden turns at exercise are the most common causes of fracture of the lateral or medial condyle. Intercondylar fractures usually re-

sult from road traffic accidents. Lateral and medial condylar fractures affect predominantly immature dogs (peak age incidence, 4 months) whilst intercondylar fractures are more evenly distributed between skeletally mature and immature dogs. Condylar fractures are articular fractures and as such require surgical treatment with accurate anatomical reduction and stable internal fixation if normal joint function is to be restored.

Spaniel breeds appear to be more prone to condylar fractures. Incomplete ossification of the humeral condyle predisposing to fracture has been demonstrated in Cocker Spaniels and Brittany Spaniels and it has been suggested in the Cocker Spaniel that incomplete ossi-

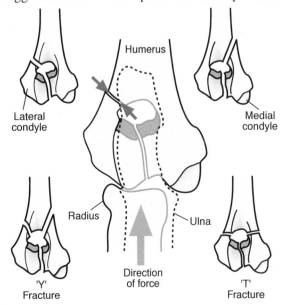

Figure 15.9: *Condylar fractures of the humerus.*

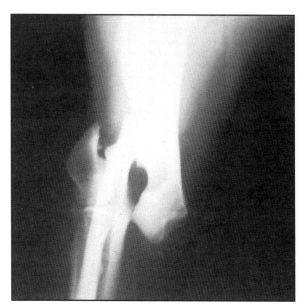

Figure 15.10: Lateral condylar fracture in a 1-year-old Springer Spaniel.

fication of the humeral condyle may be a genetic disease with a recessive mode of inheritance (Marcellin-Little *et al.*, 1994).

In the radiographic assessment of condylar fractures it is essential to take both lateral and craniocaudal views of the elbow. A lateral condylar fracture can be missed on the lateral view but should be obvious on the craniocaudal view (Figure 15.10).

Lateral condylar fractures

Lateral condylar fractures are stabilized with a transcondylar lag screw and anti-rotational K-wire (Operative Technique 15.8). The K-wire is also used for initial fixation.

Lateral condylar fractures carry a good prognosis provided they are correctly reduced and stabilized. Some 77% go on to regain full limb function and the average recovery time is 4 weeks (range 2–8 weeks). Failure to treat the fracture surgically results in medial luxation of the elbow because lateral support for the joint is lost. Malunion or non-union of the lateral condyle causes permanent joint deformity. The range of elbow movement remains limited and varying degrees of lameness persist. The prognosis is obviously better in immature dogs because of their ability to remodel the malunion. In these cases the functional end results can be surprisingly good, despite permanent joint deformity.

Closed reduction using a condyle clamp and a single transcondylar lag screw placed through a stab incision is possible if the animal is presented within a few hours of injury. However, in the majority of cases an open surgical reduction is carried out.

Medial condylar fractures

The same considerations discussed under lateral condylar fractures apply (Operative Technique 15.9). Post-

operative care and prognosis are the same as for lateral condylar fractures.

Fractures of the medial epicondyle

Fractures of the medial epicondyle are also occasionally encountered in immature dogs. They must be distinguished from developmental non-fusion of the medial epicondyle (Figure 15.11a). With fractures, the onset of lameness is acute. In both developmental and traumatic lesions the epicondylar fragment tends to be distracted by the attached antebrachial flexor muscles. If the bone fragment is large enough, it is lagged into place with a screw (Figure 15.11b). Smaller fragments causing persistent lameness are removed and the muscles reattached to the adjacent fascia.

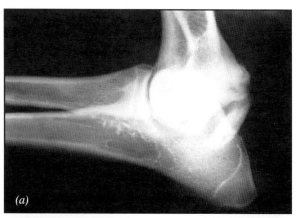

(a)

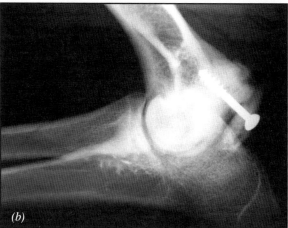

(b)

Figure 15.11: (a) Un-united medial epicondyle in a 1-year-old Golden Retriever. (b) Post-operative radiograph of (a), showing lag screw fixation with a 4 mm cancellous screw.

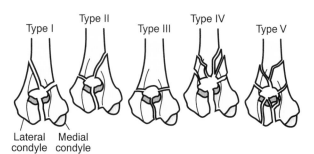

Figure 15.12: Classification of intercondylar humeral fractures, after Bardet et al. (1983).

Intercondylar ('Y' or 'T') fractures

The humeral intercondylar fracture is referred to as a 'Y' fracture if the supracondylar ridges are fractured obliquely, or as a 'T' fracture if the ridges are fractured transversely. Although intercondylar fractures are traditionally divided into these two broad groups, they can be further divided into five types (Bardet *et al.*, 1983) (Figure 15.12).

Successful treatment of these fractures can be difficult and may present a real challenge, even to the most experienced orthopaedic surgeon. Good exposure of the fracture is essential to achieve accurate anatomical reduction of the fragments. A caudal approach with osteotomy of the olecranon and dorsal reflection of the triceps muscle mass is used. Reconstruction and fixation of the condyles is achieved with a transcondylar lag screw in combination with a K-wire. The condyles are then attached to the shaft with a plate applied to the medial supracondylar ridge of the humerus (Operative Technique 15.10).

Prognosis is favourable for return to reasonable function in the majority of animals (64–70%) provided accurate anatomical reduction and good stability are achieved, thus allowing early pain-free elbow mobility (Denny, 1983; Anderson *et al.*, 1990).

REFERENCES

Anderson TJ, Carmichael LS and Miller A (1990) Intercondylar humeral fracture in the dog: a review of 20 cases. *Journal of Small Animal Practice* **31**, 437–442.

Bardet JF, Hohn RB, Rudy RL *et al.* (1983) Fractures of the humerus in dogs and cats. A retrospective study of 130 cases. *Veterinary Surgery* **12**(2), 73–77.

Braden TD (1975) Surgical correction of humeral fractures. In: *Current Techniques in Small Animal Surgery*, ed. MJ Bojrab, pp. ???. Lea & Febiger, Philadelphia.

Brinker WO (1974) Fractures of the humerus. In: *Canine Surgery, 2nd edn*, ed. J. Archibald, p. 1019. American Vet Publications Inc., Santa Barbara, California.

Dejardin LM, Bennett RL and Flo GL (1995) Salter Harris Type III fracture of the proximal humerus in a dog. *Veterinary Comparative Orthopaedics and Traumatology*, **8**, 66–69.

Denny HR (1983) Condylar fractures of the humerus in the dog: a review of 133 cases. *Journal of Small Animal Practice* **24**, 185–197.

Holt PE (1990). In: *Canine Orthopaedics, 2nd edn*, ed. WG Whittick, p. 363. Lea & Febiger, Philadelphia/London.

Johnson JA, Austin C and Breur GJ (1994) Incidence of canine appendicular musculoskeletal disorders in 16 veterinary teaching hospitals from 1980 through 1989. *Veterinary Comparative Orthopaedics and Traumatology* **7**, 56–69.

Marcellin-Little DJ, DeYoung DJ, Ferris KK and Berry CM (1994) Incomplete ossification of the humeral condyle in spaniels. *Veterinary Surgery* **23**, 475–487.

Marti JM and Miller A (1994) Delimitation of safe corridors for the insertion of external fixator pins in the dog. 2: Forelimb. *Journal of Small Animal Practice* **35**, 78–85.

Piermattei DL and Greeley RG (1979) *An Atlas of Surgical Approaches to the Bones of the Dog and Cat, 2nd edn*. WB Saunders, Philadelphia.

OPERATIVE TECHNIQUE 15.1

Salter-Harris I and II fractures of the proximal humerus

Positioning
Lateral recumbency – restraining band placed under axilla and secured to tabletop to help with traction.

Assistant
Ideally.

Tray Extras
Appropriate size K-wires or intramedullary pins; chuck; drill; pin cutters; Gelpi and Hohmann retractors; pointed reduction forceps; Kern or Burns bone holding forceps. Appropriate screw set, drill bits etc. in dogs over 7 months of age if using lag screw technique.

Surgical Approach
A longitudinal incision is made over the craniolateral aspect of the proximal humerus. The deep fascia is incised along the caudal border of the brachiocephalicus muscle; the muscle is reflected cranially to expose the fracture (Piermattei and Greeley, 1979). Additional exposure of the proximal shaft can be achieved by incision of the periosteum between the cranial border of the deltoideus muscle and the superficial pectoral muscle.

Reduction and Fixation
The epiphysis is grasped with pointed AO reduction forceps and the proximal metaphysis with Kern bone holding forceps. Reduction can be difficult but is achieved by a combination of steady direct traction using the Kern forceps while a periosteal elevator is interposed between the fracture surfaces and used to lever the metaphysis forward until reduction is achieved (Figure 15.13). Stability is usually good and can be maintained in animals under 7 months of age by the insertion of two K-wires or a Steinmann pin (Figure 15.14a,b). The implants are introduced from the greater tubercle and driven down into the shaft of the humerus. A cancellous bone screw can be used for fixation in animals over 7 months of age (Figure 15.14 c).

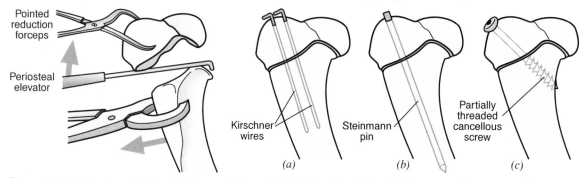

Figure 15.13: Reduction of Salter-Harris Type I/II fracture.

Figure 15.14: Salter-Harris Type I/II fractures of the proximal humerus: methods of fixation.

Wound Closure
Routine. Periosteum and deep fascia can be closed as one layer.

Post-operative Care
Bandage is optional; exercise is restricted for 4 to 6 weeks. In growing animals, implants should be removed once fracture union is complete (4 to 8 weeks), but in practice they are generally left *in situ* unless loosening causes soft tissue problems.

OPERATIVE TECHNIQUE 15.2
Salter-Harris III fractures of the proximal humerus

Positioning
Lateral recumbency – restraining band placed under axilla and secured to tabletop to help with traction.

Assistant
Yes.

Tray Extras
Appropriate size K-wires or intramedullary pins; wire for tension band; chuck; drill; pliers/wire twisters; pin/wire cutters; Gelpi and Hohmann retractors; pointed reduction forceps; Kern or Burns bone holding forceps; small hand-saw or bone cutters.

Surgical Approach
(See also Operative Technique 14.2.)
Tenotomy of the tendon of insertion of the infraspinatus muscle is necessary to give good exposure of the shoulder and also to allow the humeral shaft to be pulled distally using Kern forceps (positioned as in Figure 15.13) during exposure of the fracture surfaces. The joint capsule or its remains are reflected to allow inspection of the articular surfaces. The fractured humeral head usually loses all soft tissue attachments and is found impacted in the soft tissues caudal to the shoulder.

Reduction and Fixation
At this stage the proximal humeral shaft is rotated out of the incision; the humeral head is picked up and placed in its correct position on the metaphysis. It can then be held in place by one of two methods. In the first, K-wires are driven down from the articular surface through the head into the metaphysis; the wires are cut flush with the joint surface and then countersunk. Alternatively, two or three K-wires can be driven in normograde fashion from the cranial, craniolateral and craniomedial aspect of the metaphysis up into the humeral head (Figure 15.15a). To allow maximum purchase in the head, each K-wire is advanced until its point just penetrates the articular surface; the wire is then retracted until the tip lies just below the surface.

The distal ends of the wires are cut close to the surface of the metaphysis. If there is fracture of the lesser tuberosity and the fragment is unstable, K-wire fixation can be carried out at this stage. The humeral head is placed back into the glenoid. The avulsed greater tuberosity of the humerus is grasped with pointed AO reduction forceps and reattached to the metaphysis with diverging two or three K-wires driven from the craniolateral surface of the tubercle into the caudal aspect of the metaphysis (Figure 15.15b).

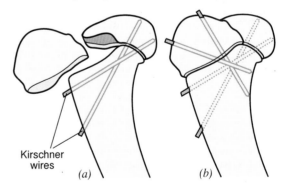

Figure 15.15: Salter-Harris Type III fractures of the proximal humerus: method of fixation.

Wound Closure
Remnants of joint capsule are sutured. The infraspinatus tenotomy is repaired with Bunnel or a 'locking loop' suture reinforced with two mattress sutures. The rest of the wound closure is described in Operative Technique 14.2.

Post-operative Care
Bandage is optional; exercise is restricted for 4 to 6 weeks. Ideally implants are removed once healing is complete, but in practice they are generally left *in situ* unless loosening causes soft tissue problems.

OPERATIVE TECHNIQUE 15.3
Bone plating: craniolateral approach to the humerus for cranial or lateral plate fixation

Positioning
Lateral recumbency – restraining band placed under axilla and secured to tabletop to help with traction.

Assistant
Essential.

Tray Extras
Appropriate plate and screw set, drill bits, etc. (3.5 DCP and screw set used most often in medium sized dogs; 2.7 DCP and screw set in small breeds; 4.5 DCP and screws in large or giant breeds; 2.7 screw set useful for lag screw fixation of small fragments in all sizes of dog). Drill; plate benders and/or bending press; pointed reduction forceps; self-locking bone holding forceps; Hohmann retractors and self-retaining retractors (West's or Gelpi).

Surgical Approach
A craniolateral skin incision is made from the greater tuberosity to the lateral condyle (Figure 15.16a). The cephalic vein is identified and ligated; the brachiocephalicus and the brachialis muscles are separated to expose the shaft of the humerus (Figure 15.16b). The radial nerve can be easily identified in the mid-shaft region by separating the brachialis muscle from the lateral head of the triceps muscle: once the nerve has been identified between these two muscles, follow it distally as it runs around the caudal border of the brachialis muscle to emerge on its lateral aspect at the level of the extensor carpi radialis muscle. The brachialis muscle can be retracted caudally and used to protect the radial nerve (Figure 15.16c).

> **WARNING**
> **The radial nerve should be identified and protected throughout the surgery.**

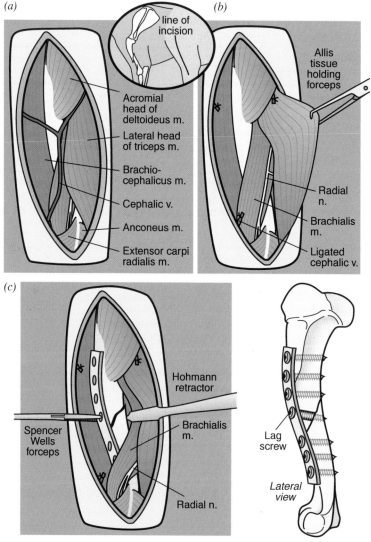

Figure 15.16: Craniolateral approach for application of a plate to the cranial aspect of the humeral shaft.

→

OPERATIVE TECHNIQUE 15.3 (CONTINUED)

Bone plating: craniolateral approach to the humerus for cranial or lateral plate fixation

Additional exposure for lateral plating

Exposure of the humeral shaft is as described above, but in addition the brachialis muscle and the radial nerve are mobilized so that the plate can be slid beneath them on the lateral side of the humerus (Figure 15.17). The origin of the extensor carpi radialis muscle is freed from the lateral condyle to complete exposure of the distal humerus.

WARNING

Fracture reduction and insertion of implants, especially in comminuted fractures, is not easy and the inexperienced surgeon should consider referring such cases to a specialist for treatment.

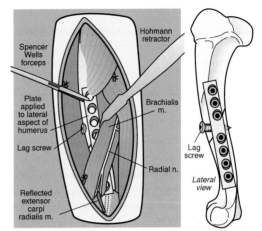

Figure 15.17: Additional exposure for application of a plate to the lateral side of the humerus.

Wound Closure

Suture the brachiocephalicus to the brachialis muscle. The deep brachial fascia, subcutaneous tissue and skin are closed in layers.

Post-operative Care

Strict exercise restriction for 6 to 8 weeks. Plates on the humerus are generally left *in situ*. It is often difficult to identify the radial nerve in scar tissue resulting from the initial surgery and therefore plate removal carries a risk of iatrogenic damage to the radial nerve.

OPERATIVE TECHNIQUE 15.4

Bone plating: medial approach to the humerus for medial plate fixation

---

Positioning
Lateral recumbency, with affected leg down. The upper forelimb is pulled well caudally.

Assistant
Essential.

Tray Extras
As for Operative Technique 15.3.

Surgical Approach
The skin incision is made over the medial aspect of the humerus from mid-shaft to medial condyle (Figure 15.18). The median nerve and biceps muscle are retracted cranially, while the ulnar nerve and the medial head of the triceps muscle are retracted caudally to expose the humeral shaft. Branches of the brachial artery and vein accompany the nerves and all these vital structures should be protected. In the cat, it is important to note that the median nerve runs through the epicondyloid fossa of the humerus (Figure 15.19). Exposure of the more proximal regions of the humerus is possible by mobilizing the vessels and subperiosteal elevation of the superficial pectoral and brachiocephalicus muscles.

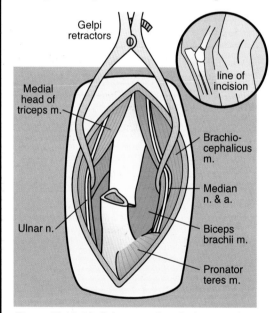

Figure 15.18: Medial approach to the humerus for application of a plate.

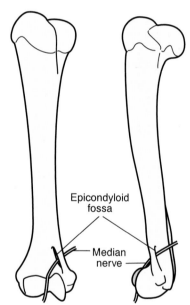

Figure 15.19: Medial aspect of feline humerus showing the epicondyloid fossa.

Wound Closure
The deep fascia, subcutaneous tissue and skin are closed in layers.

Post-operative Care
Strict exercise restriction for 6 to 8 weeks. Plates on the humerus are generally left *in situ*.

OPERATIVE TECHNIQUE 15.5

Intramedullary pinning: humerus

Pre-operative Planning
Radiographs are taken of both the fractured and the normal humerus. The normal is used as a guide to select a pin of the correct diameter to fit the medullary cavity as tightly as possible. The author's preference is to transect the pin partially with a hacksaw (cut around the entire outer circumference) so that the pin can then be broken off flush with the surface of the greater tuberosity after insertion (see also Chapter 9).

Positioning
Lateral recumbency – restraining band placed under axilla and secured to tabletop to help with traction.

Assistant
Yes, but surgery can often be done single-handed in the cat.

Tray Extras
Pointed reduction forceps; Kern or Burn's bone holding forceps; Gelpi and Hohmann retractors; appropriate intramedullary pins; chuck; pin cutters (or hacksaw); wire for cerclage; ± appropriate external fixator set if type I fixator is to be used as adjunct.

Surgical Approach
A craniolateral approach is used as described in Operative Technique 15.3.

Reduction and Fixation
After exposing the fracture, apply self-locking bone holding forceps to the bone just proximal and distal to the fracture site (protect the radial nerve); the bone ends are toggled against each other until reduction is achieved. The method of introduction of the intramedullary pin is a matter of personal preference. Using a Jacobs chuck, the pin can be introduced from the proximal end of the humerus: the correct point of entry is just lateral to the ridge of the greater tuberosity. The pin is then directed to glide down the medial cortex of the humerus towards the fracture site. Reduction of the fracture is maintained by an assistant with the bone holding forceps. When the tip of the pin can be felt approaching the fracture, the bone fragments should be bowed slightly medially to help to direct the tip of the pin down into the medial condyle.

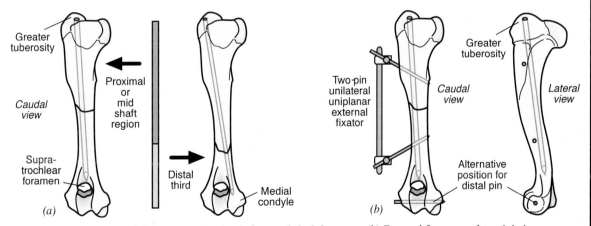

Figure 15.20: *(a) Intramedullary pin positioning in humeral shaft fractures. (b) External fixator used to minimize rotation following intramedullary pinning.*

OPERATIVE TECHNIQUE 15.5 (CONTINUED)

Intramedullary pinning: humerus

The alternative method of pin introduction is retrograde pinning. The pin is driven up the shaft from the fracture site, keeping the shoulder flexed and the pin directed towards the lateral side of the greater tuberosity. Once the tip of the pin has emerged, it is grasped with the Jacobs chuck and drawn up the shaft sufficiently to permit reduction of the fracture. Reduction is maintained with the bone holding forceps while the pin is driven into the distal shaft. The position of the fracture influences the length of pin required. For fractures involving the proximal or mid-shaft region, the pin is driven down the shaft to a point just proximal to the supratrochlear foramen (Figure 15.20a). For fractures involving the distal third, a smaller diameter pin is used. The pin should be directed towards the medial side of the shaft so the tip bypasses the supratrochlear foramen and is embedded in the medial condyle (Figure 15.20a). When the pin has been inserted to the correct depth, it is broken off flush with the bone. If it has not already been pre-cut, the pin is cut with pin cutters (or a hacksaw) just proximal to the tuberosity.

A two-pin unilateral/uniplanar external fixator (Figure 15.20b) can be used to supplement the intramedullary pin to minimize rotation and the risk of non-union. Alternatives to the external fixator for preventing rotational instability following intramedullary fixation include cerclage and hemi-cerclage wires or stack pinning.

Wound Closure
As for Operative Technique 15.3. If external fixation pins have been placed, they are clamped to the external connecting bar and routine wound closure is undertaken.

Post-operative Care
Exercise restriction until fracture union is complete. The fixator is removed after about 3 weeks, before problems with soft tissues are encountered. The intramedullary pin can then be removed once fracture healing is complete. Pre-cut pins in cats often remain *in situ* but in dogs the pins eventually have a tendency to migrate dorsally because of the looser pin fit. If this happens, the pin is easily removed.

OPERATIVE TECHNIQUE 15.6

External fixation: humerus

Pre-operative Considerations

The humerus is surrounded by muscle and, with the exception of two small areas on the proximal and distal ends of the bone (Figure 15.21), there are no safe corridors for the introduction of the pins (Marti and Miller, 1994). Transfixion of large muscle masses by pins results in pain and stiffness due to muscle fibrosis. In addition, pin tract infections are more likely to occur. These problems can be minimized by using a standard craniolateral approach to the fracture. Once the fracture is aligned the pins can be introduced either through the main incision or, preferably, through stab incisions close to the main incision. The pins are then directed between muscle bellies, avoiding the radial nerve, and are driven into the bone, penetrating both cortices.

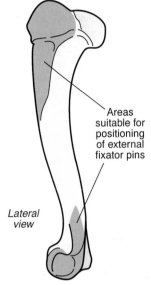

Areas suitable for positioning of external fixator pins

Lateral view

Figure 15.21: *External fixator: safe areas for pin introduction. (After Marti and Miller, 1994.)*

Positioning

Lateral recumbency – restraining band placed under axilla and secured to tabletop to help with traction.

Tray Extras

Appropriate external fixator set; pin cutters; variable-speed drill; chuck; pointed reduction forceps; bone holding forceps; drill bits and tissue guards if pre-drilling pin holes.

Surgical Approach

A craniolateral approach is used as described in Operative Technique 15.3.

Reduction and Fixation

In comminuted fractures of the diaphysis, the intact shaft on either side of the comminuted area is grasped with self-locking bone holding forceps. Traction is exerted until satisfactory length and alignment of the bone are achieved. The fracture site is disturbed as little as possible, with the fragments being left *in situ* (see Chapter 10). A unilateral external fixator is applied to the craniolateral surface of the bone generally with three pins in the proximal fragment and two in the distal fragment. The distal pin is placed first. If the distal segment is very short then the pin is placed in the transcondylar position; this pin can be safely introduced through a stab incision over the condyle (Figure 15.22a). If the distal segment is long enough, the pin can be placed just proximal to the supratrochlear foramen but this should be done as an open approach so as to identify the radial nerve (Figure 15.16b). The most proximal pin is placed just distal to the greater tuberosity (stab incision). Five clamps are placed on a connecting bar. The proximal and distal clamps are attached to the pins already in place (Figure 15.22b). Fracture alignment is re-checked and, once it is satisfactory, the clamps are tightened to maintain reduction. The three centre pins are then driven into the humerus, using the clamps as guides (Figure 15.22c).

→

OPERATIVE TECHNIQUE 15.6 (CONTINUED)

External fixation: humerus

PRACTICAL TIP
The three central pins are introduced through the main incision or stab incisions adjacent to it, allowing the pins to be safely guided between muscle bellies into the bone.

Final adjustment of the clamps is made and the wound is closed. In potentially infected grade 2 or 3 open fractures, after thorough wound debridement and application of the fixator the wound is only partially closed to allow drainage.

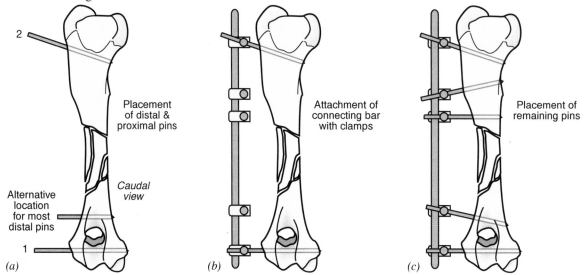

Placement of distal & proximal pins

Caudal view

Alternative location for most distal pins

Attachment of connecting bar with clamps

Placement of remaining pins

(a)   (b)   (c)

Figure 15.22: External fixator used in open and comminuted fractures.

Wound Closure
As in Operative Technique 15.3.

Post-operative Care
Exercise restriction while fixator is in place. Check the frame at weekly intervals to ensure that clamps and/or pins have not loosened and that pin tract infection has not occurred. A loose pin is accompanied by an increase in pin tract discharge and lameness. Replace or remove the pin if necessary. Radiography at 4 and 8 weeks. Remove fixator once healing is complete.

OPERATIVE TECHNIQUE 15.7

Supracondylar fractures of the distal humerus

Positioning
Dorsal recumbency, with the fractured leg pulled cranially.

Assistant
Yes.

Tray Extras
Appropriate intramedullary pins; K-wires; wire for cerclage; pliers/wire twisters; pin/wire cutters; drill; chuck; self-locking bone holding forceps; pointed reduction forceps.

Surgical Approach
A medial approach is used to expose the fracture (Operative Technique 15.4).

> **WARNING**
> **Protect the median and ulnar nerves.**

The skin incision should be made towards the caudal aspect of the elbow to allow skin to be reflected from both sides of the joint.

Reduction and Fixation
The humeral condyles are grasped with pointed reduction forceps; the distal humeral shaft is held with self-locking bone holding forceps; the bone fragments are tilted caudally, toggled against each other, and then pushed cranially until reduction is achieved. If there is a medial oblique supracondylar fragment, small pointed reduction forceps can be used to hold this fragment in reduction with the shaft (Figure 15.23).

Having checked that reduction is possible, the fracture site is hinged open to expose the medullary cavity of the medial supracondylar ridge. An intramedullary pin is retrogradely introduced into the cavity and directed laterally up the humeral shaft to emerge on the lateral side of the greater tuberosity. The Jacobs chuck is then attached to the proximal end of the pin, which is pulled up until just the tip is visible at the fracture surface.

The fracture is reduced and then, with the elbow extended, the pin is driven down into the medial condyle. Finally a K-wire is driven up through the lateral condyle obliquely across the fracture and into the medial cortex of the humerus (Figure 15.23). This second point of fixation prevents rotation. Both pins are cut close to the bone after insertion.

Skeletally immature animals
In skeletally immature animals, the medial cortex is usually fractured obliquely and a lag screw or K-wire can be placed proximal to the growth plate. Crossed K-wires are then inserted to complete fixation (Figure 15.24).

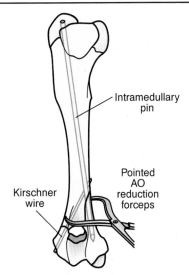

Figure 15.23: Supracondylar fracture of the humerus: fixation using an intramedullary pin and K-wire.

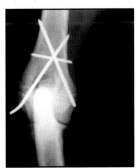

Figure 15.24: Post-operative radiograph of the case shown in Figure 15.8: three K-wires have been used for fixation.

→

OPERATIVE TECHNIQUE 15.7 (CONTINUED)
Supracondylar fractures of the distal humerus

Wound Closure
The deep brachial fascia, subcutaneous tissue and skin are closed in layers.

Post-operative Care
Exercise restriction until fracture healing is complete and pins can be removed.

OPERATIVE TECHNIQUE 15.8

Lateral condylar fractures

Positioning
Lateral recumbency – restraining band placed under axilla and secured to tabletop to help with traction.

Assistant
Optional.

Tray Extras
Appropriate sized bone screw set, drill bits, etc.; K-wires; pin/wire cutters; drill; Gelpi self-retaining retractor; pointed reduction forceps; Vulsellum forceps.

Surgical Approach
A skin incision is made directly over the lateral condyle. The lateral head of the triceps muscle is exposed and the deep fascia along its cranial border is incised (Figure 15.25a). The muscle is retracted to expose the fractured condyle (Figure 15.25b).

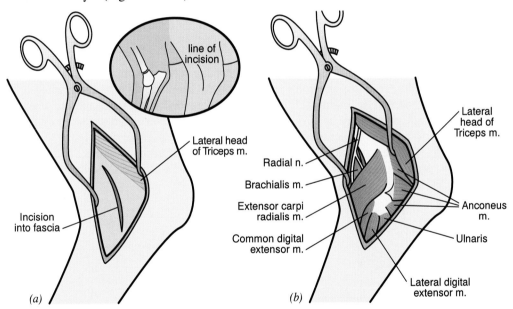

Figure 15.25: Surgical approach for exposure in lateral condylar fractures.

> **WARNING**
> The radial nerve emerges between the lateral head of the triceps and the brachialis muscle just proximal to the incision, but provided dissection is limited to the soft tissues over the lateral condyle and its supracondylar ridge there should be little risk of nerve damage during exposure.

Using a periosteal elevator, any remaining muscle attachments are cleared from the adjacent surfaces of the fractured supracondylar ridge. The condyle is then rotated laterally to allow removal of haematoma and granulation tissue from the intercondylar fracture site.

Reduction and Fixation
The simplest method of reducing the condyle is to exert pressure on the condyle with finger and thumb and then maintain reduction with pointed reduction forceps (Figure 15.26a). The lateral condyle does have a tendency to rotate caudally and application of Allis tissue forceps across the fractured supracondylar ridge helps to prevent this (Figure 15.26b). Alternatively, a K-wire can be used (Figure 15.26c,d).   →

OPERATIVE TECHNIQUE 15.8 (CONTINUED)

Lateral condylar fractures

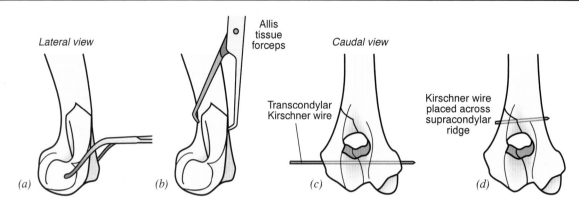

Figure 15.26: Methods of maintaining reduction of lateral condylar fractures during insertion of the transcondylar lag screw.

A transcondylar lag screw and anti-rotational K-wire are used for fixation. There are two methods of preparation of the drill hole for the transcondylar lag screw: outside-in, or inside-out.

Outside-in method

After reduction of the condyle, the drill hole for the transcondylar lag screw is commenced from a point immediately below and just in front of the most prominent point on the lateral condyle and is directed at the corresponding spot on the medial condyle (Figure 15.27a). A cortical screw is usually used; and with this type of screw, the hole in the lateral condyle must be overdrilled to the same diameter as the screw to ensure that the lag effect is achieved as the screw is tightened, giving compression of the fracture site (Figure 15.27b,c). In very young puppies with soft bone, a partially threaded cancellous screw is used for fixation. With this type of screw, only a transcondylar pilot hole is drilled. Provided *all* the threads of the screw grip in the medial condyle, the lag effect will be achieved (Figure 15.27d).

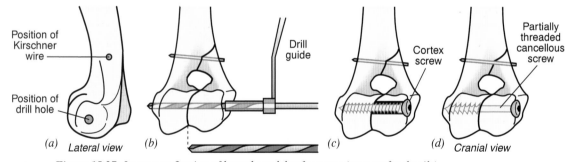

Figure 15.27: Lag screw fixation of lateral condylar fractures (see text for details).

Inside-out method

This is the most accurate. After exposure of the fracture site, completely rotate the lateral condyle out of the incision on its collateral ligament to allow exposure of the fractured trochlea surface. The glide hole for the screw can then be accurately drilled "inside-out', starting in the centre of the fractured trochlea and drilling from this point to the lateral surface of the lateral condyle (Figure 15.28b). The appropriate sized drill sleeve is introduced into the glide hole from the lateral side and the condyle is rotated back into position. A K-wire can now be placed across the supracondylar fracture to maintain reduction and prevent rotation while the lag screw is inserted (Figure 15.28c). The glide hole has already been prepared in the lateral condyle and the drill sleeve is *in situ*. Next, the smaller drill bit, which will be used to prepare the pilot hole, is passed through the sleeve and used to drill the pilot hole in the medial condyle (Figure 15.28c). Length of screw is assessed with a depth gauge, a thread is cut in the pilot hole with a tap (unless a self-tapping screw is used) and then the appropriate size screw is inserted. The K-wire in the supracondylar portion of the fracture is cut off flush with the bone. It is important to have this second point of fixation to prevent rotation of the condyle on the screw (Figure 15.28d).

→

OPERATIVE TECHNIQUE 15.8 (CONTINUED)
Lateral condylar fractures

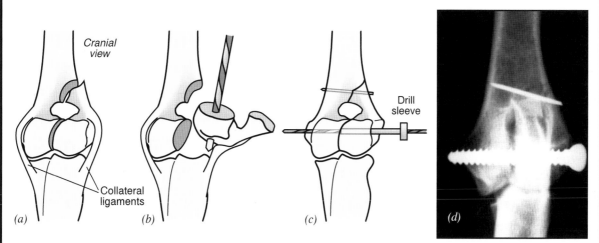

Figure 15.28: *'Inside-out' method of preparing transcondylar screw hole. (a) Fractured condyle. (b) Condyle rotated out laterally on collateral ligament; glide hole drilled from medial to lateral. (c) Fracture is reduced and stabilized with a K-wire; drill sleeve is inserted in glide hole to allow accurate placement of pilot hole through medial condyle. **(d)** Post-operative radiograph of fracture shown in Figure 15.10: fixation with transcondylar lag screw (4.5 mm cortex screw) plus K-wire across supracondylar fracture line to prevent rotation of the condyle.*

PRACTICAL TIP
Provided the fracture of the supracondylar ridge is accurately reduced, it can be assumed that reduction of the intercondylar fracture is also adequate.

Wound Closure
The deep fascia, subcutaneous tissue and skin are closed in layers.

Post-operative Care
A support bandage is applied for 5 days. Movement of the joint is important following repair of any articular fracture – to minimize stiffness and encourage nutrition and healing of articular cartilage. Gentle passive flexion and extension of the joint and controlled exercise should be recommended. Restrict exercise to 10-minute walks on a leash only for 4 to 6 weeks. Implants are generally left *in situ*.

OPERATIVE TECHNIQUE 15.9
Medial condylar fractures

Positioning
Lateral recumbency with affected leg down. The upper forelimb is pulled well caudally.

Assistant
Optional.

Tray Extras
As for Operative Technique 15.8.

Surgical Approach
As for Operative Technique 15.4.

Reduction and Fixation
The comments for lateral condylar fractures apply here also. However, the medial fragment is often large enough to accept two lag screws placed from medial to lateral; one transcondylar and one proximal to the supratrochlear foramen (Figure 15.29a,b).

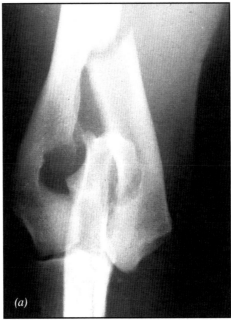 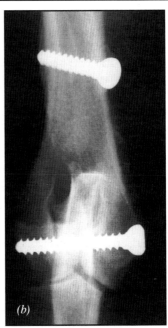

Figure 15.29: (a) Pre-operative radiograph of 4-year-old German Pointer with medial condylar fracture. (b) Follow-up radiograph taken 3 months after the fracture was stabilized with two lag screws (4.5 cortex screws).

Wound Closure
The deep brachial fascia, subcutaneous tissue and skin are closed in layers.

Post-operative Care
As for Operative Technique 15.8.

OPERATIVE TECHNIQUE 15.10
Intercondylar fractures

Positioning
Dorsal recumbency with the affected leg pulled cranially.

Assistant
Essential.

Tray Extras
Appropriate sized plate and screw set, drill bits, etc.; K-wires; tension-band wire; pin/wire cutters; pliers/wire twisters; drill; Gelpi and Hohmann retractors; self-locking bone holding forceps; pointed reduction forceps; Vulsellum forceps; hacksaw or gigli wire.

Surgical Approach
A skin incision is made over the caudolateral aspect of the elbow; the subcutaneous fat and fascia are incised and undermined to allow reflection of skin from both sides of the elbow. Fascia along the cranial border of the medial head of the triceps are incised and the ulnar nerve is identified and retracted from the olecranon (Figure 15.30a). The cranial margin of the lateral head of the triceps is also freed from its fascial attachments. The proximal shaft of the ulna is exposed by separating the flexor carpi ulnaris and extensor carpi ulnaris muscles.

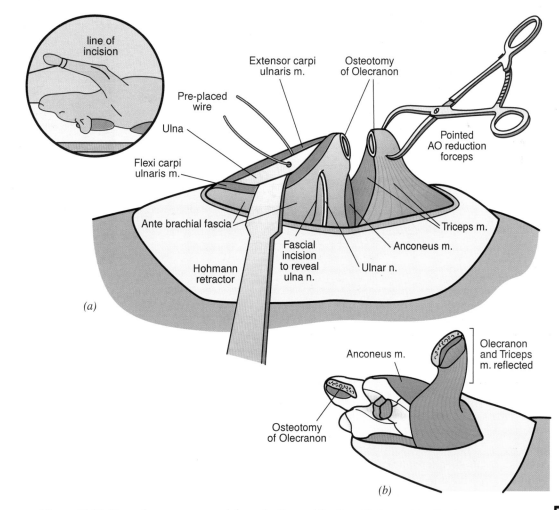

Figure 15.30: *Transolecranon approach for reduction and fixation of intercondylar fractures.*

→

OPERATIVE TECHNIQUE 15.10 (CONTINUED)
Intercondylar fractures

A hole is drilled tranversely through the ulna with a 2 mm drill just distal to the elbow; a length of orthopaedic wire (18 or 20 gauge) is passed through the hole, and fashioned into a loop. This wire will be used later as a tension band but at this stage it makes a useful handle for an assistant to exert traction on the ulna during exposure and reduction of the humeral condyles (Figure 15.30a). If a screw is to be used to repair the olecranon osteotomy, the screw hole should be prepared and tapped prior to osteotomy.

Transverse osteotomy of the olecranon is performed with a saw or gigli wire distal to the tendon of insertion of the triceps on the olecranon and proximal to the anconeal process. Protect the ulnar nerve during this procedure. The olecranon is reflected dorsally with the attached triceps muscle mass; remnants of the anconeus and joint capsule are refected from the caudal aspect of the elbow to complete exposure of the condyles (Figure 15.30b).

Reduction and Fixation
The condyles are reduced, ensuring accurate reconstruction of the articular surface. The assistant exerts traction on the ulnar wire to steady the elbow. The medial condylar fragment is held with small bone holding forceps while the lateral condyle is aligned in its normal position with the medial condyle and held in reduction with pointed reduction forceps. The proximal ends of the condylar fragments are transfixed with a K-wire (Figure 15.31b). In fracture types I and II, a lag screw can be used instead, if the fragments are large enough. Once this area has been stabilized, the articular margins of the fracture can be checked again and final adjustments in reduction made before inserting a transcondylar lag screw from lateral to medial (see lateral condylar fracture repair) (Figure 15.31c).

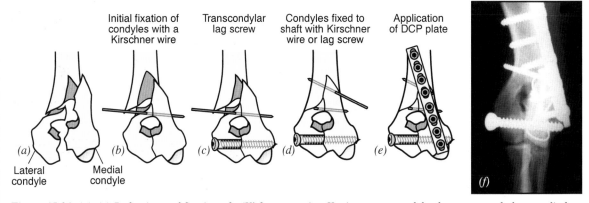

Figure 15.31: (a)–(e) Reduction and fixation of a 'Y' fracture using K-wires, transcondylar lag screw and plate applied to medial supracondylar ridge of the humerus. (f) Three-month follow-up craniocaudal radiograph of a Springer Spaniel that had a 'Y' fracture. Fixation had been achieved using a transcondylar lag screw (4.5 cortex screw), supracondylar lag screw (2.7 cortex) and a plate (8-hole 3.5 DCP) applied to medial supracondylar ridge.

The distal shaft of the humerus is grasped with self-locking bone holding forceps while the condyles are grasped with pointed reduction forceps. Reduction of the supracondylar portion of the fracture is then achieved by a combination of direct traction and toggling the fracture surfaces against each other. If possible, the condyles are temporarily attached to the shaft at this stage with a K-wire placed obliquely across the supracondylar fracture line (Figure 15.31d).

A plate (3.5 or 2.7 DCP) is then applied to the caudal aspect of the medial supracondylar ridge. This is a flat surface and the plate should require little or no contouring (Figure 15.31e,f). If a K-wire is not used: having ensured that it is possible to reduce the supracondylar fracture site, disengage the fragments and rotate the medial condyle laterally so that the medial supracondylar ridge is easily visible. Attach the distal end of the plate to the caudal aspect of the medial condylar ridge. It is usually possible to place three screws, especially if a 2.7 DCP is used for fixation, but take care that the most distal screws do not penetrate

→

OPERATIVE TECHNIQUE 15.10 (CONTINUED)
Intercondylar fractures

the articular surface. Having attached the plate, the free proximal end of the plate can be used as a lever arm to complete reduction of the fracture site: hold the plate against the bone with self-locking bone holding forceps while the first two screws are inserted proximal to the fracture site. Once stability is achieved, the forceps can be removed and the rest of the screws placed. In large dogs a second, smaller plate can be applied to the lateral supracondylar ridge to improve stability (Figure 15.32). In young puppies, pins or K-wires can be used to attach the condyles to the shaft, but plate fixation gives the best results.

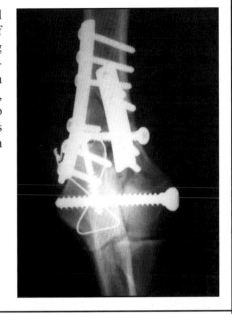

Figure 15.32: Post-operative craniocaudal radiograph of a 4-year-old German Shepherd Dog with a "T" fracture. The fracture has been stabilized with a transcondylar lag screw (4.5 mm cortex screw) and two plates on the supracondylar ridges (6-hole 2.7 DCP medially, 4-hole 2.7 DCP laterally).

Wound Closure
The olecranon osteotomy is repaired with a lag screw (Figure 15.33) or two K-wires are used in combination with the pre-placed ulna wire which is used as a tension band. The lag screw is preferred as it causes less soft tissue interference and can usually be left *in situ*. The K-wires, by contrast, may loosen – causing local soft tissue problems – and will require removal.

The olecranon is reduced and the lag screw is inserted down the long axis of the olecranon, using the prepared drill hole. The screw is not fully tightened at this stage. The proximal end of the ulna wire loop is cut off; the two ends of the wire are crossed in a figure-of-eight and brought over the caudal edge of the olecranon. One end of the wire is passed through the insertion of the triceps, keeping close to the bone and taking care to ensure that the wire will be anchored under the screw head. The wire is then brought down to one side of the olecranon, where it is twisted tight with the other free end of wire

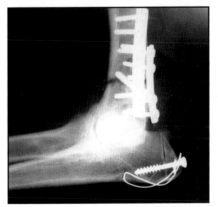

Figure 15.33: Lateral view of Figure 15.32 showing a 4 mm cancellous screw + tension-band wire used for repair of the olecranon osteotomy.

to complete the proximal loop of the tension band. (Because the wire tension band is bridging such a short osteotomy, it is possible to get good tension by placing twists in one side only rather than placing twists on either side of the olecranon.) After the tension band has been completed, the lag screw is tightened. The triceps fascia is repaired on both lateral and medial sides (avoid the ulnar nerve in sutures on the medial side). The rest of the wound closure is routine.

Post-operative Care
A Robert Jones bandage is applied for 5 days post-operatively to provide support and to control post-operative swelling; otherwise management is as described for lateral condylar fractures. Implants are generally left *in situ* unless loosening causes soft tissue problems. The proximal ends of K-wires used for repair of olecranon osteotomy are the most common problem but once these wires have been removed any associated lameness tends to resolve.

CHAPTER SIXTEEN

Radius and Ulna

Warrick J. Bruce

INTRODUCTION

Fractures of the radius and ulna constitute 8.5% to 17.3% of all fractures seen in the dog and cat (Sumner-Smith and Cawley, 1970; Phillips, 1979). They result from many types of trauma, including road traffic accidents, gunshot accidents, falls from heights, kicks, bites and crushing injuries. In some small breeds, they can be seen following minimal trauma. Pathological fractures secondary to neoplasia or metabolic bone disease may also occur.

Fractures of the radius and ulna are associated with a relatively high incidence of complications (Vaughan, 1964; DeAngelis *et al*, 1973). These include delayed union, non-union, malunion, osteomyelitis, and angular deformities due to growth plate damage. The radius and ulna account for around half of all cases of long bone fracture non-union recorded in the dog (Vaughan, 1964; Sumner-Smith and Cawley, 1970; Atilola and Sumner-Smith, 1984). Toy and miniature breeds have a disproportionately high incidence of delayed and non-unions (Sumner-Smith, 1974). Problems are also encountered in large and giant breeds of dog due to the large forces placed on fractures and fixation devices in the antebrachium.

PROXIMAL ULNA

All fractures in this area require open reduction and internal fixation to counteract the powerful traction of the triceps group of muscles. These forces are equalized by use of the tension-band principle (Chapter 9).

Simple fractures through the semi-lunar notch
See Figure 16.1 and Operative Technique 16.1.

Avulsion fracture of the olecranon
See Figure 16.2 and Operative Technique 16.1.

Comminuted fracture of the proximal ulna with fracture of the anconeal process
See Figure 16.3 and Operative Technique 16.2.

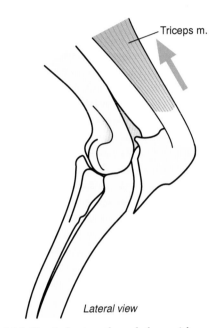

Figure 16.1: *Simple fracture through the semi-lunar notch of the ulna.*

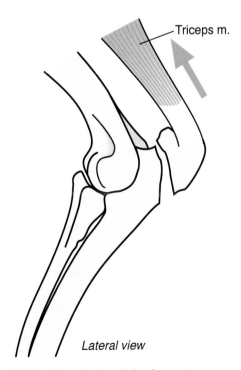

Figure 16.2: *Avulsion fracture of the olecranon.*

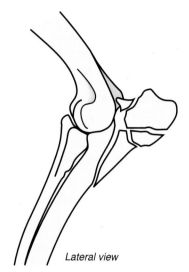

Figure 16.3: Comminuted fracture of the proximal ulna.

Fractures of the ulna with concurrent dislocation of the radial head

Fracture of the proximal third of the ulna and anterior dislocation of the proximal epiphysis of the radius (Figure 16.4) was first described in humans by Monteggia (1814). A spectrum of injuries (Monteggia lesion) can result in dislocation of the elbow joint and fracture of the ulna and these have been classified on the basis of direction of the dislocation and the angulation of the ulnar fracture (Bado, 1962; Schwarz and Schrader, 1984).

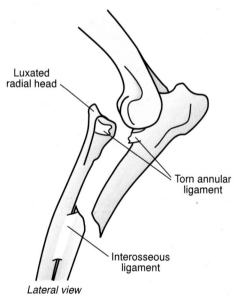

Figure 16.4: Type I Monteggia fracture.

All fracture-dislocations of this nature are rare, but cranial dislocation of the radial head, with cranial angulation of the fractured ulna (type I Monteggia lesion) was found to be the most common in dogs and cats (Schwarz and Schrader, 1984). It has been proposed that this injury is caused by a direct blow to the olecranon when the antebrachium is extended and weightbearing (Wadsworth, 1981). Displacement of

the radial head occurs as a result of tearing of the annular ligaments and contracture of the biceps brachii and brachialis muscles. In some cases separation of the radius and ulnar diaphysis occurs secondary to rupture of the interosseous ligament.

In recent injuries, where the interosseus ligament remains intact, a closed reduction and closed normograde insertion of a pin in the ulna may be attempted. However, this is frequently difficult to achieve and open reduction with internal fixation is required (see Operative Technique 16.3).

PROXIMAL RADIUS

These fractures are uncommon as the weaker lateral humeral condyle often fractures first, thus sparing the proximal radius. When they do occur, they are often articular and can be associated with fractures of the ulna and dislocation of the elbow joint.

Salter–Harris Type I fracture

Fractures through this metaphyseal growth plate (Figure 16.5) require open reduction if there is significant fracture displacement and reduction cannot be accomplished by closed means (Operative Technique 16.4).

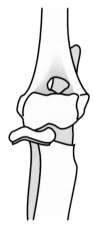

Figure 16.5: Salter–Harris Type 1 fracture of the proximal radius.

Articular fractures

These generally require accurate anatomical reduction and fixation with lag screws and K-wires, depending on the size of the fracture fragments (Operative Technique 16.4).

Comminuted fractures of the proximal radius

Comminuted fractures in this area are difficult to manage and require a wide dissection (Bloomberg, 1983). Salvage procedures such as ostectomy of the radial head (Prymak and Bennett, 1986) and elbow joint arthrodesis have been advocated for non-reconstructable fractures of the radial head (Bloomberg, 1983).

The prognosis depends on the type of fracture and the accuracy of reconstruction. Metaphyseal growth plate fractures heal quickly and carry the best prognosis. However, premature closure of the growth plate and short radius syndrome is a potential complication. Elbow joint osteoarthritis is a common sequel to fractures of the proximal radius.

RADIAL AND ULNAR DIAPHYSES

These fractures most commonly affect the middle and distal third and frequently involve both bones. Isolated fractures affecting the shafts of either bone are less common (Phillips, 1979; Ness and Armstrong, 1995). Table 16.1 suggests appropriate treatments.

Procedure	Comments
Casts or splints	Treatments with casts or splints should be reserved for closed fractures involving only one bone, incomplete fractures, or minimally displaced transverse, spiral or oblique fractures that are relatively stable.
Bone plating Operative Technique 16.5	Plate fixation can be used for most radial diaphyseal fractures in dogs and cats. It is the preferred method of treatment for non-unions, delayed unions and distal fractures in miniature and toy breeds of dogs.
External fixation Operative Technique 16.6	The external fixator is appropriate for the repair of nearly all diaphyseal fractures of the radius and ulna. It is particularly suitable for the treatment of severely comminuted fractures and open fractures with soft tissue loss.
Intramedullary pinning	This method of fixation is not recommended for fractures of the radius.

Table 16.1: Decision making in the management of radial and ulnar diaphyseal fractures.

External support

Many fractures of the radius and ulna of the dog and cat are amenable to treatment with casts or splints if adequate closed reduction can be attained and maintained. The surgeon should aim for at least 25% end-to-end fracture segment contact with no angulation (Lappin *et al.*, 1982). In some cases a limited open approach may be required to align the fragments adequately. Best results are achieved in young (less than 1 year) medium-sized dogs (Lappin *et al.*, 1983).

> **WARNING**
> **Casts and splints should not be used as the sole means of support in giant breeds, nor should they be used for distal fractures of the radius and ulna in miniature and toy breeds of dogs.**

Care must be taken in small dogs and cats as fracture alignment is often difficult due to small bone diameter, poor soft tissue support, and tension in the carpal and digital flexor muscles which tend to displace the fragments. In addition there are technical difficulties in applying lightweight casts of suitable strength that do not slip distally in these animals (Chapter 7).

Bone plating

Bone plating is a popular method of fixation for fractures of the radius and ulna. The natural flattening and cranial curvature of the radius make its dorsal (tension) surface ideal for plate application. Both compression and neutralization plates have been used with success (Lappin *et al.*, 1983).

In most dogs and cats only the radius is plated and fixation of the ulna is unnecessary. Plating both the radius and ulna is recommended in large and giant breeds of dog because of their large size and the extreme forces placed on the fixation devices (Lappin *et al.*, 1983; Brinker *et al.*, 1990).

External fixation

The external fixator can be applied following closed or limited open reduction. It may be used alone or as an adjunct to some form of internal fixation such as lag screws or cerclage wires.

All configurations (unilateral, bilateral, biplanar) have been used successfully in the antebrachium. The unilateral uniplanar design is the simplest to apply, has the lowest complication rate and is adequate for the majority of cases.

Intramedullary pinning

Intramedullary pinning of the radius is not recommended due to the high complication rates associated with this technique (Lappin *et al.*, 1983). The radius is less amenable to pinning compared with the ulna and other long bones as it has a relatively straight oval-shaped medullary canal which is bounded by articular cartilage at both ends.

This means that both the elbow and the antebrachiocarpal joints are endangered when pinning and only small diameter pins may be used. An intramedullary pin poorly resists rotational instability and axial compression and potentially damages the endosteal vessels to a bone with a tenuous distal blood supply. There are better methods of radial fracture fixation available.

Fractures of the distal third of the radius and ulnar diaphyses in miniature and toy breeds

These fractures are associated with a disproportionately high incidence of delayed and non-unions (Sumner-Smith, 1974). The main reason for this phenomenon is thought to be inadequate immobilization, but factors such as infection, delays in fracture stabilization and the tenuous blood supply to the bones may also be contributory (Sumner-Smith and Cawley, 1970; Hunt *et al.*, 1980; Bartels, 1987; Eger, 1990).

Rigid stabilization is mandatory and plating with mini plates or mini T-plates is recommended (Figure 16.6). Bone plate removal is also recommended as a number of cases have been observed where the radius has re-fractured at the proximal end of the plate several years later as a result of local loss of bone strength. It is the author's policy to remove these plates between 6 months and 1 year post-operatively. Earlier plate removal and cancellous bone grafting has been recommended (Lesser, 1986). The limb must be supported in a Robert Jones bandage for 1 to 2 weeks following plate removal and the dog's activity restricted for 4 weeks.

An effective and economical alternative to bone plating is to use transfixation pins and acrylic cement (Figure 16.7) (Eger, 1990; Tomlinson and Constantinescu, 1991). To ensure accurate reduction, a limited open approach is recommended. K-wires are driven transversely through the radius above and below the fracture and the exposed ends of the wires are

bonded together on either side of the limb. Staged disassembly may be performed from 9 to 12 weeks post-operatively.

DISTAL RADIUS AND ULNA

Fractures of the distal radius and ulna are common and frequently occur following falls from heights. Open fractures tend to occur in this area as there is little soft tissue protection.

Many fixation methods have been used to repair distal antebrachial fractures, including external coaptation alone or in combination with lag screws, crossed K-wires or pins and cerclage wire (Gambardella and Griffiths, 1984), internal fixation with Rush pins, T-plates, hook plates (Bellah, 1987) and external fixation. The ultimate choice of fixation technique depends on the size of the bone, the nature of the fracture, the facilities available and the financial resources of the owner.

Salter–Harris Type I fractures

Fractures of the distal radial and ulna metaphyseal growth plates are common in the immature animal and can result in premature closure of these growth plates (Chapter 11). Fracture through the distal radial growth plate is usually accompanied by fracture of the distal ulna or its growth plate (Figure 16.8). Early closed reduction should be attempted and stable fractures can

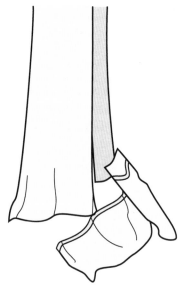

Figure 16.8: Salter–Harris Type I fracture of the distal radius with concurrent fracture of the distal ulna.

be managed with external coaptation for three weeks. Less stable or irreducible fractures require open reduction and the fracture should be stabilized using cross or parallel pinning techniques (Operative Technique 16.7).

Styloid fractures

Avulsion fractures of the radial or ulnar styloid processes give rise to instability of the antebrachiocarpal

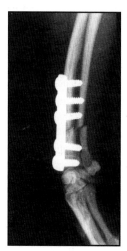

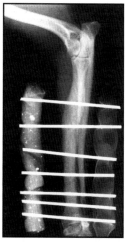

Figure 16.6: Distal antebrachial fracture in a 1.2kg Chihuahua repaired with a 5 hole 2 mm plate on the cranial radius.

Figure 16.7: Distal antebrachial fracture in a 4.5kg Poodle repaired with a bilateral external fixator comprising full non-threaded pins and methylmethacrylate connecting bars.

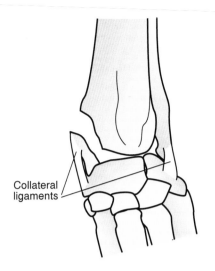

Collateral
ligaments

Figure 16.9: Avulsion fracture of radial styloid process with resultant instability of the antebrachiocarpal joint.

joint as the collateral ligaments originate on the styloid processes (Figure 16.9). These fractures may occur in association with subluxation or luxation of this joint and should be accurately repaired by internal fixation (Operative Technique 16.8).

Articular fractures

Articular fractures require perfect anatomical reduction to minimize secondary osteoarthritis. The articular surface is repaired with lag screws or K-wires, depending on the size of the fragment(s). In comminuted fractures the distal fragments are then aligned and reattached to the radial metaphysis by means of a bone plate. Hook and T-plates are most useful in this location. A cranial approach is used as described in Operative Technique 16.7.

REFERENCES AND FURTHER READING

Atilola MAO and Sumner-Smith G (1984) Non-union fractures in dogs. *Journal of Veterinary Orthopaedics* **3**, 21.

Bado JL (1962) *The Monteggia Lesion.* CC Thomas, Springfield.

Bartels KE (1987) Non-union. *Veterinary Clinics of North America* **17**, 799.

Bellah JR (1987) Use of a double hook plate for treatment of a distal radial fracture in a dog. *Veterinary Surgery* **16**, 278.

Bloomberg MS (1983) Fractures of the radius and ulna. In: *Current Techniques in Small Animal Surgery*, 2nd edn, ed. MJ Bojrab. Lea and Febiger, Philadelphia.

Brinker WO, Piermattei DL and Flo GL (1990) Fractures of the radius and ulna. In: *Handbook of Small Animal Orthopaedics and Fracture Treatment*, 2nd edn. WB Saunders, Philadelphia.

DeAngelis MP, Olds RB, Stoll SG *et al.* (1973) Repair of fractures of the radius and ulna in small dogs. *Journal of the American Animal Hospital Association* **19**, 436.

Denny HR (1990) Pectoral limb fractures. In: *Canine Orthopaedics*, 2nd edn, ed. WG Whittick. Lea and Febiger, Philadelphia.

Eger CE (1990) A technique for the management of radial and ulnar fractures in miniature dogs using transfixation pins. *Journal of Small Animal Practice* **31**, 377.

Egger EL (1990) External skeletal fixation. In: *Current Techniques in Small Animal Surgery*, 3rd edn, ed. MJ Bojrab, SJ Brichard and JL Tomlinson Jr. Lea and Febiger, Philadelphia.

Gambardella PC and Griffiths RC (1984) A technique for repair of oblique fractures of the distal radius in dogs. *Journal of the American Animal Hospital Association* **20**, 429.

Hunt JM, Aitken ML, Denny HR and Gibbs C (1980) The complications of diaphyseal fractures in dogs: a review of 100 cases. *Journal of Small Animal Practice* **21**, 103.

Lappin MR, Aron DN, Herron HL and Malnati G (1983) Fractures of the radius and ulna in the dog. *Journal of the American Animal Hospital Association* **19**, 643.

Lesser AS (1986) Cancellous bone grafting at plate removal to counteract stress protection. *Journal of the American Veterinary Medical Association* **189**, 696.

Marti JM and Miller A (1994) Delimitation of safe corridors for the insertion of external fixator pins in the dog. 2: Forelimb. *Journal of Small Animal Practice* **35**, 78.

Miller A (1994) The carpus. In: *Manual of Small Animal Arthrology*, ed. JEF Houlton and RW Collinson, pp. 211–233. British Small Animal Veterinary Association, Cheltenham, Gloucestershire.

Monteggia GB (1814) *Instituzioni Chirurgiche*, 2nd edn. G. Masper, Milan.

Ness MG and Armstrong NJ (1995) Isolated fracture of the radial diaphysis in dogs. *Journal of Small Animal Practice* **36**, 252.

Phillips IR (1979) A survey of bone fracture in the dog and cat. *Journal of Small Animal Practice* **20**, 661.

Piermattei, DL (1993) *An Atlas of Surgical Approaches to the Bones and Joints of the Dog and Cat, 3rd edn.* WB Saunders, Philadelphia.

Prymak C and Bennett D (1986) Excision arthroplasty of the humeroradial joint. *Journal of Small Animal Practice* **27**, 307.

Schwarz PD and Schrader SC (1984) Ulnar fracture and dislocation of the proximal radial epiphysis (Monteggia lesion) in the dog and cat: a review of 28 cases. *Journal of the American Veterinary Medical Association* **184**, 190.

Sumner-Smith G (1974) A comparative investigation into the healing of fractures in miniature Poodles and mongrel dogs. *Journal of Small Animal Practice* **15**, 323.

Sumner-Smith G and Cawley AJ (1970) Non-union fractures in the dog. *Journal of Small Animal Practice* **11**, 311.

Tomlinson JL and Constantinescu GM (1991) Acrylic external skeletal fixation of fractures. *Continuing Education Article No. 6*, **13**, 2, 235.

Vaughan LC (1964) A clinical study of non-union fractures in the dog. *Journal of Small Animal Practice* **5**, 173.

Wadsworth P (1981) Biomechanics of the luxation of joints. In: *Pathophysiology in Small Animal Surgery*, ed. MJ Bojrab. Lea and Febiger, Philadelphia.

OPERATIVE TECHNIQUE 16.1
Fractures through the semi-lunar notch and avulsion fractures of the olecranon

Positioning
Dorsal recumbency with the affected limb extended cranially (Figure 16.10).

Assistant
Ideally.

Tray Extras
K-wires; chuck; air or electric drill and bits; pin/wire cutters; pliers; Kern bone holding forceps (or pointed reduction forceps); periosteal elevator; ± appropriate bone plating and screw set; ± ASIF 2.0 mm parallel drill guide.

Surgical Approach
Making a caudomedial incision over the olecranon has several advantages: it allows for identification of the ulnar nerve; the skin is thinner in this area and therefore heals with less scarring; and the incision is hidden from view. The skin is reflected laterally and the underlying flexor carpi ulnaris, anconeus and ulnaris lateralis muscles are elevated from the ulna (Figure 16.10).

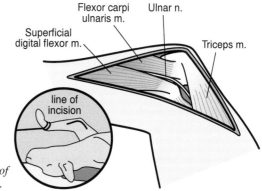

Figure 16.10:
Caudal exposure of the proximal ulna.

Reduction and Fixation
The proximal ulna is held with Kern bone holding forceps and the first pin is driven in a retrograde fashion from the fracture surface to emerge at the point of the elbow (Figure 16.11a). The pin is then backed out until its tip is level with the fracture surface. With the patient's elbow held **in extension**, the fracture is accurately reduced and the pin is driven in a normograde direction to anchor in the cranial cortex of the ulna (Figure 16.11b). A second, more caudal pin may be placed parallel to the first using a parallel drill guide (Figure 16.11c).

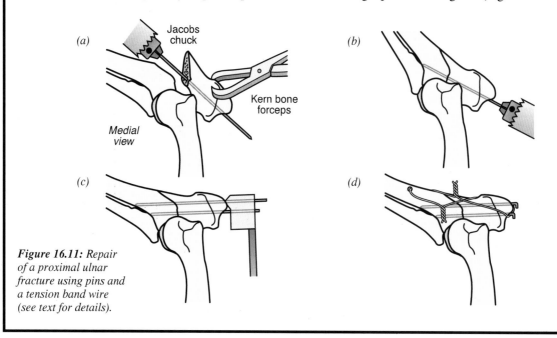

Figure 16.11: Repair of a proximal ulnar fracture using pins and a tension band wire (see text for details).

→

OPERATIVE TECHNIQUE 16.1 (CONTINUED)
Fractures through the semi-lunar notch and avulsion fractures of the olecranon

PRACTICAL TIPS
It is easiest to power-drive small diameter arthrodesis or K-wires using an air or electric drill. Larger Steinmann pins may be placed by hand, using a Jacobs chuck.

When placing larger diameter pins by hand it is often easier, and more precise, to pre-drill a pilot hole using a smaller diameter drill bit.

A hole is then drilled transversely through the ulna 1 to 2 cm distal to the fracture. A length of stainless steel wire is passed through the hole and its free ends are crossed. Similarly, a length of wire is passed around the caudal aspect of the olecranon cranial to the pins. The ends of the two wires are then twisted together alternately until the tension band is tight.

WARNING
The proximal loop of the tension-band wire must pass as close as possible to the bone to avoid pressure necrosis at the triceps tendon insertion.

Finally, the pins are bent in a caudal direction close to the end of the olecranon and are cut, leaving a small hook. Each pin is twisted 180° cranially so that the bent end of the cranial pin lies over the tension-band wire (Figure 16.11d).

The diameter of the pins is based on the size of the animal and the ability to place two pins parallel to each other in the ulna. In small dogs and cats, a single pin placed within the intramedullary canal and a wire tension-band is often sufficient. However, if this technique is used, the fracture should be oblique and interlocking to prevent rotational instability, and the pin should extend the length of the proximal third of the ulnar diaphysis.

Stainless steel wire of 0.8 mm diameter is sufficient in cats and toy dogs; larger dogs require wire of 1–1.2 mm diameter.

WARNING
Note the lateral curvature and narrow intramedullary canal of the proximal ulna. Care must be taken to avoid exiting through the side of the ulna or entering the elbow joint when driving pins in this area.

Care must be taken to identify and protect the branch of the ulnar nerve that courses near the medial humero-ulnar articulation.

Wound Closure
Routine. Periosteum and deep fascia can be closed as one layer.

Post-operative Care
A light dressing is applied for a few days and passive elbow flexion/extension exercises should be encouraged post-operatively. Exercise should be controlled for 4 to 6 weeks. On occasions the pins may loosen, or their protruding ends may cause soft tissue irritation; this would necessitate removal once fracture healing is complete.

Alternative Technique
In medium-sized to large breeds of dogs, place the fragments under compression using a lagged cortical or cancellous screw in combination with a pin and tension-band wire (see Figure 15.33).

OPERATIVE TECHNIQUE 16.2
Comminuted fractures of the proximal ulna and fractures of the anconeal process

Positioning
Dorsal recumbancy with the affected limb extended cranially. The contralateral limb is pulled caudally and secured.

Assistant
Ideally.

Tray Extras
Air or electric drill and bits; Kern bone holding forceps; pointed reduction forceps; periosteal elevator; West or Gelpi self retaining retractors; Hohmann retractor; semitubular plate or DCP (3.5 for large and medium-sized dogs, 2.7 for small breeds, 4.5 for giant breeds); appropriate bone plating and screw set; plate benders.

Approach
A caudomedial approach to the ulna is made (see Operative Technique 16.1). The incision may need to be extended distally to allow plate application to the ulnar diaphysis.

Reduction and Fixation
The anconeal process should first be reduced and fixed to the olecranon in cases complicated by its fracture. A screw is placed in a lagged fashion, either from the caudal aspect of the olecranon into the anconeal process, or by countersinking an intra-articular screw caudal to the articular surface of the anconeal process. Alternatively it may be excised if it cannot be lag screwed back (Denny, 1990).

A DCP or semitubular plate may be applied to the caudal aspect, or tension-band surface of the ulna. In this position, the plate acts as a tension band and resists the pull of the triceps muscle. In cases where accurate anatomical reduction is impossible, the plate acts as a buttress preventing fracture collapse. Bone plates can be applied to the caudolateral surface in cases where the width of the ulna is too small to accommodate bone screws.

A bone plate is then contoured and applied to the proximal fragment first. At least two bone screws should be placed in the proximal fragment (see Figure 16.14). Where there is a small proximal fragment, the plate is contoured around the point of the elbow. In giant breeds a hook plate may be useful.

The fracture is reduced with the elbow joint extended and bone holding forceps are used to fix the plate to the distal fragment prior to screw placement. Smaller fragments are held in position with lag screws or small K-wires.

Accurate anatomical reduction of any articular components is essential to minimize secondary osteoarthritis.

> **WARNING**
> **Care must be taken to avoid placing screws through the articular surface of the semi-lunar notch.**

Wound Closure
Routine. Periosteum and deep fascia can be closed as one layer.

Post-operative Care
A Robert Jones bandage is used for a few days to limit swelling. Early use of the elbow should be encouraged with passive range of motion exercises and controlled walking. If fixation is tenuous or bony defects remain at the fracture site then it is safest to maintain elbow motion without weight bearing by using a carpal flexion bandage.

→

OPERATIVE TECHNIQUE 16.3

Fractures of the ulna with concurrent dislocation of the radial head (Monteggia lesion)

Positioning
The patient is positioned in dorsal recumbency with the affected limb extended cranially.

Assistant
Ideally.

Tray Extras
Periosteal elevator, pointed reduction forceps, Gelpi self-retaining retractors, Hohmann retractors; chuck; K-wires, pliers, pin cutters, ± drill, ± appropriate plate and screw set, drill bits etc.

Surgical Approach
A combination of a lateral approach to the elbow joint (see Operative Technique 16.4) and caudal approach to the ulna (see Operative Technique 16.1) is made to expose the fracture–dislocation.

Reduction and Fixation
The radial head is reduced by sliding it medially over the lateral humeral condyle with the elbow held in flexion. Reduction of the radial head is frequently complicated by the interposition of soft tissues, bone fragments, or an organized blood clot. Reduction is maintained using pointed reduction forceps (Figure 16.12). Where possible, the torn annular ligaments are sutured with polydiaxanone. In adult animals, the author prefers to fix the radial head securely to the ulna using a bone screw (medium to large size dogs) (see Figure 16.13a) or small pin (small dogs and cats) (see Figure 16.13b). An alternative means of fixation is to use a full or hemicerclage wire to maintain anatomical reduction of the radius. The ulna may be stabilized by a number of methods depending on the location and type of pin; more proximal fractures require pin and tension-band wire fixation (see Figure 16.13b). Comminuted fractures usually require bone plate fixation (see Figure 16.14).

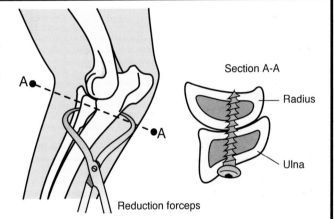

Figure 16.12: Managing Monteggia fractures. Once reduced, the radial head can be temporarily held in position using pointed reduction forceps. The cross-section shows the position of a transfixing screw to maintain the reduction during healing.

WARNING
Neurological injuries are commonly associated with this type of fracture in man and have been reported in dogs (Schwarz and Schrader, 1984).

WARNING
Transfixing the radial head to the ulna in an immature animal may interfere with the independent growth of the radius and ulna and result in elbow joint incongruity and angular limb deformities.

→

OPERATIVE TECHNIQUE 16.3 (CONTINUED)
Fractures of the ulna with concurrent dislocation of the radial head (Monteggia lesion)

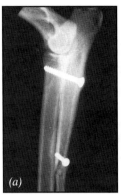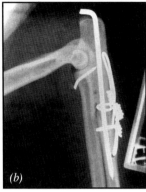

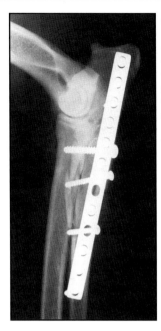

Figure 16.14: Repair of a Type I Monteggia fracture in a 35 kg Deerhound. The radius has been secured to the ulna using transfixion screws (most proximal). The comminuted ulnar shaft fracture has been partially reconstructed with lag screws and buttressed with a caudolateral plate.

Figure 16.13: (a) Repair of a Type I Monteggia fracture in a 16 kg Border Collie using a transfixing screw to maintain reduction of the radial head. The oblique fracture of the ulnar diaphysis was repaired with a lag screw. (b) Repair of a Type I Monteggia fracture in a cat. The radius has been secured to the ulna using a K-wire and the ulnar shaft has been repaired using an intramedullary pin and a tension band wire with two additional cerclage wires.

Wound closure
Routine. Periosteum and deep fasia can be closed as one layer.

Post-operative care
The limb should be supported in a padded dressing or cast in slight flexion for 2 to 3 weeks post-operatively. Transfixing screws and pins should be removed 3 to 4 weeks post-operatively.

Prognosis
Guarded due to the high incidence of post-operative complications, such as non-union of ulna, reluxation of radial head, traumatic periarticular ossification, osteoarthritis, reduced elbow joint range in motion, nerve damage, osteomyelitis, implant migration and synostosis (Schwarz and Schrader, 1984). The prognosis is better in cases where the interosseus attachments of the radius to the ulna are preserved.

OPERATIVE TECHNIQUE 16.4

Fractures of the proximal radius

Positioning

Dorsal recumbency with the affected limb extended caudally. The contralateral limb is pulled caudally and secured (Figure 16.15).

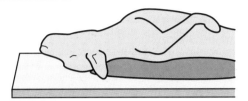

Figure 16.15: Repair of proximal radial fractures: patient positioning.

Assistant

Ideally.

Tray Extras

Periosteal elevator; pointed reduction forceps; Hohmannn retractor; Gelpi self-retaining retractors; chuck; pin/wire cutters; pliers; wire benders; ± air or electric drill and bits; K-wires; ± appropriate bone plating and screw set.

Approach

A lateral approach to the elbow joint is used to expose the radial head (Figure 16.16). The origin of the common digital extensor muscle may be incised and retracted and the supinator muscle may be elevated off the radius for better exposure.

For articular fractures, the origins of the three extensor muscles may be included in an osteotomy of the lateral humeral condyle (Piermattei, 1993). Transection of the annular and collateral ligaments may also be necessary to gain adequate exposure.

Comminuted fractures require a wide dissection and a bilateral approach to the elbow joint can be used.

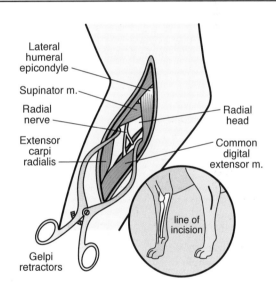

Figure 16.16: Repair of proximal radial fractures: lateral exposure of the proximal radius.

Reduction and Fixation

Fractures in this area are reduced with the elbow flexed. Metaphyseal growth plate fractures are stabilized with a K-wire driven from the proximolateral surface of the radial head near the articular surface, across the fracture, to anchor in the medial cortex of the radius. A second K-wire inserted in a similar direction or from the medial side may further improve stability (Figure 16.17).

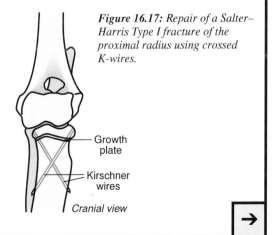

Figure 16.17: Repair of a Salter–Harris Type I fracture of the proximal radius using crossed K-wires.

→

OPERATIVE TECHNIQUE 16.4 (CONTINUED)
Fractures of the proximal radius

Simple articular fractures are repaired with lag screws and K-wires. For more complex fractures, the articular surface is repaired first with lag screws and then aligned and reattached to the radial metaphysis by means of a bone plate. Small non-reducible articular fragments, which would otherwise cause mechanical irritation to the joint, should be removed.

> **WARNING**
> **The radial nerve lies deep to the supinator muscle and must be protected during surgery.**

Wound Closure
Routine separate layer closure. Transected portions of the collateral ligament are sutured with polydioxanone. Transected extensor muscles are sutured with a horizontal mattress or cruciate suture pattern. An osteotomized lateral humeral epicondyle is reattached with a lag screw or pins and tension-band wire.

Post-operative Care
Proximal radial growth plate fractures require support in a Robert Jones bandage for 1 to 2 weeks and exercise is restricted for 3 to 4 weeks. Healing is usually rapid and K-wires are removed from 4 weeks post-operatively.

Articular and more complicated fractures may require support in a Robert Jones bandage or cast for 2 to 6 weeks depending on the rigidity of fixation and the speed of healing.

OPERATIVE TECHNIQUE 16.5
Bone plating diaphyseal fractures of the radius

Positioning
Dorsal recumbency with the limb pulled either caudally (see Figure 16.5) or cranially depending on the approach. The contralateral limb is pulled caudally and secured.

PRACTICAL TIPS

Use a beanbag to support the patient rather than a high-sided plastic cradle as a beanbag is more compliant and tends to be less intrusive.

Hanging the animal from the affected limb whilst preparing for surgery fatigues the muscles and aids in fracture reduction.

Assistant
Ideally.

Tray Extras
Periosteal elevator; Hohmannn retractor; Gelpi self-retaining retractors; pointed reduction forceps (or bone holding forceps of choice); bone cutters; plate benders; air or electric drill and bits; appropriate bone plating and screw set.

Approach
The craniomedial approach is classically used to expose the diaphysis of the radius (Figure 16.18). For fractures of the proximal to middle radial diaphysis, a lateral approach between the extensor carpi radialis muscle and the common digital extensor muscle is preferred (Figure 16.19) (Piermattei, 1993).

The diaphysis of the ulna is exposed by a caudal approach.

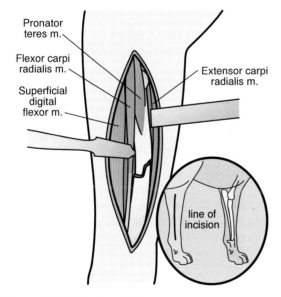

Figure 16.18: Craniomedial exposure of the radial diaphysis.

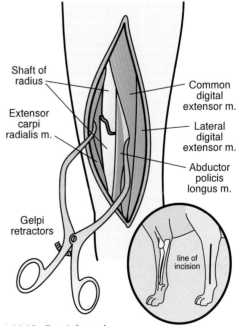

Figure 16.19: Craniolateral exposure of the radial diaphysis.

→

OPERATIVE TECHNIQUE 16.5 (CONTINUED)
Bone plating diaphyseal fractures of the radius

Reduction and Fixation

Fracture reduction may be accomplished by bending the limb caudally at the fracture site, toggling the bone ends against each other and then straightening the limb. Where there is significant overriding of the fracture a Hohmannn retractor may be used to lever the distal fragment into alignment. Sometimes the radius cannot be reduced without first reducing the ulna. In these cases, it is useful to cut back the ulnar fragment.

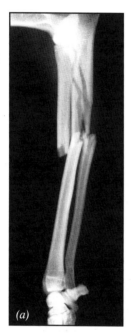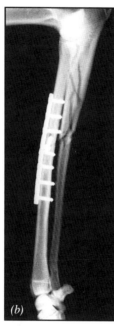

Figure 16.20: (a) Oblique fracture of the radial shaft with a comminuted ulnar fracture.
(b) The fractured radius was repaired using an interfragmentary lag screw and a cranial neutralization plate. Open reduction of the radius had realigned the ulnar diaphysis and the radial fixation should provide sufficient support for uncomplicated healing of the ulna.

PRACTICAL TIP
Beware of soft tissue interposition at the ulnar fracture site preventing accurate radial fracture alignment.

When a plate is applied to the cranial surface of the radius (see Figure 16.20), it should first be prestressed to allow for the natural cranial curvature of the radius and to ensure compression at the transcortex (see Chapter 9). It is best to apply the plate to the distal radial fragment first so that it may be used as a lever to aid in reduction. Once the fracture is reduced, bone holding forceps are used to fix the plate to the proximal fragment prior to screw placement. Oblique fractures are stabilized with pointed reduction forceps, and where possible a lag screw, or alternatively a K-wire, is placed across the fracture. This will prevent the fragments from slipping past each other during plate application.

PRACTICAL TIP
When using a craniomedial approach, the extensor muscles are forced laterally during plate application, which often results in varus angulation of the distal fragment. A cranial approach (see Figure 16.22) to the distal screw holes may help to avoid this.

WARNING
When drilling holes in the proximal radial diaphysis, care must be taken not to burst through the transcortex and strike the side of the ulna. This would inevitably result in a broken drill bit.

Screws should not be allowed to penetrate both the radius and ulna. In the young animal this will interfere with the normal growth and may result in elbow incongruity and angular limb deformity. In older animals it may result in complications such as implant failure and synostosis.

Wound Closure

Routine. Periosteum and deep fascia can be closed as one layer.

Post-operative Care

A Robert Jones bandage is applied for a few days to limit swelling. Exercise should be controlled for 4 to 6 weeks.

OPERATIVE TECHNIQUE 16.6

External fixation of radial diaphyseal fractures

Positioning
Dorsal recumbency with the contralateral limb pulled caudally and secured. When working alone, or in cases where a closed or limited open approach is planned, it is easiest to suspend the patient from the affected limb throughout the operation.

Assistant
Ideally.

Tray Extras
Appropriate external fixator set; Ellis pins (2 mm for cats and small dogs, 3 mm for medium dogs, 4 mm for large and giant breeds); clamps; connecting bars; large pin cutters (or hack saw); spanners; air or electric drill and bits; chuck and key; drill guides; periosteal elevator; pointed reduction forceps; Gelpi self-retaining retractors.

Approach
A craniomedial approach to the fractured radius is used, if required.

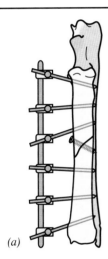
(a)
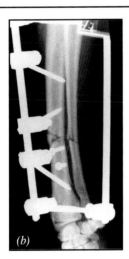
(b)

Figure 16.21: (a) Schematic view of the radius to show placement of a unilateral medial external fixator. A lag screw has also been placed across the oblique radial fracture. This would be inserted following fracture reduction via a limited craniomedial approach. (b) Repair of a comminuted radius and ulnar fracture in a 20 kg Border Collie. The radius was reduced via a limited craniomedial approach and interfragmentary lag screws inserted. The two major fragments were then supported with a bilateral uniplanar fixator (modified type II, see Chapter 9).

Reduction and Fixation
The fracture is reduced using similar techniques to those described in Operative Technique 16.5.

External fixation is usually applied to the medial radius as the distal two-thirds of the medial aspect of the radius represent a safe corridor for pin insertion (Marti and Miller, 1994). However, the radius is flattened in the mediolateral plane, making pin insertion from this direction more difficult. Maximum bone purchase is achieved by directing pins in an oblique craniomedial to caudolateral plane.

Open pin placement is recommended for the medial aspect of the proximal radius as pin insertion in this area can be difficult and unsafe (Marti and Miller, 1994). The pins should be placed between the flexor muscle bellies and this is achieved by directing the pins slightly obliquely in a caudomedial to craniolateral plane.

A unilateral external fixator is applied to the medial aspect of the radius generally with three pins in the proximal fragment and three pins in the distal fragment (Figure 16.21a). If the proximal fragment will not accommodate three pins then the proximal part of the connecting bar may be bent caudally so that pins can be placed in the proximal ulna. Where there is a short distal fragment a biplanar frame may be constructed and distal pins may be driven between the extensor tendons in a cranial orientation. Bilateral uniplanar frames may also be used with this type of fracture.

Unstable comminuted or open fractures often require bilateral (Figure 16.21b) or biplanar frames. Other designs, such as lateral frame orientation for proximal radial fractures and cranial orientation for small bones, have also been advocated (Egger, 1990).

→

OPERATIVE TECHNIQUE 16.6 (CONTINUED)
External fixation of radial diaphyseal fractures

Wound Closure
Routine.

Post-operative Care
Non-adhesive, semi-occlusive dressings should be placed around the fixator pins. The area between the skin and connecting bar is padded out with cotton wool and a Robert Jones bandage is applied over the limb and fixator, including the foot. The bandage is left in position for 2 to 3 days to control swelling. When the bandage is removed the clamps and pin ends should be protected with Vetrap. Controlled exercise is required while the fixator is in place. The frame should be checked weekly and the limb radiographed at 6 weeks. The fixator may be removed or destaged at this time, depending on fracture healing (see Chapter 5).

OPERATIVE TECHNIQUE 16.7

Salter–Harris fractures of the distal metaphyseal growth plates

Positioning
Dorsal recumbency with the affected limb free and the contralateral limb pulled caudally and secured.

Assistant
Not essential.

Tray Extras
Pin/wire cutters; chuck and key (or air/electric drill and bits); wire bender; Gelpi self-retaining retractors; K-wires.

Approach
A cranial approach to the distal radius is made (Figure 16.22).

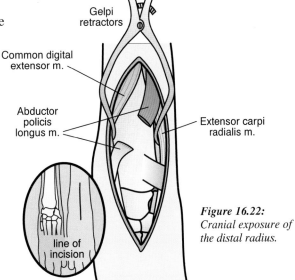

Figure 16.22:
Cranial exposure of the distal radius.

Reduction and Fixation
The antebrachium is grasped whilst the carpus is flexed and is used as a handle. Traction is exerted and the fracture ends are toggled together and manipulated until alignment is achieved.

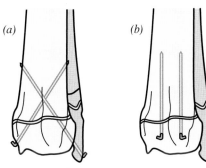

(a)   *(b)*

WARNING
Care should be taken to minimize trauma to the growth plate during reduction.

Figure 16.23: Two configurations for K-wire repair of a Type I Salter–Harris fracture of the distal radius: (a) crossed; (b) parallel.

The fracture is stabilized with a small K-wire driven from the medial styloid process, across the fracture, to anchor in the lateral cortex of the radial metaphysis. Often this is sufficient to provide fracture stability. However, when the ulna is involved, a second K-wire directed across the fracture from the lateral styloid process may further improve stability (Figure 16.23a). An alternative method is to place the K-wires parallel and perpendicular to the fracture surface (Figure 16.23b).

→

OPERATIVE TECHNIQUE 16.7 (CONTINUED)
Salter-Harris fractures of the distal metaphyseal growth plates

Wound Closure
Routine.

Post-operative Care
The limb should be supported in a Robert Jones bandage for 1 to 2 weeks and exercise is restricted for 3 to 4 weeks. Healing is usually rapid and K-wires are removed from 4 weeks post-operatively.

OPERATIVE TECHNIQUE 16.8
Styloid fractures

Positioning
Dorsal recumbency with the affected limb free and the contralateral limb pulled caudally and secured.

Assistant
Not essential.

Tray Extras
Pin/wire cutters; chuck and key (or air/electric drill and drill bits); wire bender; Gelpi self-retaining retractors; K-wires; cerclage wire for tension band; ± plating equipment.

Approach
A lateral or medial approach is made depending on the fracture site.

Reduction and Fixation
These fractures are usually reduced easily by applying a varus or valgus angulation towards the fracture site.

Pin and tension-band wire techniques are used to stabilize these fractures. One or two K-wires are used, depending on the size of the avulsed fragment. The K-wires are hand- or power-driven across the fracture site into the far cortex. For ulnar avulsions a single K-wire is either inserted into the ulna or directed obliquely into the distal radius (Figure 16.24). For the radius, pins are driven obliquely to engage the lateral cortex. The tension-band wire is placed around the pin end(s) and through a hole 1 or 2 cm proximal to the fracture site. The wire is tightened and the pins are cut, bent over, and buried in the collateral ligament.

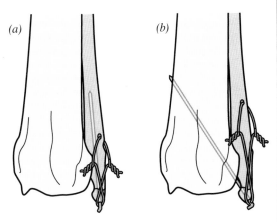

Figure 16.24: *Two options for pin positioning in the repair of ulnar styloid fractures: (a) into the ulna; (b) obliquely into the distal radius.*

If the fragments are too small to permit pin insertion, the ligament may be reattached to the bone using a screw and spiked plastic washer. Alternatively, the small fragments are removed and the ligament is sutured to a screw and washer placed in the styloid process. The ligament repair is further buttressed with wire or non-absorbable suture placed through bone tunnels or around screws and washers in the styloid processes and ulnar/radial carpal bones (Miller, 1994).

Wound Closure
Routine.

Post-operative Care
The limb should be supported in a Robert Jones bandage for 1 to 2 weeks, or longer, depending on the strength of the repair. Exercise is restricted for 4 to 6 weeks. Pin and wire removal is indicated if they become loose or irritate the soft tissues once the fracture has healed.

CHAPTER SEVENTEEN

The Pelvis and Sacroiliac Joint

Marvin L. Olmstead

INTRODUCTION

About 25% of all fractures in dogs and cats involve the pelvis (Brinker, 1975). The high prevalence of fractures involving this bone means veterinary surgeons must be able to select satisfactory treatment options for many different types of fracture. The choices range from non-surgical patient management to the reconstruction of specific pelvic fractures.

The treatment plan adopted will depend on:

- The convalescent care needed
- The comfort of the patient
- The severity of fragment displacement
- The location of the fracture
- The degree of pelvic canal compromise present.

Pelvic fractures are most commonly associated with motor vehicle trauma (Betts, 1993; Denny, 1978). The forces creating a pelvic fracture can come from many different angles and have varied magnitudes; therefore pelvic fractures can occur with many different configurations. It is almost impossible to have a single fracture in the pelvis because of its interconnected, box-like configuration. An animal hit directly from behind may have shear fractures in both ilial wings or bilateral sacroiliac luxations, or a combination of an ilial fracture and a sacroiliac luxation. A force from the side may drive the head of the femur into the acetabulum, creating fractures in the acetabulum, ilium and pelvic floor with medial displacement of the fragments. Since the possible combinations of fracture configurations are many it is critical to assess the pelvis fully, through physical and radiographic examination. However, total patient evaluation is paramount.

> **WARNING**
> **Almost half of all dogs with pelvic trauma caused by a motor vehicle will have thoracic injuries.**

CONSIDERATIONS IN PATIENT EVALUATION

Dogs and cats with pelvic fractures generally present with a history of an acute onset of lameness, usually non-weight-bearing, in one or both hindlimbs (Betts, 1993; Brinker *et al.*, 1990). In some animals the lameness is mild even though the fractures appear radiographically to be moderate or severe. Following a general physical examination to establish the patient's current health status, a complete orthopaedic examination should be performed. Careful digital rectal palpation of the pelvic canal is indicated when a pelvic fracture is suspected. This should be performed as an isolated examination and in conjunction with a passive range of motion manipulations of the coxofemoral joint. The degree of canal narrowing and the location of fractures and bone fragments should be carefully assessed throughout the canal's circumference.

External palpation may also provide useful information. Sacroiliac luxations and iliac fractures may be palpated as unstable bone segments or may cause disruption of normal anatomical relationships between the spine, pelvis and proximal femur. If an acetabular fracture is present, the relationship between the ischium and greater trochanter is often abnormal. The femoral head may have been driven into the acetabulum, displacing the trochanter medially, or if a concomitant ilial shaft fracture exists there may be cranial displacement of the trochanter.

> **WARNING**
> **An acetabular fracture can be present without a pain response to manipulation of the hip joint.**

Definitive diagnosis is established through radiographs of the pelvis. The two standard radiographic views of the pelvis for evaluating fractures are the ventrodorsal and lateral views. Sometimes, an oblique view of the hemi-pelvis is necessary for better definition of fracture lines and fragment position. It may reveal fragment displacement not seen on standard views.

MANAGEMENT

Surgical or non-surgical?

The decision to treat these injuries non-surgically or surgically is based on:

- Factors relating to the fracture
- The effect that malpositioned fragments will have on the patient
- The length and quality of the expected convalescent period
- The patient's comfort.

Fractures that are relatively non-displaced, stable and not painful, and that do not affect a vital structure or body function, may be treated with cage rest and proper nursing care. Compared with the surgically treated patient, a non-surgically treated patient might have more extensive nursing care needs, require additional physical therapy and have a prolonged recovery period.

The objectives of surgical treatment of pelvic fractures are:

- To re-establish normal load transmission pathways between the limb and the spine
- To restore the pelvic canal
- To re-establish the acetabulum's articular surface
- To shorten the patient's convalescent time.

SACROILIAC LUXATIONS

Sacroiliac luxations are treated surgically if they are very unstable, markedly displaced or painful (Tarvin and Lenehan, 1990). A minimally displaced sacroiliac luxation will stabilize adequately with fibrous tissue after 2 or 3 weeks of cage rest. If the ilial wing is markedly displaced the locomotive capability of the hindlimb and the load transmission between the pelvis and spine can be directly affected (Figure 17.1). The patient's convalescent period will be greatly reduced if an unstable or painful sacroiliac luxation/fracture is surgically stabilized. Either a lag screw or a trans-ilial pin can be used to stabilize a sacroiliac luxation (Operative Technique 17.1).

ILIAL SHAFT FRACTURES

Ilial fractures are more frequently treated surgically than are sacroiliac luxation/fractures. The ilium is often displaced medially, compromising the pelvic canal and endangering the sciatic nerve and other structures in the canal (Figure 17.2). The ilium is important in transmitting loads between the hindlimb and the spine during weight bearing. Repair of ilial fractures decreases pain and thus reduces convalescent time (Operative Technique 17.2). Patients will recover locomotor function more quickly if fractures of the ilium or acetabulum are stabilized. Only in patients with minimal or non-displaced ilial or acetabular fractures and already walking should non-surgical treatment be considered.

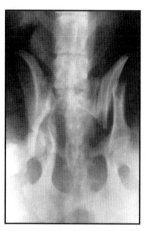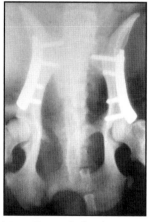

Figure 17.2: Ventro-dorsal pelvic radiograph showing bilateral ilial fractures in a dog. The pelvic canal and limb load transmission from the pelvis to the spine have both been compromised. The dog could not bear weight on either limb. In the post-operative radiograph, the fractures have been reduced via lateral approaches and stabilized using bone plates. Although on this view the left-hand plate appears to be compromising the acetabulum, the lateral view showed this was not the case.

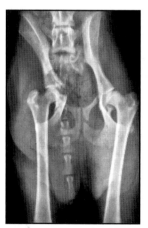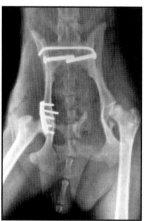

Figure 17.1: A pre-operative ventrodorsal pelvic radiograph showing bilateral sacroiliac luxation and a right acetabular fracture. There is marked displacement of the iliac wings. The dog was unable to bear weight on either limb. The post-operative radiograph shows reduction of the sacroiliac luxations and stabilization using lag screws and a trans-ilial pin. The acetabular fracture was stabilized with a dorsally positioned bone plate.

ACETABULUM

The acetabulum contains one of the articular surfaces of the coxofemoral joint. The principles of joint fracture repair dictate that the joint surface must be anatomically reconstructed to minimize the risk of the joint developing osteoarthritis (Figure 17.1). The weight-bearing surface of the acetabulum (its cranial two-thirds) must be reconstructed if its integrity is to be maintained (Operative Technique 17.3). Repair of fractures in the caudal one-third of the acetabulum is controversial. Although unrepaired fractures in this area will result in coxofemoral osteoarthritis (Boudrieau and Kleine, 1988), it has not been definitively proved that repairing fractures in this area will improve the patient's recovery. Osteoarthritis may be present but limb function may be unaffected. Due to their small size, fractures of the caudal one-third of the acetabulum can be difficult to stabilize adequately. With a caudal fracture the sciatic nerve is at greater risk of injury during surgery than when the fracture is located more cranially.

CONCURRENT ILIAL AND ACETABULAR FRACTURE

When a fracture of both the ilium and the acetabulum are present, it is preferable to repair the ilial shaft first. Repair of the ilium is often done with a stronger fixation system than is used on the acetabulum because usually more screws and a longer, stronger plate can be applied to the ilium. The reconstruction of the ilium does not have to be as anatomically exact as reconstruction of the acetabulum. When the acetabulum is repaired last, it will be fixed to a solidly stabilized ilial segment. Also, its fixation will not be subjected to addition loads that would be generated during manipulation of the ilial fragments if the ilium were fixed last.

ISCHIUM AND PUBIS

The pubis and ischium do not directly transmit loads during weight bearing and are surrounded by muscles that generally hold any bone fragments in relative position. Fragments are seldom displaced in a manner that compromises vital structures. If there is marked ischial fragment rotation or displacement due to muscle pull or wide separation of pubic fragments with an unstable pelvic floor, surgical stabilization with wire, pins and/or lag screws may be needed.

REFERENCES AND FURTHER READING

Betts CW (1993) Pelvic fractures. In: *Textbook of Small Animal Surgery*, *2nd edn*, ed. D Slatter, p. 1769. WB Saunders, Philadelphia.

Boudrieau RJ and Kleine LJ (1988) Nonsurgically managed caudal acetabular fractures in dogs: 15 cases (1979—1984). *Journal of the American Veterinary Medical Association* **193**, 701.

Brinker WO (1975) Fractures of the pelvis. In: *Canine Surgery, 2nd edn*, ed. J Archibald, p. 987. American Veterinary Publications, Santa Barbara.

Brinker WO and Braden TD (1984) Pelvic fractures. In: *Manual of Internal Fixation in Small Animals*, ed. WO Brinker, RB Hohn and WD Prieur, p. 152. Springer Verlag, Berlin.

Brinker WO, Piermattei DL and Flo GL (1990) Fractures of the pelvis. In: *Handbook of Small Animal Orthopedics and Fracture Treatment, 2nd edn*, p.76. WB Saunders, Philadelphia.

Decamp CE and Braden TD (1985a) The anatomy of the canine sacrum for lag screw fixation of the sacroiliac joint. *Veterinary Surgery* **14**, 131.

Decamp CE and Braden TD (1985b) Sacroiliac fracture-separations in the dog. A study of 92 cases. *Veterinary Surgery* **14**, 127.

Denny HR (1978) Pelvic fractures in the dog: a review of 123 cases. *Journal of Small Animal Practice* **19**, 151.

Olmstead ML (1990) Surgical repair of acetabular fractures. In: *Current Techniques in Small Animal Surgery, 3rd edn*, ed. MJ Bojrab, p. 656. Lea and Febiger, Philadelphia.

Piermattei DL (1993) The hind limb. In: *An Atlas of Surgical Approaches of the Bones of the Dog and Cat, 3rd edn*, p.264. WB Saunders, Philadelphia.

Slocum B and Hohn RB (1975) A surgical approach to the caudal aspect of the acetabulum and body of the ischium in the dog. *Journal of the American Veterinary Medical Association* **65**, 167.

Tarvin GB and Lenehan TM (1990) Management of sacroiliac dislocations and ilial fractures. In: *Current Techniques in Small Animal Surgery, 3rd edn*, ed. MJ Bojrab, p. 649. Lea and Febiger, Philadelphia.

OPERATIVE TECHNIQUE 17.1
Sacroiliac luxations

Positioning

On the sternum with hindlimbs straddling sandbags or a positioning pad (Figure 17.3). Positioning the animal in this manner makes manipulation and visualization of the bone fragments easier in most cases.

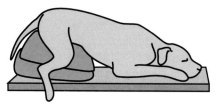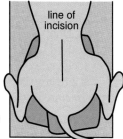

Figure 17.3: Patient positioning for surgical repair of sacroiliac luxation/fracture. The hindquarters are elevated by the pads. A dorsal midline approach is used to expose the sacroiliac area.

Assistant

Essential for maintaining exposure of the sacrum with a Hohmann retractor while the surgeon drills the thread hole for the lag screw (see below). The rest of the surgery can be done with either self-retaining retractors or assistant-held retractors.

Tray Extras

For lag-screw technique: appropriate screw set and necessary drill bits ± tap; drill; periosteal elevator; Hohmann retractor.
For trans-ilial pin technique: appropriate size pin; chuck; large pin cutters.
For both techniques: Kern bone-holding forceps; hand-held or self-retaining retractors (e.g. Gelpi).

Surgical Approach

A dorsal midline approach is used to expose sacroiliac luxation/fractures. The dorsal back muscles are reflected laterally off the spinous processes of L6, L7 and the sacrum. The lateral surface of the sacrum is exposed and the dorsal aspect of the displaced ilium is identified.

Alternatively, the lateral sacrum can be approached via an incision over the iliac spine, with subsequent dissection down between the epaxial muscles and the medial aspect of the ilium (Piermattei, 1993). The midline approach is the author's preference for both of the repair techniques described below, but either approach is equally satisfactory. The midline approach facilitates trans-ilial pinning.

Reduction and Fixation

Lag screw

The thread hole is drilled in the body of the sacrum before the ilial segment is reduced. The lateral surface of the sacrum is exposed and the ilial wing is displaced ventrally by placing the tip of a Hohmann retractor under the ventral point of the sacrum. The thread hole in the sacrum should be placed in the centre of the exposed sacral surface, thus placing the screw in the maximum available bone. A slight ventral angulation of the thread hole's position ensures the screw's position in bone and out of the neural canal (Figure 17.4) (DeCamp and Braden, 1985a,b).

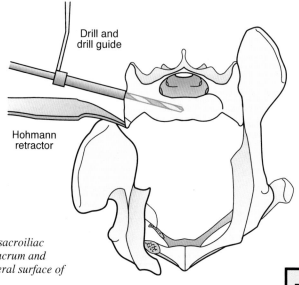

Figure 17.4: Positioning the screw hole during repair of sacroiliac luxations. The thread hole is started in the centre of the sacrum and angled slightly ventrally to miss the neural canal. The lateral surface of the sacrum is exposed by levering the ilium ventrally.

→

OPERATIVE TECHNIQUE 17.1 (CONTINUED)
Sacroiliac luxations

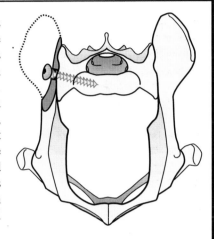

The caudal portion of the middle gluteal muscle is reflected off its origin along the caudal dorsal iliac spine and the lateral surface of the ilium is exposed. The sacral articulation on the medial iliac surface is identified visually and/or with palpation. A glide hole is drilled from lateral to medial, exiting the centre of the ilium's sacral articulation. The ilium is reduced by grasping the caudal dorsal iliac spine with a bone reduction forceps with fixation teeth, such as a Kern bone clamp, and manipulating the ilium into near anatomical position. A space is left between the ilium and the sacrum so placement of the screw in the thread hole can be visualized. The appropriate sized screw is inserted through the glide hole. The screw is manipulated into position until its tip is in the thread hole. Tightening the screw will reduce the luxation (Figure 17.5). If the sacrum is large enough, a second lag screw or small pin is inserted into the sacrum to prevent rotation of the fragments.

Figure 17.5: Screw position for fixation of sacroiliac luxations. Drill a glide hole through the ilium. Digital palpation of the articular surface on the medial ilial wall guides the position of the glide hole. The screw is pushed partially through the glide hole before the luxation is reduced, so that its engagement with the thread hole in the sacrum can be visualized. Fully tightening the screw reduces the luxation.

> **WARNING**
> **Positioning the thread hole outside the sacrum's centre may place the screw in a thin part of the bone or in the neural canal.**

Trans-ilial pin

To reduce the ilium, pointed reduction forceps are positioned with one point in the caudal sacrum and one point in the lateral ilial surface and the clamp is tightened. The fully tightened clamp will hold the ilium and sacrum in reduction while the trans-ilial pin is applied. Because this reduction technique closes the space between the ilium and sacrum it cannot be used with the lag screw technique described above.

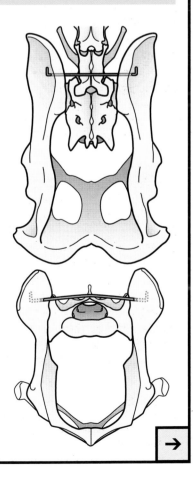

Once the luxation/fracture is reduced, the trans-ilial pin can be inserted. The pin selected for fixation should be easily bent and no larger than 3 mm in diameter. The selected pin is driven by hand lateral to medially through the ilium on the side of the injury. The pin should pass dorsal to the 7th lumbar vertebra at the level of the base of the dorsal spinous process. It can pass either through the dorsal spinous process or just caudal to it. Once the pin is past the dorsal spinous process, the hand chuck driving the pin is elevated, which lowers the pin's point. The pin is driven medial to lateral through the opposite ilium and the middle gluteal muscle until just enough of its point is exposed to be grasped. The pin should not penetrate the skin. The pin is bent dorsally as it is advanced. When the pin is advanced far enough, it is bent 90° and is cut off, leaving a bend at the end. The pin is pulled back until the bend is buried in the gluteal muscle over the ilium opposite the injured side. The pin on the injured side is bent dorsally 90° and cut off. The pin now has hooks on both ends that prevent migration (Figure 17.6). If desired, a second trans-ilial pin can be inserted in the same manner.

Figure 17.6: Trans-ilial pin stabilization of sacroiliac luxations. The trans-ilial pin passes through the wing of each ilium and dorsal to the 7th lumbar vertebra. The ends of the pin are bent to prevent migration.

→

OPERATIVE TECHNIQUE 17.1 (CONTINUED)
Sacroiliac luxations

Post-operative Care
The animal should be placed on limited activity for 4 to 8 weeks. No activity more strenuous than a walk is allowed during this period. Towel or sling support of the hindquarters is provided as necessary. Supply soft bedding to prevent pressure sores developing. Urine and faecal soiling of the patient are cleaned as required.

PRACTICAL TIP
If the sacroiliac luxation/fracture is accompanied by an ilial fracture on the opposite side, the ilial fracture should be stabilized first as this alone may result in reduction and adequate stability of the sacroiliac joint, because of the box configuration of the pelvis.

OPERATIVE TECHNIQUE 17.2
Ilial shaft fractures

Positioning
Lateral recumbency.

Assistant
Helpful for maintaining exposure and reduction of the ilium while the surgeon implants the bone plate.

Tray Extras
Appropriate bone plate and screw set including drill bits ± taps; drill; bone-holding forceps; self-retaining and hand-held retractors; periosteal elevator.

Surgical Approach
A lateral approach is used. The ventral margin of the middle and deep gluteal muscles is isolated and the muscles are elevated off the face of the ilium to the extent needed in the fracture repair (Figure 17.7).

Figure 17.7: Exposure of the lateral surface of the ilium.

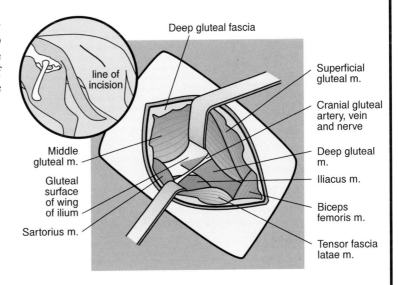

Reduction

> **WARNING**
> **Ilial fragment reduction can be the most difficult part of the surgery.**

Often the free segment of the pelvis is displaced cranially and/or medially. The fragment should be lateralized first and, if necessary, moved caudally. If the fracture segments are collapsed medially, either a Lahey retractor or a pair of Kern bone forceps is helpful in repositioning the fragments laterally. A Lahey retractor, which is blunt, strong, and bent 90° at its end, is passed along the medial wall of the free segment. The retractor's tip is maintained on the bone's surface as it is passed along the medial wall to avoid compromising the sciatic nerve. Pulling laterally with the retractor's handle moves the fracture segments laterally (Figure 17.8).

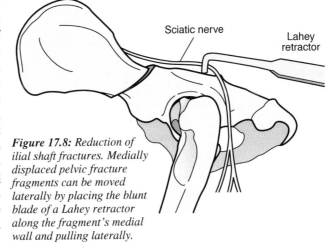

Figure 17.8: Reduction of ilial shaft fractures. Medially displaced pelvic fracture fragments can be moved laterally by placing the blunt blade of a Lahey retractor along the fragment's medial wall and pulling laterally.

→

OPERATIVE TECHNIQUE 17.2 (CONTINUED)
Ilial shaft fractures

If the fragment is large enough, Kern bone-holding forceps can be clamped along the ventral edge of the free ilial shaft, allowing the fragment to be manipulated (Figure 17.9). If an ilial segment is cranially displaced then a self-centring reduction clamp can be placed with one holding surface of the clamp on the secure cranial fragment and the other holding surface on the free caudal fragment. Closing this clamp will move the free fragment caudally (Figure 17.10). Some reduction techniques discussed for reducing acetabular fractures are also helpful in reducing ilial shaft fractures when no acetabular fracture exists. Ilial shaft alignment can be slightly off and still give a satisfactory final result. Reduction of the ilial fracture can almost always be maintained temporarily by positioning self-centring or Kern bone clamps dorsal to ventral across the fracture segments.

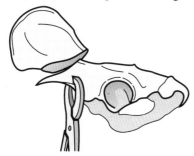

Figure 17.9: Reduction of ilial shaft fractures. The Kern bone clamp's configuration provides two points of fixation in the caudal free ilial fragment. This allows the fragment to be manipulated into proper alignment.

PRACTICAL TIP
After the ilial fracture has been reduced, the most effective way of stabilizing the fracture is bone plating.

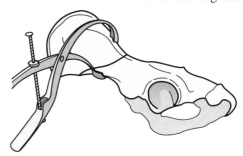

Figure 17.10: Reduction of ilial shaft fractures. A self-centring clamp can be used to reduce free ilial segments. One blade of the clamp is placed on the ilium's dorsal rim while the other blade is placed on the ventral rim of the free fragment. Closing the clamp will bring the free segment to the fixed segment. Reduction is maintained with the self-centring clamp while a bone plate is applied.

Fixation
Several types of plates developed by the AO/ASIF group can be used, depending on the size of the animal and the degree of comminution of the fracture. For ilial fractures, mini-fragment T or L plates or standard Dynamic Compression Plates, which accept 3.5, 2.7 or 2.0 mm screws, are available. The size of fragments will govern the size of implant used.

For ilial shaft fractures the plates must be contoured to the concave shape of the lateral surface of the ilium. If possible at least three screws should be placed in each fracture segment. If the screws are placed in the caudal fragment first, the plate will aid in reduction of the fracture when the screws are tightened in the cranial segment (Figure 17.11) (Brinker and Braden, 1984). If the fracture is reduced and minimal collapse is present, the screws nearest the fracture line are placed first, one each in the caudal and cranial fragments. The remaining screws are inserted alternately on either side of the fracture from nearest to furthest from the fracture line.

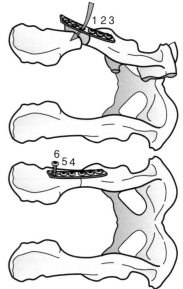

Figure 17.11: Plate fixation of ilial fractures. Screws placed in the bone plate in the order indicated will move the free caudal ilial segment laterally.

Post-operative Care
As for Operating Technique 17.1. The activity levels of these patients must be strictly limited to reduce the chance that the fragments will change position during the convalescent period.

OPERATIVE TECHNIQUE 17.3
Acetabular fractures

Positioning
Lateral recumbency.

Assistant
In most cases, an assistant is required to maintain exposure and reduction of the acetabular fracture while the surgeon implants the bone plate.

Tray Extras
Appropriate bone plate and screw set, including drill bits ± taps; drill; bone-holding forceps; self-retaining and hand-held retractors; periosteal elevator.

Surgical Approaches
Acetabular fractures are approached either by a trochanteric osteotomy or by a caudal approach (Slocum and Hohn, 1975; Olmstead, 1990; Piermattei, 1993). The author only uses the trochanteric osteotomy when wider exposure of the cranial pelvis is needed for fracture repair, as when the ilial shaft and the acetabulum are both fractured on the same side.

> **WARNING**
> **The sciatic nerve must be protected.**

Trochanteric osteotomy
The superficial gluteal muscle is isolated, incised at its insertion and reflected dorsally. The osteotomy of the greater trochanter is performed starting at the level of the third trochanter and extending dorsally to the junction of the greater trochanter and the femoral neck. The middle and deep gluteal muscles, still attached to the greater trochanter, are reflected dorsally (Figure 17.12). The caudal portion of the deep gluteal and the gemellus muscles are elevated with a periosteal elevator from their origin over the dorsal rim of the acetabulum, exposing the fracture site.

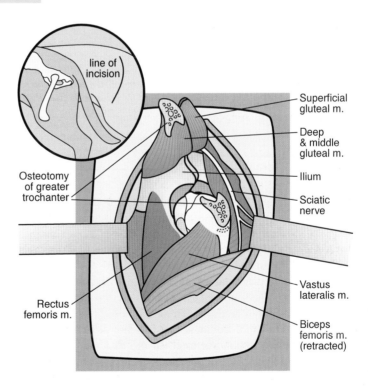

Figure 17.12: The trochanteric osteotomy exposes fractures of the acetabulum. The sciatic nerve should be isolated before the osteotomy is performed. Following repair of the acetabulum, the trochanter is reattached with two pins and a tension-band wire (Figure 17.17).

→

OPERATIVE TECHNIQUE 17.3 (CONTINUED)
Acetabular fractures

Caudal approach

Usually, the caudal approach is preferable. It provides exposure of the acetabulum equal to the trochanteric osteotomy, does not require creation of a fracture site in the femur and is more quickly closed.

The caudal approach also starts with tenotomy of the superficial gluteal muscle at its insertion point on the third trochanter. The muscle is tagged with suture and retracted dorsally. The internal obturator and gemelli muscles are incised at their insertion in the trochanteric fossa, tagged, and retracted caudodorsally, providing exposure of the caudal acetabulum and protection for the sciatic nerve.

The caudal portion of the deep gluteal and gemellus muscles are elevated until the entire dorsal rim of the acetabulum is exposed. The caudal aspect of the ilium can be exposed by inserting the tip of a Hohmann retractor just cranial to the ventral border of the ilium under the middle and the deep gluteal muscles. The retractor displaces the middle and deep gluteal muscles distally. Maintaining the hip in an extended and internally rotated position provides maximal exposure to the acetabular rim (Figure 17.13).

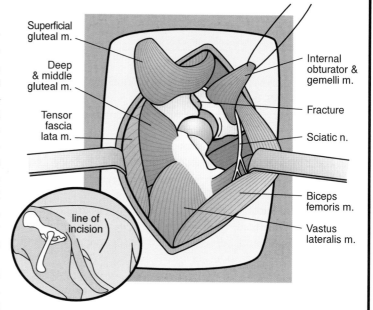

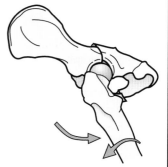

Figure 17.13: Caudal approach to the acetabulum. The external rotators of the hip are incised at their trochanteric fossa insertion. These muscles are retracted caudally to protect the sciatic nerve. Extension and internal rotation of the femur enhances the exposure. A Hohmann retractor placed under the middle and deep gluteal muscles and hooked on the ventral edge of the ilium retracts these muscles ventrally.

Reduction

Because the acetabulum is a joint surface, it must be completely reduced anatomically if a successful outcome is to be achieved. In addition to the techniques discussed below, some of the techniques used for reducing ilial fractures (Operative Technique 17.2) can also be used for reducing acetabular fractures.

The caudal bone segment of an acetabular fracture is often displaced cranially. The fragment can be brought into a more caudal position by two different methods. These methods are also used to provide traction on an ilial fragment that is being difficult to move when the acetabulum is not fractured. In the first method, an intramedullary pin is driven with a pin chuck ventral to dorsal through the ischium just cranial to the ischial rim. During this procedure, the hip joint should be flexed. The pin should penetrate the skin on either side of the ischium. If a second pin chuck is attached to the portion of the pin exposed dorsally, the two pin chucks can be used as handles to pull the fracture segment caudally (Figure 17.14). Rotation of the segment can also be provided with this method, although since there is only a single point of fixation in the fragment the amount of rotation achieved is limited.

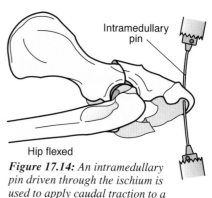

Figure 17.14: An intramedullary pin driven through the ischium is used to apply caudal traction to a free pelvic segment. Flexing the hip while driving the pin moves the hamstring muscles out of the way.

→

OPERATIVE TECHNIQUE 17.3 (CONTINUED)
Acetabular fractures

The second method for providing caudal traction uses a large Kern bone-holding clamp. An incision wide enough to allow insertion of the end of the Kern bone-holding clamp is made parallel with the ischial rim. Because the fixation teeth of the Kern clamp provide four points of fixation, this instrument can be used for both caudal retraction and rotation of the segment (Figure 17.15). Large Kern clamps are used in most moderate and all large dogs because small Kern clamps do not have a long enough lever arm to manipulate the fracture segment easily.

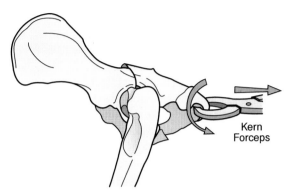

Figure 17.15: A Kern bone-holding clamp is applied to the ischium through an incision over the tuber ischia allowing the free segment to be rotated and retracted caudally.

Acetabular fracture reduction is maintained with pointed reduction bone forceps, or by manually holding the fragments in place until the permanent stabilization procedure is completed. Reduction of an acetabular surface can be checked by placing ventral traction on the greater trochanter. This will pull the femoral head out of the acetabulum enough for the articular rim of the acetabulum to be observed through an incision in the joint capsule or an existing tear.

Fixation

Although non-plating surgical techniques have been described for repair of acetabular fractures, none of them has proved to be as effective as bone plates or has provided the clinical results that bone plates have. Two different sizes of C-shaped acetabular plates from the AO/ASIF group (Synthes Ltd) are effective in the treatment of simple acetabular fractures. Miniature fragment plates and standard Dynamic Compression Plates® (Synthes, Ltd) have been used to stabilize acetabular fractures. Some surgeons prefer to use the reconstruction plate for acetabular fractures because it can be bent in several different planes.

> **PRACTICAL TIP**
> **The bone fragments will shift in position as the screws are tightened if the plate is not perfectly contoured to the dorsal surface of the acetabulum.**

The C-shaped acetabular plates are easy to contour to the acetabulum's dorsal bone surface because of their shape. Mini plates are easy to bend because they are thin. However, this makes them relatively weak and limits the size of animal in which they can be used. The dorsal surface is used for plate placement because adequate bone is present there and this is the tension surface of the bone (Figure 17.16). In all acetabular fractures at least two screws should be located on either side of the fracture line, and they should be angled so that they do not penetrate the articular cartilage surface (Figure 17.16). It is sometimes helpful to bend the plate before surgery, using a model of an intact pelvis that is approximately the same size as the pelvis that needs repair. The pre-bent plate can be sterilized and minor contouring adjustments made during surgery. This technique reduces surgical time.

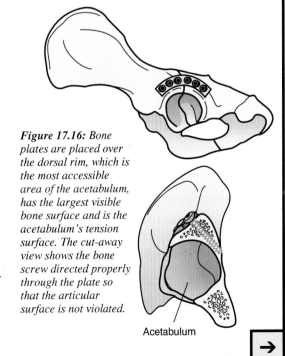

Figure 17.16: Bone plates are placed over the dorsal rim, which is the most accessible area of the acetabulum, has the largest visible bone surface and is the acetabulum's tension surface. The cut-away view shows the bone screw directed properly through the plate so that the articular surface is not violated.

Acetabulum

→

OPERATIVE TECHNIQUE 17.3 (CONTINUED)
Acetabular fractures

One of the most difficult fractures to stabilize is one that has a component of the medial wall of the acetabulum fractured out. If a large section of this wall is involved, the femoral head will displace medially into the pelvic canal. If the fracture segment containing the medial wall extends far enough cranially, lag screw and/or intramedullary pin fixation of the ilial segment should be done to stabilize the fragment. If the fragment cannot be stabilized, a slight over-bending of the plate closing the diameter of the articular surface makes it more difficult for the femoral head to displace medially. If the femoral head cannot be prevented from displacing medially, a salvage procedure, the excision arthroplasty, should be considered. Excision arthroplasty may also be performed for severe fractures where reconstruction is not possible. This procedure is done only as a last resort as it sacrifices joint function but is intended to save limb function. If an acetabular malunion from an untreated acetabular fracture has resulted in osteoarthritis in a dog over 14 kg, a total hip replacement may be considered.

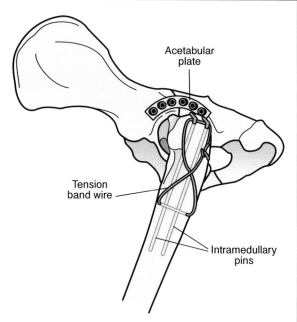

Figure 17.17: *Fixation of a trochanteric osteotomy using two pins and a tension-band wire.*

Closure
If osteotomy was performed, the greater trochanter is reattached to the proximal femur with the tension-band technique (Figure 17.17). After caudal approach, the internal obturator and gemelli muscles are sutured to fascial tissue near their original insertion point. The remaining tissues are routinely closed.

Post-operative Care
As for Operative Technique 17.1.

CHAPTER EIGHTEEN

The Femur

A. Colin Stead

INTRODUCTION

Femoral fractures are common in small animal practice, mostly the result of road accident trauma and less commonly as pathological fractures in juveniles with nutritional osteodystrophies and mature animals with bone tumours.

PROXIMAL FEMUR

An appreciation of the blood supply of the femoral head and neck is vital to treatment of fractures in this area (Figure 18.1). Fractures within the joint capsule will disrupt the blood supply and avascular necrosis

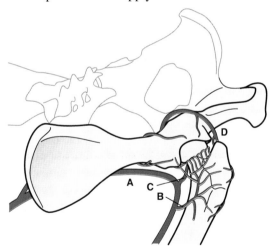

Figure 18.1: *Arterial blood supply to the femoral head and neck of a dog. A, femoral artery: B, lateral circumflex femoral: C, medial circumflex femoral; D, caudal gluteal.*

may be a consequence. However, several reported series of fracture repairs in this area have indicated no cases of avascular necrosis (Daly, 1978; De Camp *et al.*, 1989; Jeffery, 1989) but thinning and remodelling of the femoral neck is common. The proximal femoral growth plate or physis closes between 6 and 12 months in the dog (Sumner-Smith, 1966) and between 7 and 10 months in the cat (Smith, 1969). Early closure of this growth plate may cause a varus deformity of the hip, while closure of the greater trochanteric growth plate may lead to a valgus deformity of the hip and subluxation. Daly (1978) reported cases of early closure with no apparent clinical problems.

Fractures of the femoral head and neck
These fractures can be classified into five types (Figure 18.2): epiphyseal, physeal, subcapital, intertrochanteric and trochanteric.

Epiphyseal
The treatment for this is surgical (Vernon and Olmstead, 1983) and should be done promptly to minimize damage to the hip joint and the risk of avascular necrosis (Operative Technique 18.1).

Physeal, subcapital and intertrochanteric
Prompt surgical treatment is necessary and various techniques have been used:

- Lag screws (2.0 mm) inserted retrograde from the articular surface (Kuzma *et al.*, 1989; Tillson *et al.*, 1994). In a small series reported by Miller and Anderson (1993) some dogs

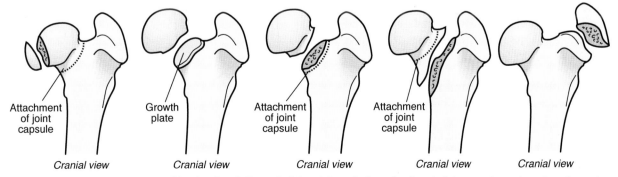

Attachment of joint capsule	Growth plate	Attachment of joint capsule	Attachment of joint capsule	
Cranial view	*Cranial view*	*Cranial view*	*Cranial view*	*Cranial view*

Figure 18.2: *Fractures of the femoral head and neck. From the left, epiphyseal, physeal, subcapital, intertrochanteric and trochanteric.*

Intramedullary pinning (Operative Technique 18.4)	• Simple transverse or short oblique fractures in cats and small to medium sized dogs • Selected comminuted shaft fractures in cats
Bone plating (Operative Technique 18.5)	• Fractures of the femoral diaphysis from the subtrochanteric area distally which are either comminuted, long oblique, oblique spiral or segmental. • Transverse or short oblique fractures in medium to larger dogs
External fixation (Operative Technique 18.6)	As with the humerus, the femoral shaft is not ideally suited for using an external fixator because of its muscle coverage. However, in situations where anatomical reconstruction is decided against and in open fractures, external fixation may be used as part of a minimally invasive strategy (see Chapter 10)

Table 18.1: Decision making in the surgical management of femoral diaphyseal fractures.

remained lame and required an excision arthroplasty
• Three K-wires inserted from the subtrochanteric area, described by Jeffery (1989)
• Lag screws with or without an anti-rotation K-wire from a similar approach (Nunamaker, 1973; Hulse *et al.*, 1974).

Lambrechts *et al.* (1993) showed experimentally that the latter two techniques were the strongest of the subtrochanteric techniques. In skeletally mature dogs, the preferred technique is a subtrochanteric lag screw. In cats and skeletally immature dogs, K-wires are used [Operative Technique 18.2].

Trochanteric
Trochanteric fractures are uncommon and they usually occur in association with separation of the proximal femoral epiphysis or dislocation of the hip. The technique of choice is two K-wires and a wire tension-band (Operative Technique 18.3).

FEMORAL DIAPHYSIS

Fractures of the femoral diaphysis are common and normally require internal fixation, the exceptions being undisplaced and impacted shaft fractures and pathological fractures associated with nutritional bone dystrophies in immature animals, which will heal with rest alone.

The method of fixation depends on the age and size of the animal and the nature of the fracture (Table 18.1).

Comminuted diaphyseal fractures in cats
In many instances, the use of buttress and neutralization plates is indicated; however, Denny (1993) advocates the use of an intramedullary pin plus cerclage wire to tie in the fragments for most comminuted fractures (see Figure 18.12). An external fixator may also be used.

DISTAL FEMUR

Three fracture types occur in this area (Figure 18.3):

• Fractures involving the distal growth plate
• Fractures of the distal femoral metaphysis or epiphysis
• Intercondylar fractures.

Fractures involving the distal femoral growth plate
These fractures are common; they are normally Salter–Harris type II in the dog and type I in the cat. Surgical treatment is necessary.

Various treatments have been used, but the recommended technique employs either two Rush pins (Lawson, 1959) or crossed K-wires (Milton *et al.*, 1980) (Operative Technique 18.7). Raiha *et al.* (1993) described the use of biodegradable polylactic acid rods used as cross pins, but the technique is not widely used at present. There is a chance that if the implants are removed within 4 weeks an open growth plate may continue to grow, especially if Rush pins are used (Stone *et al.*, 1981). In some instances where early growth plate closure has occurred, compensatory lengthening of other bones in the affected limb has been reported (Alcantara and Stead, 1975).

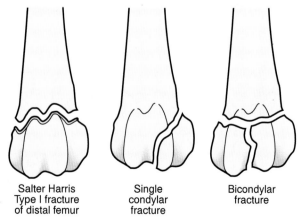

Salter Harris Type I fracture of distal femur   Single condylar fracture   Bicondylar fracture

Figure 18.3: Fractures of the distal femur.

Fractures of the distal femoral metaphysis in skeletally mature animals

A fracture of this type may also be treated with Rush pins or crossed K-wires, as above. An alternative is to use a lag screw into the medial condyle (Denny, 1993) (Operative Technique 18.7).

> **WARNING**
> **A lag screw should not be used in an immature animal.**

Intercondylar fractures

These are rare. Single or bicondylar fractures occur, and are articular fractures requiring anatomical reduction.

If the fracture involves one condyle, or a part of one, fixation is by a single lag screw and anti-rotation K-wire (Carmichael *et al.*, 1989) (Operative Technique 18.8). With bicondylar fractures, the articular fracture is fixed first using a lag screw and then the condyles are re-attached to the femur using two Rush pins or crossed K-wires (Operative Technique 18.7).

REFERENCES AND FURTHER READING

Alcantara P and Stead AC (1975) Fractures of the distal femur in the dog and cat. *Journal of Small Animal Practice* **16**, 649-659.

Bassett FH, Wilson J, Allen B and Azuma H (1969) Normal vascular anatomy of the head of the femur in puppies with emphasis on the inferior retinacular vessels. *Journal of Bone and Joint Surgery* **51A**, 1139-1153.

Carmichael S, Wheeler SJ and Vaughan LC (1989) Single condylar fractures of the distal femur in the dog. *Journal of Small Animal Practice* **30**, 500-504.

Chaffee VW (1977) Multiple stacked intramedullary pin fixation of humeral and femoral fractures. *Journal of the American Animal Hospital Association* **13**, 599-601.

Daly WR (1978) Femoral head and neck fractures in the dog and cat. A review of 115 cases. *Veterinary Surgery* **7**, 29-38.

De Camp CE, Probst CW and Thomas MW (1989) Internal fixation of femoral capital physeal injuries in dogs, 40 cases 1979-1987. *Journal of the American Veterinary Medical Association* **194**, 1750-1754.

Denny HR (1971) Simultaneous epiphyseal separation and fracture of the neck and great trochanter in the dog. *Journal of Small Animal Practice* **12**, 613-621.

Denny HR (1993) *Orthopaedic Surgery in the Dog and Cat*, 3rd edn. Blackwell Scientific.

Hulse DH, Wilson JW and Butler HC (1974) Use of the lag screw principle for stabilization of femoral neck and femoral capital epiphyseal fractures. *Journal of the American Animal Hospital Association* **10**, 29-36.

Hulse DH, Abdelbaki YZ and Wilson, J (1981) Revascularisation of femoral capital physeal fractures following surgical fixation. *Journal of Veterinary Orthopaedics* **2**, 50-57.

Jeffery ND (1989) Internal fixation of femoral head and neck fractures in the cat. *Journal of Small Animal Practice* **30**, 674-677.

Kaderly RE, Anderson BG and Anderson WD (1983) Intracapsular and intraosseous vascular supply to the mature dog's coxofemoral joint. *American Journal of Veterinary Research* **44**, 1805-1812.

Kuzma A, Sumner-Smith G, Miller C and McLaughlin R (1989) A technique for repair of femoral capital epiphyseal fractures in the dog. *Journal of Small Animal Practice* **30** 444-448.

Lambrechts NE, Verstraete FJM, Sumner-Smith G *et al.* (1993) Internal fixation of femoral neck fractures in the dog – an *in vitro* study. *Veterinary and Comparative Orthopaedics and Traumatology* **6**, 188-193.

Lawson DD (1959) The technique of Rush pinning in fracture repair. *Modern Veterinary Practice* **40**, 32-36.

Lee R (1976) Proximal femoral epiphyseal separation in the dog. *Journal of Small Animal Practice* **11**, 669-679.

Marti JM and Miller A (1994) Delimitation of safe corridors for the insertion of external fixator pins in the dog. 1: Hindlimb. *Journal of Small Animal Practice* **35**, 16-23.

Miller A and Anderson TJ (1993) Complications of articular lag screw fixation of femoral capital epiphyseal separations. *Journal of Small Animal Practice* **34**, 9-12.

Milton JL, Horne RD and Goldstein GM (1980) Cross pinning. A simple technique for treatment of certain metaphyseal and physeal fractures of long bones. *Journal of the American Animal Hospital Association* **16**, 891-906.

Nunamaker DM (1973) Repair of femoral head and neck fractures by interfragmentary compression. *Journal of the American Veterinary Medical Association* **162**, 569.

Olsson SE, Poulos PW Jr and Ljungren G (1985) Coxa plana vara and femoral capital fractures in the dog. *Journal of the American Animal Hospital Association* **21**, 563-571.

Piermattei DL (1993) *An Atlas of Surgical Approaches to the Bones and Joints of the Dog and Cat*, 3rd edn. WB Saunders, Philadelphia.

Raiha JE, Axelson P, Skutnabb K *et al.* (1993) Fixation of cancellous bone and physeal fractures with biodegradable rods of self reinforced polylactic acid. *Journal of Small Animal Practice* **34**, 131-138.

Smith RN (1969) Fusion of ossification centres in the cat. *Journal of Small Animal Practice* **10**, 523-530.

Stone EA, Betts CW and Rowland GN (1981) Effect of Rush pins on the distal femoral growth plate of young dogs. *American Journal of Veterinary Research* **42**, 261-265.

Sumner-Smith G (1966) Observations on epiphyseal fusion of the canine appendicular skeleton. *Journal of Small Animal Practice* **7**, 303-311.

Tillson DM, McLaughlin RM and Roush JK (1994) Evaluation of experimental proximal femoral physeal fractures repaired with two cortical screws placed from the articular surface. *Veterinary and Comparative Orthopaedics and Traumatology* **7**, 140-147.

Vernon FF and Olmstead ML (1983) Femoral head fractures resulting in epiphyseal fragmentation. Results of repair in 5 dogs. *Veterinary Surgery* **12**, 123-126.

OPERATIVE TECHNIQUE 18.1

Epiphyseal fractures of the femoral head

Positioning
Lateral recumbency with affected leg uppermost.

Assistant
Often desirable to have two assistants – one to manipulate limb and one to retract.

Tray Extras
1.5 or 2.0 mm bone screw set; drill bits; Langenbeck retractors; large and small Hohmann retractors; Gelpi self-retaining retractors; small pointed reduction forceps; chuck; K-wires; pin/wire cutters; hammer and flat-ended pin.

Surgical Approach
Either a craniolateral approach or a dorsal approach via a trochanteric osteotomy can be used. The craniolateral is regarded as the least traumatic and should be used for all fracture fixations except where retrograde K-wires are used in the cat. However, Hulse *et al.* (1981) claimed that trochanteric osteotomy did not disrupt the blood supply to the femoral head and neck.

Craniolateral Approach
Centre the skin incision over the greater trochanter and continue one-third of the way down the femoral shaft (Figure 18.4). The fascia lata is incised along the cranial edge of the biceps femoris muscle. Incise the insertion of the fascia lata over the femur and proximally along its junction with the superficial gluteal muscle. Retract the fascia lata cranially and bluntly dissect along the cranial aspect of the femoral neck to clear the joint capsule. The joint capsule is incised longitudinally to minimize vascular damage, continuing into part of the origin of the vastus muscle below the greater trochanter. Reflect part of the origin of the vastus distally to expose the third trochanter. Tenotomize the cranial one-third of the deep gluteal tendon and incise along the cranial third of the muscle to reflect it and improve the exposure of the femoral neck and head (Piermattei, 1993). Outward rotation of the stifle will lateralize the intact portion of the femoral head or neck. Preserve the teres ligament if possible. If it is essential to cut the ligament, it may be done with fine curved scissors or a hip disarticulator.

> ### PRACTICAL TIP
> Applying pointed reduction forceps to the greater trochanter is helpful in manipulation.

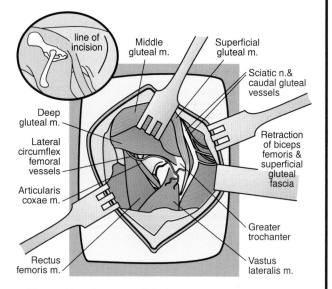

Figure 18.4: Exposure of the hip region via a craniolateral approach.

Trochanteric osteotomy approach
(See Chapter 17.) After reflecting the trochanter and the gluteal muscles dorsally, the remains of the deep gluteal muscle are cleared from the joint capsule. Incise the capsule longitudinally to expose the femoral neck and head.

→

OPERATIVE TECHNIQUE 18.1 (CONTINUED)

Epiphyseal fractures of the femoral head

Reduction and Fixation

An assistant should rotate the stifle and femoral shaft outwards to lateralize the femoral head so that the damage can be inspected. One or two Hohmann retractors are placed under the femoral neck to hold it up (Figure 18.5a). If the fragment is large enough, fixation should be done using 1.5 or 2.0 mm lag screws inserted if possible from the dorsal femoral head/neck junction. The fragment needs to be manipulated into position with a small Hohmann and grasped with forceps (on the round ligament if it is attached to the fragment) and held in place with small reduction forceps (Figure 18.5b). It may be necessary to sever the teres ligament in some cases to achieve this. The gliding hole for the lag screw is drilled from lateral to medial, angled as necessary from the femoral head/neck junction. The thread hole is drilled using a centring insert sleeve through the gliding hole. The hole is tapped and a countersink is used so that the head of the screw will be placed below the cartilage surface. Careful drill and screw measurement is necessary to avoid penetration of the articular surface. An anti-rotation K-wire should be inserted, either parallel to the screw or at an angle, also with its head countersunk (Figure 18.5c). This can be done with a hammer and a pin with a flat end. If the fragment of bone is a narrow slice, it will be necessary to insert the lag screw retrograde from the medial surface, if possible via the fovea capitis, ensuring that its head is countersunk. Small fragments may need to be removed, but assess the impact of removal on hip joint function. If it will be severely compromised, salvage surgery may be indicated (excision arthroplasty or total hip replacement).

WARNING

It is most important to minimize joint capsule damage to preserve blood supply. It is also essential that the sciatic nerve is identified and protected from damage. Do not apply pressure to it with a retractor!

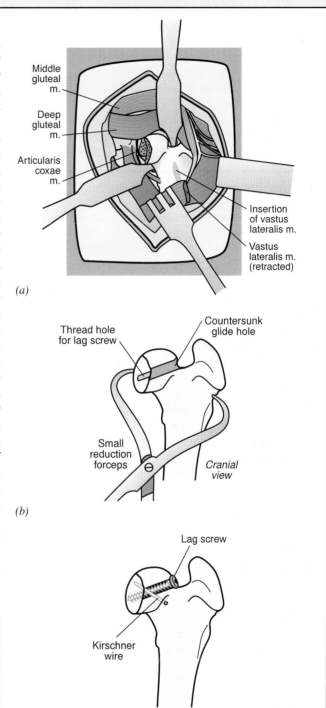

Figure 18.5: Exposure and fixation of a proximal femoral epiphyseal fracture (capital fracture in adults). (a) The femur is externally rotated and Hohmann retractors are used to elevate the distal segment to allow inspection of the fracture site. (b) Pointed reduction forceps are used to maintain reduction. (c) Lag screw and K-wire fixation.

→

OPERATIVE TECHNIQUE 18.1 (CONTINUED)
Epiphyseal fractures of the femoral head

Closure
The joint capsule should be repaired with interrupted sutures of absorbable material. The greater trochanter is re-attached using two K-wires and a wire tension-band. The gluteal tendon is sutured with mattress sutures of PDS and the vastus origin is similarly sutured to the deep gluteal. The superficial gluteal tendon is repaired with horizontal mattress sutures of PDS. The fascia lata is repaired with a continuous suture. The remainder of the closure is routine.

Post-operative Care
Six weeks of house confinement and a phased return to activity.

OPERATIVE TECHNIQUE 18.2

Physeal, subcapital and intertrochanteric fractures

Positioning
Lateral recumbency with affected leg uppermost.

Assistant
Often desirable to have two assistants – one to manipulate limb and one to retract.

Tray Extras
Appropriate bone screw set; drill bits; Gelpi, Langenbeck and small Hohmann retractors; small pointed reduction forceps; chuck; K-wires; pin/wire cutters.

Surgical Approach
Craniolateral approach as described in Operative Technique 18.1.

Reduction and fixation

Skeletally mature dogs
Assess the state of the femoral head and neck. In more chronic cases, damage due to abnormal rubbing of bone and cartilage may dictate an excision arthroplasty or hip replacement. Rotate the femoral neck out laterally and support it with Hohmann retractors (Figures 18.5 and 18.6). Drill the gliding hole for the lag screw retrograde from the neck to the subtrochanteric area (Figure 18.6). (An alternative method is to drill the hole from lateral to medial, using a C-shaped drill guide with the point of the guide centred on the lateralized femoral neck and the drill positioned over the third trochanter.) Reduce the fracture using small reduction forceps from fovea to greater trochanter after rotating the fragment into place with the aid of a small Hohmann retractor. A pair of small reduction forceps applied to the greater trochanter is also a useful aid in reduction as it allows easier mobilization of the bone. It is also possible to hold the fracture reduced by pressure against the acetabulum. Drill the thread hole for the lag screw using a centring insert sleeve through the gliding hole (Chapter 9). Before this hole is drilled, measure the depth of the fragment from the X-ray, add this to the depth of the gliding hole and set an adjustable stop on the drill bit to the required length. A thin piece of plastic tube which can be slid into place on the drill bit will suffice. This avoids penetration of the articular cartilage. An alternative is to set the drill bit in the drill to the measured total length of the gliding and thread holes. When measuring for screw size, do not add 2 mm to the screw length as is done with cortical bone. If a partially threaded cancellous bone screw is used, a gliding hole is unnecessary but careful measurement is needed to ensure that the screw threads are all within the fragment. Tap the hole. When the lag screw has been inserted, an anti-rotation K-wire of similar length, or slightly less, is inserted parallel to the screw, using a chuck or power driver (Figure 18.7). Bend over the K-wire, with the chuck attached well away from the bone, and cut it short so that the bend prevents medial migration of the wire.

An alternative technique is the use of three K-wires (below).

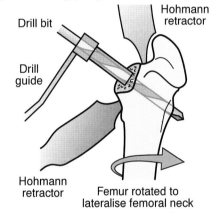

Figure 18.6: Retrograde drilling of the glide hole in the lag screw fixation of femoral neck fractures.

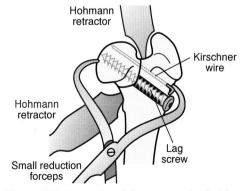

Figure 18.7: Femoral neck fracture repaired with a lag screw and anti-rotational K-wire. Pointed reduction forceps can be used to maintain reduction of a femoral neck fracture following the drilling of the screw glide hole (see text for details).

→

OPERATIVE TECHNIQUE 18.2 (CONTINUED)

Physeal, subcapital and intertrochanteric fractures

Cats and skeletally immature dogs

Two or three K-wires are used. The pins are placed retrograde from the fracture surface. Following reduction of the fracture, they are inserted the measured distance into the epiphysis before being cut (Figure 18.8). It is also possible to insert the K-wires normograde after reducing the fracture but this involves more guesswork in optimally positioning the pins.

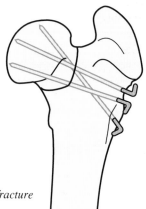

Figure 18.8: Femoral neck fracture repaired with three K-wires.

Alternative Technique

Use a trochanteric osteotomy approach. After reducing the fracture, hold it reduced by pressure against the acetabulum. Then insert two or three K-wires from the margins of the epiphysis into the femoral neck in a cruciate pattern and punch them below the articular surface using a hammer and small flat-ended pin (Figure 18.9).

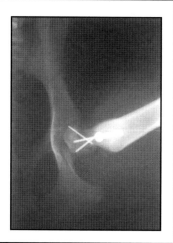

Figure 18.9: Repair of a proximal femoral physeal fracture in a dog using countersunk K-wires inserted from the articular margin (a trochanteric osteotomy was repaired with a lag screw). This is an alternative technique for the repair of physeal and neck fractures (see text for details).

Closure

See Operative Technique 18.1.

Post-operative Care

See Operative Technique 18.1.

OPERATIVE TECHNIQUE 18.3
Fracture of the greater trochanter

Positioning
Lateral recumbency with affected leg uppermost.

Assistant
Optional.

Tray Extras
Gelpi self-retaining retractors; chuck; K-wires; pin/wire cutters; wire for tension-band; drill and bit; pointed reduction forceps; pliers/wire twisters.

Surgical Approach
Incision is made over the greater trochanter directly on to the fracture.

Reduction and Fixation
The fracture is reduced by grasping the trochanter with small reduction forceps and pulling it, complete with its gluteal muscle insertions, back into position. Two K-wires are then inserted diagonally from lateral to medial through the trochanter and across the proximal femur, angled about 50° distally (see Figure 17.17). The tension-band wire should *not* be applied in a skeletally immature animal as it will close the growth plate.

Alternative technique
It is also possible to use a lag screw for this fixation in mature animals. The screw is inserted at an angle of 50° towards the medial cortex (Figure 18.9).

Post-operative Care
See Operative Technique 18.1.

OPERATIVE TECHNIQUE 18.4

Intramedullary pinning

Pre-operative Planning

The pin length is measured from the distal end of the medullary canal to the top of the greater trochanter. In a fat animal, an extra allowance for the depth of soft tissues above the trochanter has to be made. Pin size may also be assessed using a radiograph of the contralateral femur. The author prefers to pre-cut the pin to length and round off one end to make that end as atraumatic as possible; this end will be exposed to soft tissues and is less likely to cause irritation. The pin should be slightly narrower than the narrowest part of the medullary canal.

Positioning

Lateral recumbency with affected leg uppermost.

Assistant

Optional.

Tray Extras

Chuck; bone holding forceps; appropriate size intramedullary pin; wire for cerclage; pliers/wire twisters; pin/wire cutters; large pin cutters; drill and bits; Gelpi self-retaining retractors; +/- appropriate external fixator kit if type I fixator to be used as adjunct.

Surgical Approach

Make a skin incision over the cranial border of the bone from the subtrochanteric area to the femoral condyles. Retract the skin and make a small incision in the fascia lata in the same line where it is thickest, to find the muscle division between the biceps femoris caudally and the vastus lateralis cranially. The incision should lead into the gap between the two muscles. If the gap is not found, the incision is usually too caudal. Once found, extend the fascial incision with scissors and retract the biceps caudally to expose the shaft of the bone (Figure 18.10). The vastus has loose attachments to the femoral shaft which must be cut to allow its cranial retraction. The adductor muscle has firm attachments to the caudal border of the bone which include part of the femoral blood supply: these attachments should be disturbed as little as possible. This exposure allows access from the subtrochanteric area to the condyles.

Should access to the greater trochanter be necessary, the insertion of the superficial gluteal muscle may need to be tenotomized and the origin of the vastus muscle on the third trochanter has to be incised and reflected subperiosteally and distally to expose the trochanter.

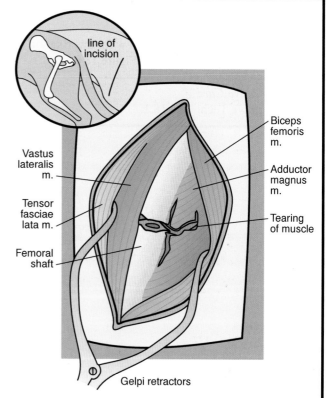

Figure 18.10: *Lateral exposure of a femoral diaphyseal fracture.*

→

OPERATIVE TECHNIQUE 18.4 (CONTINUED)

Intramedullary pinning

Reduction and Fixation

Examine the fracture ends to ensure that there are no fissure lines running longitudinally. If there are, it is essential to place cerclage wires around them before proceeding further to avoid the risk of splitting the bone during fracture reduction.

> **PRACTICAL TIP**
> It is easier to insert the pin retrograde from the fracture site up the proximal segment.

> **WARNING**
> This must be done with the hip in extension to avoid damage to the sciatic nerve.

> **PRACTICAL TIP**
> When using the larger pins, it is easier to drill a pilot hole with a narrower and sharper pin first.

The pin is drilled up the medullary canal until the point is felt to penetrate the trochanteric fossa, withdrawn and reversed to pass the blunt end up until it tents up the skin over the trochanteric fossa. Make a small incision over the head of the pin and re-attach the chuck to it. Withdraw the pin proximally to leave 1 cm protruding from the proximal fragment at the fracture site. Angle the fragments laterally (bone holding forceps may be required on the distal fragment) and hook the distal fragment on to the point of the pin (Figure 18.11a). Flatten down the fracture and drive the pin down the requisite distance (Figure 18.11b). When the chuck is removed, the pin should be at or just above the level of the trochanter and lying under the skin without tenting it up.

> **PRACTICAL TIP**
> Alignment of the edge of the adductor muscle on the caudal border of the femoral shaft is a useful check for correct alignment.

> **PRACTICAL TIP**
> If the canal is too wide for the largest pin (currently 6.25 mm), use two or three smaller pins to 'stack' the canal (Chapter 9). However, a better alternative is plate and screws (Operative Technique 18.5).

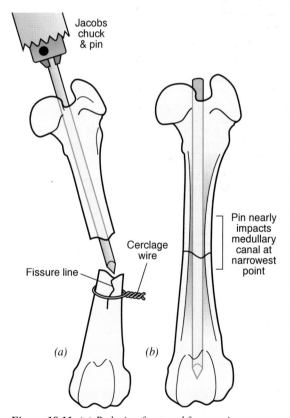

Figure 18.11: (a) Reducing fractured femur using intramedullary pin. Note cerclage wire pre-placed around a fissure line. (b) Fractured femur reduced with intramedullary pin.

OPERATIVE TECHNIQUE 18.4 (CONTINUED)
Intramedullary pinning

Preventing rotational instability in transverse and short oblique fractures
If there is rotational instability, a two-pin external fixator should be applied with the proximal pin in the subtrochanteric area and the distal in the lateral condyle, joined by a single connecting bar (Chapter 9) (Figure 18.12). An alternative in short oblique fractures is to use hemi-cerclage wire which has been pre-placed by drilling a hole through both cortices of one fragment and then tightened around the other after pin placement.

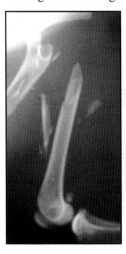 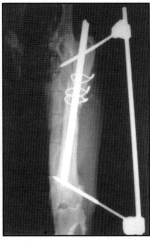

Figure 18.12: Comminuted fractured femur in a cat repaired with an intramedullary pin, three cerclage wires and an anti-rotation, two pin external fixator

Closure
The wound is closed by a continuous suture of absorbable suture in the fascia lata; thereafter closure is routine. If a wider approach has been made proximally, the origin of the vastus is sutured to the gluteal tendon insertions on the greater trochanter and the superficial gluteal is re-attached to its tendon with mattress sutures of PDS or Vicryl.

Post-operative Care
Dogs: lead exercise only for 6 weeks. Phased return to activity.
Cats (and small dogs): room confinement; cage confinement in some cases.

OPERATIVE TECHNIQUE 18.5
Bone plating

Pre-operative Planning
Plates may be positioned from the distal femoral condyles to the top of the greater trochanter. Plates are applied to the lateral surface of the femur, which is the tension side. As a plate is positioned more proximally and distally, it has to be contoured more to allow for the bone curvature.

Positioning
Lateral recumbency with affected leg uppermost.

Assistant
Useful. Essential for some fractures (see below).

Tray Extras
Appropriate size bone screw set; drill and bits; Gelpi self-retaining retractors; +/- orthopaedic wire; +/- distractor; bone holding forceps; small pointed reduction forceps; Hohmann retractors; curette for bone graft.

Surgical Approach
As for Operative Technique 18.4.

Reduction and Fixation
Oblique and spiral fractures are difficult to reduce. Assistants are essential to aid in traction on the limb and the use of several pairs of bone holding forceps is usually necessary to apply the traction and rotation manoeuvres needed to reduce the fractures. Use a distractor. Avoid glove puncture on sharp spikes of bone.

Where comminution involves the subtrochanteric area, it will be necessary to contour the plate to the top of the greater trochanter with probably two short screws angled distally through the plate and into the trochanter. (The use of a dynamic compression plate is recommended as its oval holes allow easier positioning of oblique screws.) In addition, a longer screw passing through the plate and along the femoral neck from the third trochanter area is needed (Figure 18.13). Where an intertrochanteric fracture is also present, the screw along the femoral neck has to be a lag screw. This can be supplemented by an anti-rotation K-wire, which is inserted first to hold the fracture after its reduction and before the lag screw is inserted. It is also possible to use hook plates in this situation, but this requires some special instruments and they are not widely used in small animals.

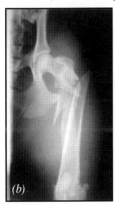
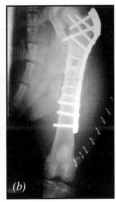

(b) (b)

Figure 18.13: Subtrochanteric comminuted fracture of femur repaired using lag screws and neutralization plate.

Closure
As for Operative Technique 18.4.

Post-operative Care
As for Operative Technique 18.4.

OPERATIVE TECHNIQUE 18.6
External fixation

Positioning
Lateral recumbency with affected leg uppermost.

Assistant
Optional.

Tray Extras
Appropriate size external fixator set; bone holding forceps; Gelpi self-retaining retractor; chuck/drill; large pin cutters.

Surgical Approach
When a fixator is used as the sole means of fracture stabilization (Figure 18.14), the pins can be inserted through stab incisions following closed reduction of the fracture. Alternatively a limited lateral approach is used (Operative Technique 18.4). Refer to the concept of a minimally invasive strategy for fracture repair discussed in Chapter 10.

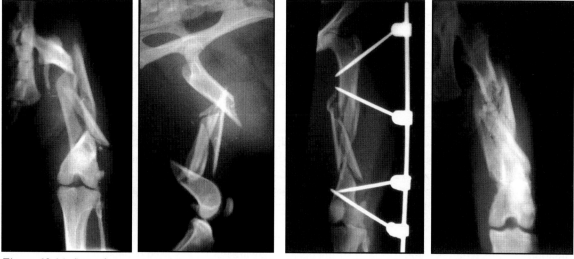

Figure 18.14: Severely comminuted femoral diaphyseal fracture in a cat. The fracture was stabilized using a unilateral uniplanar external skeletal fixator and healed uneventfully.

Post-operative Care
See Chapter 9.

OPERATIVE TECHNIQUE 18.7

Fractures involving the distal femoral growth plate

Pre-operative Planning

Rush pins may be purchased ready made, but most are too thick. It is easy to make your own from K-wires with the help of a vice and a triangular file (Figure 18.15). For cats, 1.0–1.5 mm diameter pins are used; and for dogs, 1.5–2.0 mm. The length, measured from a pre-operative radiograph, is a distance that will extend from the base of the condyle to approximately one-third to one-half the length of the diaphysis.

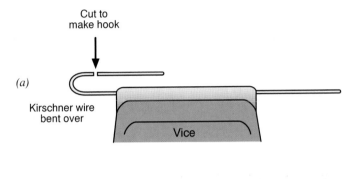

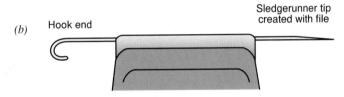

Figure 18.15: *Bend the K-wire into a loop at its measured length and clamp the loop in a vice so that the pin can be cut through the loop with the file to create a short hook which is rounded off. On the opposite side of the pin to the hook, create the sledge runner tip in a gradual tapering slope. It is unnecessary to have a point. Round off the edges with the file.*

Positioning

Lateral recumbency with affected leg uppermost.

Assistant

Optional.

Tray Extras

Langenbeck or Gelpi retractors; small Hohmann retractor; small pointed reduction forceps; implants; Rush pins/K-wires; chuck; pliers; pin/wire cutters.

OPERATIVE TECHNIQUE 18.7 (CONTINUED)
Fractures involving the distal femoral growth plate

Surgical Approach

Make a lateral parapatellar incision from the tibial tuberosity to a point 3–4 cm proximal to the patella. Continue the incision through the subcutaneous fascia and then through the dense fascia lata, ensuring that the incision is lateral to both the patella ligament and patella. Make a small stab incision in the joint capsule lateral to the patella ligament, insert the blade of a straight pair of scissors and cut proximally, parallel with the patella, to incise intermuscularly between the biceps femoris caudally and the vastus lateralis cranially. Continue proximally until the patella can be displaced medially (with the joint extended) and the joint can be explored (Figure 18.16).

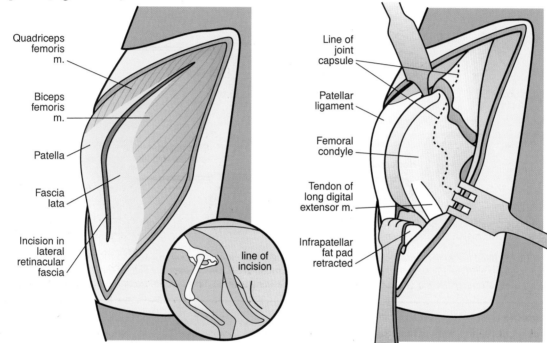

Figure 18.16: *Exposure of a distal femoral fracture.*

Reduction and Fixation

After clearing out any blood clot from the stifle and from the fracture surfaces, **the fracture is reduced with the stifle in flexion**. A pair of small reduction forceps applied transversely across the condyle may help to manipulate it. It is sometimes necessary to use a small Hohmann retractor as a lever between the condyle and the metaphysis to ease reduction. This has to be done carefully as the bone in immature animals is soft and easily damaged. Once the fracture has been reduced for the first time, it will reduce more easily thereafter.

> **WARNING**
> **Reduction should be either anatomical or stepped with the condyles slightly cranial to the metaphysis, but not underreduced.**

At this stage, the fracture may be held in reduction by inserting a K-wire obliquely from the lateral condyle into the proximal fragment. Alternatively, small reduction forceps are placed between the intercondylar fossa of the distal fragment and a small hole drilled on the cranial aspect of the distal diaphysis (Figure 18.17).

→

OPERATIVE TECHNIQUE 18.7 (CONTINUED)

Fractures involving the distal femoral growth plate

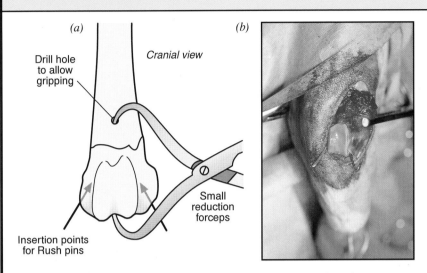

(a) Cranial view

Drill hole to allow gripping

Small reduction forceps

Insertion points for Rush pins

(b)

Figure 18.17: *(a) Position of reduction forceps to hold distal epiphyseal separation of femur reduced with insertion points for Rush pins or K-wires. (b) Reduced epiphyseal separation in a cat showing position of Rush pins before they are pushed home.*

Using a K-wire, drill a hole from the distal aspect of the lateral condyle just below the origin of the long digital extensor tendon obliquely to the mid point of the distal fragment and continue through the metaphysis into the medullary canal (Figure 18.17). Insert the first Rush pin half-way, using a pair of pliers. The Rush pin may need to be curved so that when it enters the medullary canal, it will strike the medial wall of the canal and bounce off, continuing up the canal. Check by palpation that the pin has not penetrated the medial cortex. Repeat the process on the medial condyle to insert the medial Rush pin. Remove the temporary K-wire (if used) and push both Rush pins fully home so that the bends of the distal hooks are just protruding from the bone of the condyles (Figures 18.18 and 18.19). Reduce the patella and check that joint movement is free before closure.

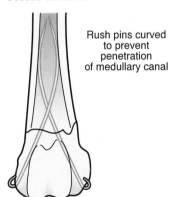

Rush pins curved to prevent penetration of medullary canal

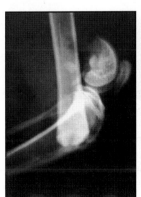
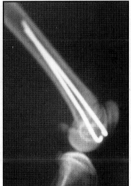
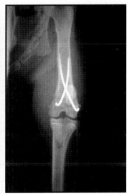

Figure 18.18: *Epiphyseal separation fixed with two Rush pins. Their hooks are above and clear of the bearing surface of the condyles.*

Figure 18.19: *Type 1 Salter-Harris distal epiphyseal separation in a cat. Pre-operative and two post-operative radiographs showing fixation with two Rush pins.*

If using crossed K-wires or arthrodesis wires for fixation, the procedure is similar, but following reduction and temporary fixation, a suitable diameter K-wire is driven obliquely from the lateral condyle to pass through the metaphysis and just penetrate the medial wall of the distal diaphysis. The distal end of the K-wire is bent over and cut short to leave a short hook. A similar wire is inserted from the medial condyle (Figure 18.20).

→

OPERATIVE TECHNIQUE 18.7 (CONTINUED)
Fractures involving the distal femoral growth plate

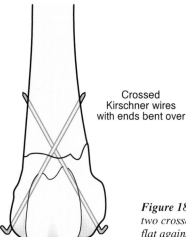

Crossed
Kirschner wires
with ends bent over

Figure 18.20: Distal epiphyseal separation of femur fixed with two crossed K-wires. Their distal ends are bent over and pushed flat against the bone.

An alternative technique for managing corresponding fractures in **skeletally mature animals** is to use a lag screw (Figure 18.21).

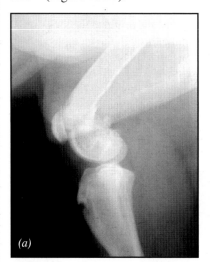

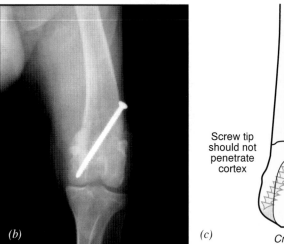

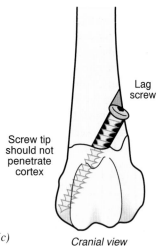

Lag
screw

Screw tip
should not
penetrate
cortex

(a)

(b)

(c)

Cranial view

Figure 18.21: Fractured distal femoral epiphysis in mature dog. Fixation by oblique lag screw (fracture healed).

Closure
The joint capsule and fascia lata are closed with interrupted cruciate sutures of Vicryl or PDS and the superficial layers of fascia and the subcutaneous layers with continuous absorbable suture.

Post-operative Care
Consider removal of the Rush pins/wires at 3 weeks if a radiograph shows the growth plate to be open, but restrict activity for a further 3 weeks.

OPERATIVE TECHNIQUE 18.8
Articular fractures of the distal femur (condylar fractures)

Positioning
Dorsal recumbency with leg extended caudally.

Assistant
Can be useful during fracture reduction.

Tray Extras
Langenbeck or Gelpi retractors; small Hohmann retractor; pointed reduction forceps; K-wires/Rush pins; chuck; pliers; pin/wire cutters; appropriate size bone screw set; drill and bits.

Surgical Approach
See Operative Technique 18.7. Increased exposure may be gained by osteotomy of the tibial tuberosity and proximal reflection of the quadriceps muscle mass (Piermattei, 1993).

Reduction and Fixation

Single condylar fractures
Reduce the condyles one to another and clamp them with small reduction forceps. Drill a gliding hole in the smaller fragment, then drill the thread hole in the larger, using an insert drill sleeve. Measure and tap the hole and insert a lag screw so that the tip of the screw is not protruding from the bone surface (Figure 18.22). Alternatively, an "inside-out' method may be used, as with the humerus (Chapter 15).

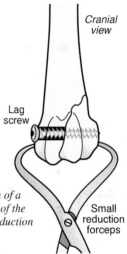

Figure 18.22: Reduction of a single condylar fracture of the distal femur held with reduction forceps and fixed with a transcondylar lag screw.

Bicondylar fractures
Reduce and fix the condyles as described above. The condyles are then reattached to the proximal fragment using Rush pins or crossed K-wires, as described in Operative Technique 18.7 (Figure 18.23).

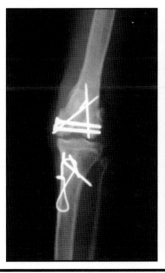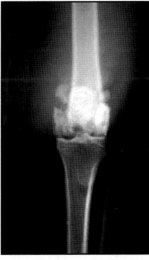

Figure 18.23: Comminuted intercondylar fracture of distal femur fixed with two lag screws and two crossed K-wires. A tibial tuberosity osteotomy used in the surgical approach has been fixed with a K-wire and wire tension band.

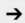

OPERATIVE TECHNIQUE 18.8 (CONTINUED)
Articular fractures of the distal femur (condylar fractures)

Closure
The joint capsule and fascia lata are closed with interrupted cruciate sutures of Vicryl or PDS. The rest of the closure is routine.

Post-operative Care
Restricted activity for 6 to 8 weeks.

CHAPTER NINETEEN

Tibia and Fibula

Steven J. Butterworth

Fractures of the tibia and fibula are commonly seen in small animal practice. In one study, they represented 14.8% of 284 canine fractures and 5.4% of 298 feline fractures (Phillips, 1979). Such injuries are usually a result of road traffic accidents but other causes include dog fights and trapping a foot whilst moving at speed.

FRACTURES OF THE PROXIMAL TIBIA AND FIBULA

In the vast majority of cases these involve physes of skeletally immature patients (Chapter 11).

Avulsion of the tibial tubercle

This injury is almost exclusively seen in animals less than about 10 months of age and the Greyhound is over-represented (Figure 19.1a,b). The tibial tubercle

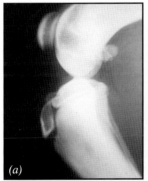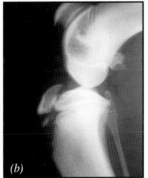

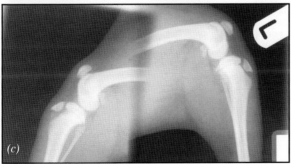

Figure 19.1: Avulsion of the tibial tubercle. (a) Mediolateral radiographs of the normal stifle of a 6-month-old Greyhound. (b) Contralateral joint of the same animal showing complete avulsion of the tubercle. (c) Partial avulsion of the right tibial tubercle in a 4-month-old Tibetan Terrier. Left included for comparison.

forms as a separate centre of ossification and serves as the point of insertion for the straight patellar ligament. Avulsion of the tubercle renders the dog unable to fix the stifle during weightbearing. Swelling will be present on the cranial aspect of the joint, the tubercle may be palpated proximal to its normal position and the patella will be positioned proximally in the trochlear groove. Radiography provides a definitive diagnosis.

If radiography shows only a partial avulsion (Figure 19.1c), then the patient may be treated conservatively. Casting or splinting is unlikely to be effective and management should comprise strict cage rest and monitoring in case the avulsion should become complete. Alternatively, surgery may be considered.

In all cases where complete avulsion has occurred, open reduction and internal fixation using the tension-band principle are required to re-establish the integrity of the quadriceps complex (Operative Technique 19.1).

Separation of the proximal tibial physis

This is an uncommon injury seen only in immature patients (Figure 19.2). It is associated with caudal rotation of the tibial plateau and craniomedial displacement of the proximal tibial metaphysis. Such rotational deformity is severely disabling since the stifle cannot be fully extended. Marked lameness will be seen, associated with pain and swelling about the stifle.

Figure 19.2: Mediolateral radiograph of the stifle of a 6-month-old Shetland Sheepdog showing a Salter–Harris type 2 fracture of the proximal tibial physis with caudal rotation of the epiphysis.

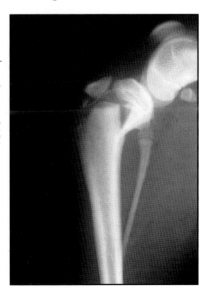

If there is only minimal displacement then the patient may be treated conservatively. Casting or splinting may be beneficial but management should also include strict cage rest.

In all cases where caudal displacement of the plateau has occurred, early open reduction and internal fixation are required to re-establish joint congruity. The plateau may be secured in place using crossed K-wires or a single intramedullary pin in larger patients (Operative Technique 19.2). If the tubercle remains attached to the plateau, this may be used to seat the implants so that they remain away from the articular margins.

Fracture of the proximal fibula

These fractures occur rarely in isolation. If they do result from a lateral blow then there may be pain or swelling on the lateral aspect of the stifle and pain on joint manipulation. The majority of these rare events are not associated with separation of the fibular head from the tibia and can be treated conservatively. If there is lateral instability of the stifle due to weakening of the insertion of the lateral collateral ligament, the fibular head could be re-attached to the tibia using either a lagged bone screw or a pin and tension-band wire.

Technique	Indications	Contraindications
Bone Plating (Operative Technique 19.3)	• As compression plates in medium to large breed, skeletally mature dogs with transverse or short oblique fractures where axial compression can be achieved • As neutralization plates in medium to large breed dogs with oblique or reconstructable, comminuted fractures where interfragmentary compression can be created using lagged bone screws • As buttress plates in any size of patient with a non-reconstructable, comminuted fracture • Proximal or distal fractures where specially designed plates (e.g. T-plates) may help to overcome problems of limited bone stock.	• When an alternative method of fixation would provide adequate stability whilst causing less iatrogenic soft tissue damage and a reduction in the cost of management, or would avoid leaving implants *in situ*.
Intramedullary pinning (Operative Technique 19.4)	• Transverse fracture (axially stable) and interdigitation of the two fragments creates rotational stability • Skeletally immature, so that early callus formation will create rotational stability to counteract the instability resulting from resorption of the fracture ends • Where augmentation with cerclage wires or an ESF may counteract rotational instability.	• When the tibial conformation is such that placement of a straight IM pin would not regain a semblance of normal anatomy, e.g. in some of the chondrodystrophoid breeds, where this might cause delayed healing and/or clinically significant malunion • When the fracture is open • When the age and/or size of the patient, together with the configuration of the fracture, makes it likely that auxillary fixation may fail or need repeated adjustments before healing is adequate and use of a bone plate and screws might be considered more appropriate in reducing post-operative management and complications.
External skeletal fixation (Operative Technique 19.5)	• Minimally displaced or stable fractures, particularly in skeletally immature patients, when an external cast might be insufficient or difficult to maintain • To protect implants used to create compression at the fracture surfaces, e.g. cerclage wires or lagged bone screws, especially in chondrodystrophoid breeds where the medullary canal is not straight, making the use of an IM pin inappropriate, and the contour of the bone's surface would make contouring of a plate difficult. • Ancillary stability for the primary method of fixation (e.g. IM pin) • Open fractures • Severely comminuted, non-reconstructable fractures*. An ESF can be used as part of a minimally invasive strategy (see Chapter 10) • Very proximal or distal, comminuted, non-reconstructable diaphyseal fractures where the option of bridging the adjacent joint with the frame can be utilized when there is insufficient bone stock adjacent to the joint to allow adequate stabilization to be achieved using other methods.	
Interlocking nails	• Not in widespread veterinary use • An alternative to ESF or plating for buttressing comminuted mid-diaphyseal fractures (see Chapter 9)	
External coaptation	• Fracture lines are hairline or minimally displaced • Skeletally immature animal • Inherent fracture stability	• When fracture is simple but rotationally unstable, comminuted or open • When patient is middle aged or old.

Table 19.1: Decision making in the management of diaphyseal fractures of the tibia and fibula.
* In non-reconstructable, comminuted or open fractures the alternatives of applying an external skeletal fixator or a bone plate exist and the choice between these options may come down to surgeon's preference. The author would tend to favour the use of bone plates, with minimal fragmentary interference in the severely comminuted fractures and external skeletal fixators in cases with open fractures.

FRACTURES OF THE TIBIAL AND FIBULAR DIAPHYSES

These injuries usually occur in combination and it is the tibial fracture that is the more important. The fibula bears little weight and shaft fractures of this bone alone may be treated conservatively. In cases where both are fractured, reduction and stabilization of the tibia will amply realign and protect the fibula during fracture healing. Where the fibula remains intact in the face of a tibial fracture, the support offered by the intact bone will greatly support the tibial repair. The sparsity of soft tissue cover in the mid and distal diaphysis results in an increase in the likelihood of such fractures being open and may also lead to a reduced rate of fracture healing. However, surgical exposure of fractures is relatively straightforward. Owing to the natural twist in the tibia, fractures tend to spiral along the shaft and hairline fissures that extend beyond the radiographically visible fracture lines are not uncommon.

The anatomy of the crus makes it feasible to employ a number of methods to stabilize tibial shaft fractures, namely casts, intramedullary pins, external skeletal fixators and bone plates and screws (Table 19.1).

DISTAL TIBIA AND FIBULA

In skeletally immature patients the 'weak points' in this region are the distal physes whereas in the older patient it is more likely that trauma will result in avulsion of the medial and/or lateral malleolus, which are the points of origin for the tarsocrural collateral ligaments. The importance of these fractures revolves around their influence on tarsocrural joint alignment and stability.

Distal physeal separation
The injury is seen in skeletally immature patients (Figure 19.3) and most often results from a medially directed blow to the lateral aspect of the distal crus which causes medial displacement of the distal tibial metaphysis and valgus deformity of the pes. Abrasions may be present or the distal tibial metaphysis might have actually broken through the skin.

If closed reduction is possible, and the fracture then feels relatively stable, external coaptation may be employed with casting of the limb as far proximal as the stifle. If reduction cannot be achieved or the site is considered unstable then open reduction and internal fixation is mandatory (Operative Technique 19.6).

Fractures of the lateral or medial malleolus
Such injuries are usually seen in skeletally mature patients and result from road traffic accidents where shearing injuries may be caused by the distal limb being trapped under the wheel of a braking car. Apart from swelling and possible displacement of the pes, the

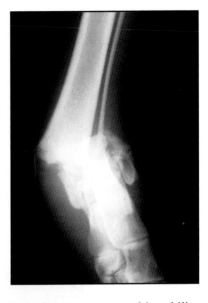

Figure 19.3: Dorsoplantar radiograph showing a displaced Salter–Harris type 1 fracture of the distal tibial physis and fibula in a 5-month-old Dobermann Pinscher.

main clinical finding relates to tarsocrural instability due to loss of collateral support (Figure 19.4a). Radiography may show gross displacement (Figure 19.4b,c) but, in some cases, stressed views may be necessary to demonstrate the instability.

In younger patients, the periosteum may not be disrupted with minimal displacement of the fragments. Such cases can be managed satisfactorily by application of a cast for 4 to 6 weeks. Cases with gross

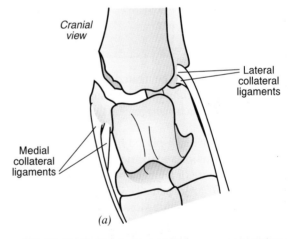

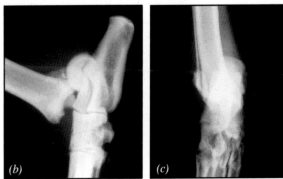

Figure 19.4: Malleolar fractures. (a) Fracture of the medial malleolus resulting in loss of collateral ligament support. (b) Mediolateral and (c) dorsoplantar radiographs showing caudal luxation of the tarsocrural joint associated with fracture of the lateral malleolus in a dog.

Figure 19.5:
(a) Dorsoplantar radiograph of a hock showing complete loss of the lateral malleolus, as a result of a shearing injury, in a 4-year-old Cavalier King Charles Spaniel. (b) Management of the injury by application of a Rudy boot fixator (see Chapter 9) to the medial aspect of the distal limb. This confers stability on the joint and allows good access to the wound whilst soft tissue healing takes place.

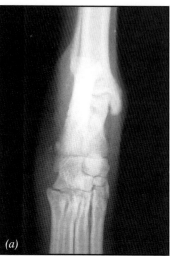

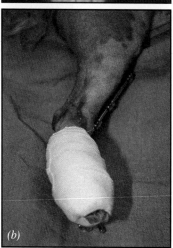

(a)

(b)

displacement can also be treated in this way if closed reduction can be achieved. Lateral malleolar fractures respond better to such management than medial malleolar fractures.

Most cases with displaced malleolar fractures require open reduction and fixation with either a pin and tension-band wire or a lagged bone screw (Operative Technique 19.7). In patients with shearing injuries (Figure 19.5a) the resulting loss of tissue may preclude anatomical reconstruction and the degree of contamination may make the use of a collateral prosthesis

inadvisable in the early stages. Management may take the form of a transarticular external skeletal fixator (possibly incorporating a 'Rudy boot' for fixation distally) to support the joint whilst soft tissue healing takes place (Figure 19.5b). Although a second procedure to create a collateral prosthesis once the wound has granulated may be planned, it is often found that satisfactory joint stability is present by the time the ESF is removed, especially if the injury involved the lateral collateral support.

REFERENCES AND FURTHER READING

Aron DN, Johnson AL and Palmer RH (1995) Biologic strategies and a balanced concept for repair of highly comminuted long bone fractures. *Compendium of Continuing Education for the Practising Veterinarian* **17**, 35.

Brinker WO, Piermattei DL and Flo GL (1990) Fractures of the tibia and fibula. In: *Handbook of Small Animal Orthopaedics and Fracture Treatment*, 2nd edn. WB Saunders Company, Philadelphia.

Butterworth SJ (1993) Use of external fixators for fracture treament in small animals. *In Practice* **15**, 183.

Carmichael S (1991) The external skeletal fixator in small animal orthopaedics. *Journal of Small Animal Practice* **32**, 486.

Eaton-Wells RD, Matis U, Robins GM and Whittick WG (1990) The pelvis and the pelvic limb. In: *Canine Orthopaedics*, 2nd edn. Lea & Febiger, Philadelphia.

Egger EL and Whittick WG (1990) Principles of fracture management. In: *Canine Orthopaedics*, 2nd edn. Lea & Febiger, Philadelphia.

Leighton RL (1994) Hindlimb. In: *Small Animal Orthopaedics*. Wolfe, London.

Lipowitz AJ, Caywood DD, Newton CD and Finch ME (1993) Tibia. In: *Small Animal Orthopaedics Illustrated – Surgical Approaches and Procedures*. Mosby, St Louis.

Marti JM and Miller A (1994) Delimitation of safe corridors for the insertion of external fixator pins in the dog 1: Hindlimb. *Journal of Small Animal Practice* **35**, 16.

Muir P, Parker RB, Goldsmid SE and Johnson KA (1993) Interlocking intramedullary nail stabilisation of a diaphyseal tibial fracture. *Journal of Small Animal Practice* **34**, 26.

Phillips IR (1979) A survey of bone fractures in the dog and cat. *Journal of Small Animal Practice* **20**, 661-674.

Piermattei DL (1993) *An Atlas of Surgical Approaches to the Bones and Joints of the Dog and Cat*, 3rd edn. WB Saunders Company, Philadelphia.

Raiha JE, Axelson P, Skutnabb K, Rokkanen P and Tormala P (1993) Fixation of cancellous bone and physeal fractures with biodegradable rods of self-reinforced polylactic acid. *Journal of Small Animal Practice* **34**, 131.

Raiha JE, Axelson P, Rokkanen P and Tormala P (1993). Intramedullary nailing of diaphyseal fractures with self-reinforced polylactide implants. *Journal of Small Animal Practice* **34**, 337.

Richardson EF and Thacher CW (1993) Tibial fractures in cats. *Compendium of Continuing Education for the Practising Veterinarian* **15**, 383.

OPERATIVE TECHNIQUE 19.1
Avulsion of the tibial tubercle

Positioning
Dorsal recumbency with the affected limb extended caudally.

Assistant
Optional.

Tray Extras
Pointed reduction forceps; Hohmann retractor; Gelpi self-retaining retractor; chuck; pliers/wire twisters; K-wires; wire for tension-band; pin/wire cutters.

Surgical Approach
A craniolateral incision extending from just below the level of the patella to about two-thirds of the way down the tibial crest. Soft tissue dissection allows identification of the tibial tubercle. Removal of organizing haematoma will expose the fracture surfaces. If a tension-band wire is to be applied, then reflection of the cranial tibialis muscle from the lateral aspect of the tibia is required to expose the site for drilling of the transverse tibial tunnel.

Reduction and Fixation
Reduction of the fracture is most easily achieved with the stifle extended; however maintaining reduction whilst implants are placed can be difficult since the fragment is often too small to be held with forceps. The traction created by the quadriceps muscle can be counteracted by the application of pointed forceps to the patella, or Allis tissue forceps to the patellar ligament, and using these to draw the fragment distally (Figure 19.6a,b).

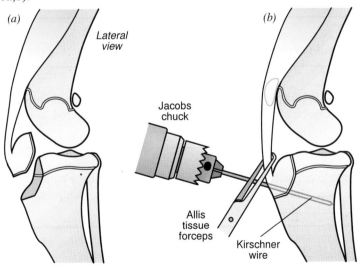
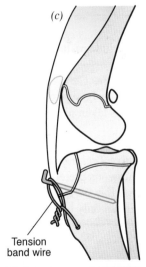

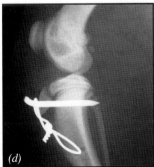

Figure 19.6: Surgical management of an avulsed tibial tuberosity. (a) Avulsed tibial tuberosity. (b) Allis tissue forceps encircling the straight patellar ligament are used to apply traction to the avulsed fragment and reduce the fracture; one or two K-wires are then driven across the fracture site to maintain reduction. (c) A figure-of-eight tension-band wire is added to counteract the pull of the quadriceps muscle group. (d) Post-operative radiograph showing a repaired tibial tuberosity avulsion in a 7-month-old Border Terrier. The fracture was stabilized using a single K-wire and figure-of-eight tension-band wire.

→

OPERATIVE TECHNIQUE 19.1 (CONTINUED)
Avulsion of the tibial tubercle

The recommended method of internal fixation involves the placement of two K-wires through the tubercle and into the proximal tibia, to prevent rotation, with a figure-of-eight tension-band wire (Figure 19.6c). In some patients, owing to their size, it is difficult to pass two pins through the tubercle. A single pin will suffice in such circumstances (Figure 19.6d). Pins should be bent over to prevent migration. In patients approaching skeletal maturity, by the time the fracture has healed (i.e. 8 to 10 months of age), the implants may be left in place; but in much younger patients implants should be removed after about 5 weeks to try to prevent early closure of the physis and subsequent drifting of the tubercle distally relative to the tibial shaft. Alternatively, in these young patients, absorbable implants may be used (e.g. biodegradable pins and/or figure-of-eight PDS sutures in place of the tension-band wire). Premature closure of the physis may result from the injury itself and deformity may be seen whatever treatment method is chosen, even if a tension band is avoided or removed early (Figure 19.7).

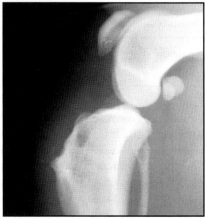

Figure 19.7: Distal migration of the tibial tuberosity due to premature growth plate closure following repair of a tibial tuberosity avulsion. The implants were removed after 4 weeks.

PRACTICAL TIP
In cases where only a small part of the tubercle has become avulsed, reattachment of the patellar ligament to the tibia is best achieved by placement of tendon sutures through the ligament and through transverse bone tunnels in the tibial tuberosity/crest.

Closure
Should include reattachment of the fascia of the cranial tibialis muscle to the cranial aspect of the tibia.

Post-operative Care
The joint may be supported in a padded dressing for 5 to 10 days and the patient should be rested until fracture healing has taken place, usually by 4 to 6 weeks. Implant removal may have to be considered, as discussed above.

Alternative Technique
Some surgeons prefer to secure the tubercle in position with a lagged bone screw, with or without an anti-rotational K-wire and/or tension-band wire. Since such a technique will create static compression of the physis it can only be recommended in patients already approaching skeletal maturity.

OPERATIVE TECHNIQUE 19.2
Separation of the proximal tibial physis

Positioning
Dorsal recumbency with the affected limb extended caudally.

Assistant
Optional.

Tray Extras
Pointed reduction forceps; Hohmann retractor; Gelpi self-retaining retractor; chuck; pliers; K-wires; wire; pin/wire cutters.

Surgical Approach
A craniomedial incision extending from just below the level of the patella to about two-thirds of the way down the tibial crest. Soft tissue dissection should allow identification of the tibial plateau and removal of any organizing haematoma will expose the fracture surfaces. If a tension-band wire is to be applied then reflection of the cranial tibialis muscle from the lateral aspect of the tibia is required to expose the site for drilling of the transverse tibial tunnel.

Reduction and Fixation
Reduction of the fracture is most easily achieved with the stifle extended. In most cases, reduction can be achieved by holding the stifle in extension and placing a small Hohmann retractor into the fracture space from the craniomedial aspect and gently levering the plateau forwards (Figure 19.8).

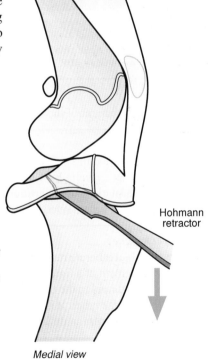

Hohmann retractor

Figure 19.8: The use of a Hohmann retractor to facilitate reduction of a proximal tibial physeal fracture.

Medial view

WARNING
The tibial plateau may split if too much leverage is applied.

→

OPERATIVE TECHNIQUE 19.2 (CONTINUED)
Separation of the proximal tibial physis

Digital pressure is usually the most practicable way of holding the plateau in reduction whilst the implants are placed. Fixation may be achieved by placement of crossed K-wires (Figure 19.9a,b). If at all possible, the pins should be bent over to avoid implant migration. Placement of implants and tension-band wires in the region of the tibial tubercle is discussed in Operative Technique 19.1.

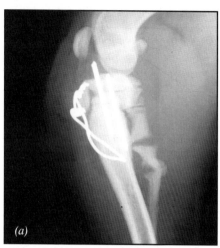 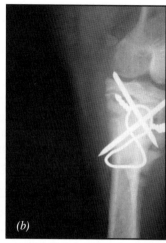 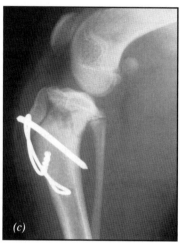

Figure 19.9: (a) Mediolateral and (b) craniocaudal post-operative radiographs of a proximal tibial physeal fracture in a 6-month-old West Highland White Terrier. The fracture was stabilized with crossed K-wires and a figure-of-eight wire. (c) Fracture of the proximal tibial physis in a 5-month-old West Highland White Terrier stabilized with a single K-wire and figure-of-eight tension-band wire.

Closure
Should include reattachment of the fascia of the cranial tibialis muscle to the cranial aspect of the tibia.

Post-operative Care
The joint may be supported in a padded dressing for 5 to 10 days and the patient should be rested until fracture healing has taken place, usually by 4 to 6 weeks. Implant removal may have to be considered as discussed above. The implants sit close to the articular margins and may interfere with normal joint function, making it necessary for them to be removed.

Alternative Techniques
In most cases the tibial tubercle remains attached to the plateau and, following open reduction, stability may be achieved by placement of a figure-of-eight wire anchored under the insertion of the patellar ligament and through a transverse tunnel in the tibial crest and/or placement of a K-wire through the tubercle and into the tibia (Figure 19.9c). If the tubercle is used to create stability then the points discussed in Operative Technique 19.1 are applicable. An intramedullary pin can also be used for fixation (see Operative Technique 19.4).

OPERATIVE TECHNIQUE 19.3

Tibia – medial bone plating

Positioning
Lateral recumbency with the affected limb down, to allow access to the medial aspect. The contralateral limb is drawn out of the surgical field and a rope or bandage sling is secured to the table, passing medial to the affected limb proximally so that traction can be applied to the fracture site by drawing on the pes without this causing movement of the patient. Alternatively, the limb may be suspended from a ceiling hook which allows 360° access to the crus.

Assistant
Useful, especially if traction is required to help maintain fragment alignment and to reduce the time taken for plate application.

Tray Extras
Pointed reduction forceps; other bone holding forceps of the surgeon's choice (e.g. Dingman or Lewin bone holding forceps); Hohmann retractor; self-retaining retractors (e.g. Gelpi or Weitlander); periosteal elevator; drill and bits; appropriate plate and screw set.

Surgical Approach (Figure 19.10)
A craniomedial skin incision is made along most (if not all) of the tibial length. If the incision is made too medially then the closure will lie directly over the plate and increase the likelihood of problems with wound healing. Dissection through the subcutaneous fascia will expose the tibial shaft easily, with the cranial tibial muscle forming the cranial margin and the long digital flexor muscle the caudal margin. The only complicating structures are those of the cranial branch of the medial saphenous artery and vein which run alongside the saphenous nerve. All three structures cross the medial aspect of the tibia in a caudoproximal to craniodistal direction about half-way along the diaphysis. Although it is preferable to try to preserve these structures, they can be ligated and sectioned in order to reduce operating time, without causing serious complications.

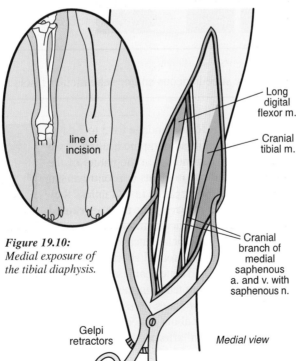

line of incision

Long digital flexor m.

Cranial tibial m.

Cranial branch of medial saphenous a. and v. with saphenous n.

Gelpi retractors

Medial view

Figure 19.10:
Medial exposure of the tibial diaphysis.

→

OPERATIVE TECHNIQUE 19.3 (CONTINUED)
Tibia – medial bone plating

Reduction and Fixation (Figure 19.11)
Common mistakes in plate application include: not exposing the tibia proximally enough where it is easy to believe the exposure must be close to the stifle when there is still one-third of the tibia further proximal (especially in obese patients); and not extending the plate distally enough for fear of compromising the tarsocrural joint. Proximal exposure is assisted by use of the groin sling described above and having an assistant to apply traction to the limb. If the bone stock is poor proximally then T- or L-plates may enable adequate screw 'grouping' and thus implant purchase, although these tend to be available in only limited lengths and are often inadequate in comminuted fractures. As long as the plate does not extend beyond the origin of the medial collateral ligament distally and the distal-most screw is angled slightly proximally, there is little chance of interfering with hock joint function.

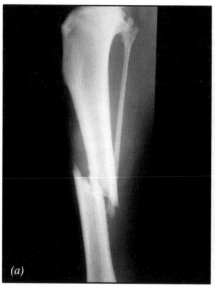
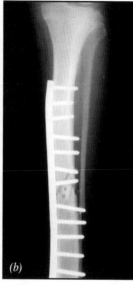

(a)

(b)

Figure 19.11: (a) Pre-operative and (b) post-operative radiographs of a short, oblique tibial diaphyseal fracture in a 1-year-old Great Dane stabilized using a dynamic compression plate.

Closure
Closure is achieved by apposition of the subcutaneous and/or subcuticular fascia and then the skin.

Post-operative Care
In most cases it is preferable to apply a Robert Jones bandage for 3 to 7 days. Exercise restriction should be implemented until radiographic healing of the fracture is apparent – usually 4 to 8 weeks, depending on the nature of the fracture and age of the patient. The need to remove implants is a controversial issue. Generally, the author prefers to leave the implants *in situ* unless they cause problems. The most common reasons for removing the plate are caused by lack of soft tissue cover in this region. The subcuticular implant may cause irritation, leading to lick granulomas (Figure 19.12), or lameness due to cooling in low environmental temperatures, leading to differential shortening of the plate and bone causing stresses within the bone and hence pain (so-called cold or thermal lameness). If any such problems are noted then the implants are removed. Following removal of a plate a Robert Jones dressing should be applied for 7 to 10 days and the patient rested for about 6 weeks whilst bone remodelling accommodates any 'stress protection' afforded by the plate.

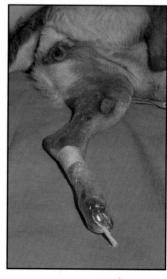

Figure 19.12: Local irritation over the tibial plate leading to lick-granuloma formation. Implant removal and resection of the affected tissue led to an uneventful recovery.

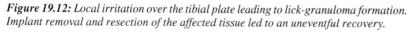

OPERATIVE TECHNIQUE 19.4
Tibia – intramedullary pinning

Positioning
Dorsolateral recumbency with the affected limb down, to allow access to the medial aspect (Operating Technique 19.3). Access to the limb should be improved by supporting the limb on a sandbag so that it can be lifted, allowing manipulation of the stifle, for intramedullary pinning.

Assistant
Optional. Most useful during reconstruction of comminuted fractures.

Tray Extras
Pointed reduction forceps; other bone holding forceps of the surgeon's choice (e.g. Dingman or Lewin bone holding forceps); Hohmann retractors; self-retaining retractors (e.g. Gelpi or Weitlander); periosteal elevator; appropriate intramedullary pins; large pin cutters; chuck; drill; orthopaedic wire for cerclage; pliers/wire twisters. External fixation equipment (see Operative Technique 19.5) if type I fixator is used as auxilliary fixation (see Figure 19.15a).

Surgical Approach
The fracture site is exposed using a limited craniomedial approach (Operative Technique 19.3).

Reduction and Fixation
In the case of reconstructable, comminuted fractures the fragments are reduced and compressed into position using cerclage wires until a two-piece fracture is achieved. When applying these it must be ensured that the fibula is not included, since this will make it impossible to achieve adequate tension in the wire. The proximal part of the tibial diaphysis is wedge-shaped and to prevent slipping of the wire it may be necessary to create a notch in the surface of the bone or apply the wire in a hemicerclage fashion (Chapter 9). If the wire is tightened by twisting the two ends around one another then it is usually necessary to bend the ends over, as there is inadequate soft tissue cover to consider the option of leaving them standing at right angles to the bone surface. It is inappropriate to place the pin first and then try to reconstruct the fragments, as some bone length will have been lost and accurate anatomical alignment will not be possible. The resulting fracture gaps will create extra strain on the wires leading to their loosening.

> **PRACTICAL TIP**
> Although, with care, retrograde pinning is possible, it is generally considered that normograde pinning is most appropriate for tibial fractures.

The pin is introduced alongside the medial border of the straight patellar ligament through a key-hole incision with the stifle held flexed. It enters the bone at the base of the tibial crest, cranial to the intermeniscal ligament (Figure 19.13). Although a Jacobs chuck can be used, a slow-speed power drill affords better control of placement and is less likely to be associated with the pin slipping off the proximal tibia. To prevent the pin slipping off the tibial plateau during insertion, a pilot hole can be made with a smaller diameter pin (a drill bit can be used but this tends to wrap up the soft tissues, and the limited access prevents satisfactory use of tissue guards). Whenever possible the notch in a pre-cut pin is protected by being kept within the chuck in order to prevent premature breakage. The pin is driven into the distal metaphysis (Figure 19.13). As the pin approaches the distal metaphysis, it is perhaps better to abandon a power drill (if used) in favour of a Jacobs chuck. The chuck provides better control, making it less likely that the hock joint will be entered.

→

OPERATIVE TECHNIQUE 19.4 (CONTINUED)
Tibia – intramedullary pinning

Figure 19.13: (a) Cranial, (b) dorsal and (c) lateral views of the tibia to illustrate the anatomical landmarks for normograde placement of a tibial intramedullary pin.

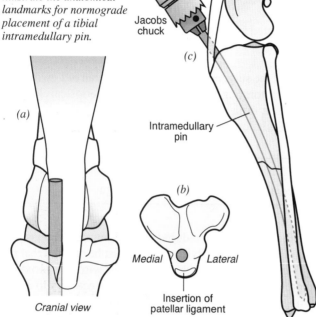

Jacobs chuck

(c)

Intramedullary pin

(a)

(b)

Medial   Lateral

Insertion of patellar ligament

Cranial view

Lateral view

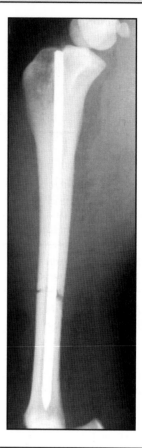

Figure 19.14: Post-operative radiograph showing repair of a transverse tibial fracture in an adult Terrier using a single intramedullary pin.

Closure
Closure is routine with the addition of a single suture in the skin at the site of pin placement.

Post-operative Care
A Robert Jones bandage may be applied for 3 to 7 days if appropriate. Exercise is restricted until radiographic healing of the fracture is apparent (usually 4 to 8 weeks, depending on the nature of the fracture and age of the patient).

Implant removal is a controversial issue. Generally, when dealing with a skeletally immature patient it may be preferable to remove the pin in case it becomes totally encased within the growing bone, making removal very difficult if problems become apparent. In such cases the pin should be left long to facilitate removal. Otherwise the pin is left *in situ* unless it causes problems by loosening or protruding too far into the stifle. There fore, in adult patients it may be better to pre-cut the pin so that it breaks close to the bone margin (Figure 19.14). In most cases cerclage wires are left in place.

OPERATIVE TECHNIQUE 19.5

Tibia – external fixation

Positioning

Lateral recumbency with the affected limb down, to allow access to the medial aspect (Operative Technique 19.3) but with allowance to lift the leg off the table if full pins are being used. Alternatively, the limb may be suspended from a ceiling hook which allows 360° access to the crus.

Assistant

Useful, especially if traction is required to help maintain fracture alignment and also to assist in the assembly of the connecting bar and clamps.

Tray Extras

Appropriate external fixation set; variable speed drill; large pin cutters (hack saw as last resort); chuck; smaller diameter pins or drill bits and appropriate soft tissue guards if pre-drilling is performed.

Surgical Approach

Closed or limited open approach (Operating Technique 19.3) to fracture site.

Reduction and Fixation

Once the fracture has been reduced – either closed using traction, or by a limited approach – the ESF may be applied. The medial aspect of the tibia is most commonly used for placement of fixation pins. Two half-pins will create a unilateral, uniplanar (type I) fixator that is adequate to control rotational forces around an intramedullary pin (Figure 19.15a), whereas four to six half-pins would be sufficient to stabilize relatively simple fractures either alone or in combination with cerclage wires or lagged bone screws (Figure 19.15b). Full pins, used to create a bilateral, uniplanar (type II) frame, are generally only required when there is axial instability due to comminution where fragments have not been or cannot be reconstructed. Bilateral, biplanar (type III) frames are rarely required. They are most often used in situations where much bone stock has been lost and the fracture is open, i.e. where healing is expected to be slow, and this situation is most commonly associated with gunshot injuries.

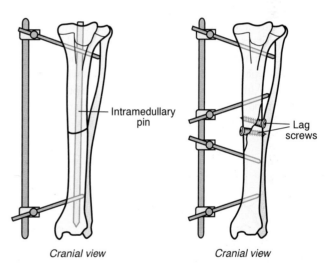

Cranial view — 2 pin unilateral, uniplanar type I external skeletal fixator

Cranial view — 4 pin unilateral, uniplanar type I external skeletal fixator

Figure 19.15: (a) Two-pin unilateral uniplanar (type I) ESF may be used as an adjunct to intramedullary pinning in order to counteract rotational forces acting at transverse or short oblique fracture lines. (b) Type I (four-pin unilateral uniplanar) ESF may be used to stabilize simple fractures either alone or in combination with interfragmentary implants such as lagged bone screws or cerclage wires. An alternative fixator configuration would be a modified type II (uniplanar bilateral) frame (Chapter 9).

Closure

Routine.

Post-operative Care

It is usually necessary to apply a padded dressing to the limb within the frame and including the foot for 7 to 10 days, otherwise swelling of the limb and foot is often seen,. Other care is routine. It is wise to restrict the patient's exercise until radiographic union is complete or until 3 to 4 weeks after frame removal.

OPERATIVE TECHNIQUE 19.6
Separation of the distal tibial physis

Positioning
Lateral recumbency with the affected limb down and the contralateral limb drawn cranially.

Assistant
Optional.

Tray Extras
Gelpi self-retaining retractor; Hohmann retractor; small periosteal elevator; self-retaining pointed reduction forceps; K-wires or small intramedullary pins; chuck; pliers; pin/wire cutters.

Surgical Approach
A medial approach is made to the distal tibia (Chapter 20).

Reduction and Fixation
Reduction is achieved by toggling the fragments (Figure 19.16a,b). This may be assisted by using a Hohmann retractor as a lever. Once reduced, the fracture will remain stable, provided the foot is not allowed to displace laterally. One or two K-wires or small Steinmann pins are then placed diagonally, at an angle of about 30 to 40° to the longitudinal axis, in normograde fashion through the medial malleolus and distal tibia (Figure 19.16c). After placement of *each* pin, movement of the tarsocrural joint should be checked so that if an implant has compromised joint function it can be removed and relocated. The ends should then be bent over to prevent migration. Whether the pins are placed through the transcortex or whether the Rush pin principle is used is a matter of personal preference. Although theoretically the Rush pin principle is superior, in practical terms crossed pins are easier to apply and produce satisfactory results. Increased stability is then achieved by suturing torn soft tissues and may be further increased by placement of a K-wire through a key-hole incision over the lateral malleolus.

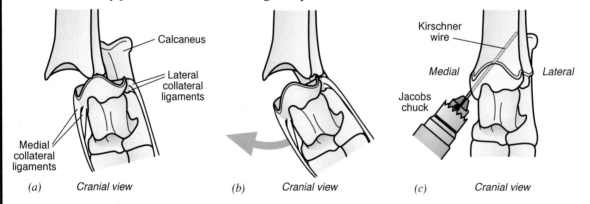

Figure 19.16: *Reduction and fixation of a distal tibial physeal separation. (a) Distal physeal separation with lateral displacement of the pes. The fracture often feels 'locked' in this position. (b) The fracture is reduced by toggling the ends (Chapter 9). A Hohmann retractor, placed in the fracture and used to lever the physis distally, is sometimes necessary. (c) Once reduced, fixation is achieved by normograde placement of one or two K-wires through the medial malleolus.*

Closure
Closure is by apposition of the subcutaneous and/or subcuticular fascia and then the skin.

Post-operative Care
See Operative Technique 19.5.

Alternative Technique
An intramedullary pin may be used but this gains very little purchase in the distal epiphysis and it restricts articular function if it is passed across the tarsocrural joint to improve security.

OPERATIVE TECHNIQUE 19.7
Fractures of the medial and lateral malleoli

Positioning
Lateral recumbency with the affected limb down and the contralateral limb drawn cranially, for exposure of a medial malleolar fracture; and with the affected limb uppermost, supported on a bolster, for exposure of a lateral malleolar fracture.

Assistant
Optional.

Tray Extras
Gelpi self-retaining retractor; Hohmann retractor; small periosteal elevator; self-retaining pointed reduction forceps; K-wires; wire for tension band; chuck; pliers/wire twisters; pin/wire cutters. Appropriate screw set, drill bits etc. if a lag screw technique is used.

Surgical Approach
A medial or lateral approach is made to the distal tibia/fibula (Chapter 20).

Reduction and Fixation
Reduction is achieved by traction on the fragment and collateral ligament. Holding the fragment in reduction can be difficult but pointed reduction forceps may assist in holding the fragment (Figure 19.17a) or Allis tissue forceps may be used to grasp the ligament. One or two K-wires are then placed diagonally, at an angle of about 30 to 40° to the longitudinal axis, through the medial or lateral malleolus and distal tibia (Figure 19.17b,c). After placement of *each* pin, movement of the tarsocrural joint should be checked so that an implant can be removed and relocated if it has compromised joint function. The ends should then be bent over to prevent migration. The tension-band wire is then placed around the pin ends and through a tunnel drilled in the distal tibia. Increased stability may be achieved by suturing torn soft tissues.

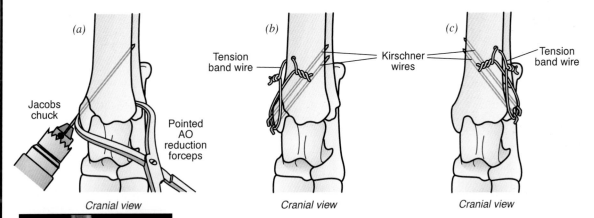

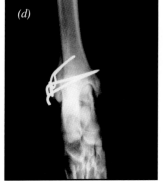

Figure 19.17: Reduction and fixation of malleolar fractures. (a) Reduced medial malleolar fracture; pointed reduction forceps can be used to maintain the malleolar fragment in position whilst a K-wire or pin is introduced. (b) A second K-wire or pin may then be placed and a figure-of-eight tension-band wire added. (c) Repaired lateral malleolar fracture. (d) Post-operative radiograph showing the use of two K-wires and a tension-band to repair a lateral malleolar fracture in a dog.

→

OPERATIVE TECHNIQUE 19.7 (CONTINUED)
Fractures of the medial and lateral malleoli

Closure
Closure is achieved by apposition of the subcutaneous and/or subcuticular fascia and then the skin.

Post-operative Care
The repair may need protection with a cast but if adequate stability has been achieved then it should be possible to avoid casting and allow early return to controlled joint function. In general, the application of a Robert Jones bandage for 2 weeks, when the skin sutures may also be removed, is sufficient as long as the patient's exercise is restricted to cage/room rest and short lead walks for 6 weeks after surgery.

Alternative Techniques
A lagged bone screw may be used instead of the pin and tension-band wire. Where the fragment is too small to accommodate implants it may be more appropriate to use a bone screw and spiked washer to reattach the avulsed collateral ligament.

CHAPTER TWENTY

Carpus and Tarsus

John E.F. Houlton

INTRODUCTION

Fractures of the carpus and tarsus often involve articular surfaces and may affect one or more bones or joints. They are frequently associated with ligamentar injuries, especially in the athletic dog, and a thorough physical examination, combined with good radiographic technique, is essential to identify the full extent of the damage. Localized soft tissue swelling, point pain, reduced range of joint movement, instability and crepitus are the usual clinical findings in carpal and tarsal fractures.

Multiple radiographic views may be necessary, including oblique and stressed projections, and high detail film is recommended.

> **PRACTICAL TIP**
> **It is often useful to view films with a bright light as well as on conventional light boxes. A magnifying glass can be helpful to identify small fragments and cortical fissures.**

A detailed knowledge of the anatomy of the area in question is a prerequisite to making the correct diagnosis, and a bony specimen is often useful when interpreting unfamiliar radiographic projections.

Surgical approaches to the carpus and tarsus are usually made directly over the area of interest and the structure is exposed by sharp dissection. Good haemostasis is essential and blood vessels should be cauterized or ligated. A relatively bloodless surgical field can generally be achieved with an Esmarch's bandage and tourniquet but there is always the risk of post-operative haemorrhage unless haemostasis is adequate. Nevertheless, a Robert Jones bandage, which is changed 24 hours later, generally provides adequate pressure to control post-operative bleeding.

THE CARPUS

The carpus is a compound ginglymus (hinge) joint that permits flexion and extension and a small amount of lateral angulation. It comprises the antebrachiocarpal, middle and carpometacarpal joints as well as the inter-

carpal joints. The antebrachiocarpal joint exists between the distal radius and ulna and the proximal row of carpal bones; the middle carpal joint between the proximal and distal rows of carpal bones; and the carpometacarpal joint between the distal row of carpal bones and the heads of the metacarpal bones. In the sagittal plane, the individual carpal bones are separated by the intercarpal joints.

There are seven named carpal bones. The proximal row comprises the radial, ulnar and accessory carpal bones and the distal row the first, second, third and fourth carpal bones. A small sesamoid bone in the tendon of insertion of the abductor pollicis longus muscle is situated medial to the distal aspect of the radial carpal bone.

The carpus relies on a series of ligaments to maintain its stability. The most important of these are the collateral ligaments and the ligaments on the palmar aspect of the joint. The radial collateral ligament arises from the styloid process of the distal radius and has two components: a straight and an oblique portion. The straight component inserts on the medial aspect of the radial carpal bone and prevents lateral angulation (valgus) of the antebrachiocarpal joint when it is extended. The oblique component inserts on the palmaromedial aspect of the radial carpal bone and prevents valgus angulation of the antebrachiocarpal joint when it is flexed.

The styloid process of the distal ulna is the origin of the short ulnar collateral ligament. This inserts on the ulnar carpal bone and prevents medial angulation (varus) of the antebrachiocarpal joint.

The palmar ligaments prevent hyperextension of the carpus. The palmar radiocarpal and ulnocarpal ligaments arise from the palmar border of the radial articular surface and the ulnar styloid process respectively and insert on the palmar aspect of the radial carpal bone. Both prevent hyperextension of the antebrachiocarpal joint. The palmar radiocarpal–metacarpal ligament and accessoro-metacarpal ligaments connect the radial and accessory carpal bones with metacarpal bones two and three, and four and five, respectively. They prevent hyperextension of the middle carpal joint. The thick, palmar carpal fibrocartilage pad which invests all the carpal bones and the heads of metacarpals two, three, four and five prevents hyperextension of the carpometacarpal joint.

Fractures of the distal radius and ulna

These fractures are discussed in Chapter 16.

Fractures of the radial carpal bone

Fractures of the radial carpal bone generally comprise chips or slabs off the dorsal articular surface. The fragments can be quite small and it may be necessary to take multiple oblique radiographic views with the joint in both flexion and extension in order to skyline them. They are generally seen in working dogs or as injuries following a jump or fall.

There is little tendency for these fractures to heal and they frequently cause chronic secondary osteoarthritis when treated conservatively. Joint thickening and a reduction in carpal flexion develop over two to three months. The initial lameness improves and may become clinically insignificant in a small sedentary animal, but active dogs generally go lame again with the resumption of exercise.

Dorsal slab or chip fractures (Figure 20.1)

In active dogs, chip fractures should be treated by excision of the fragment. Non-displaced fragments in pet dogs may be treated by casting the joint for 4–6 weeks, but owners should be warned of the possible consequences. If large enough, dorsal slabs should be re-attached using a lag screw (Figure 20.1b). Exposure is achieved via a dorsal approach to the carpus (Operative Technique 20.1).

Medial chip fractures

Medial fragments should be carefully assessed as they may represent avulsions of the insertion of the radial collateral ligament. Small isolated fragments should be excised, and the remainder re-attached using a tension-band technique. A dorsal approach is employed (Operative Technique 20.1).

Palmar fractures (Figure 20.2)

These are avulsion fractures of the origin of the palmar radiocarpal–metacarpal ligament. They should be re-attached with a small K-wire and tension-band wire via a palmaromedial approach (Operative Technique 20.2). Small fragments should be excised.

Parasagittal fractures (Figure 20.3)

Parasagittal fractures of the radiocarpal bone invariably start at the proximal articular surface and extend

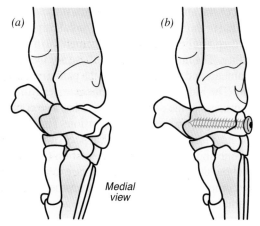

Figure 20.1: (a) Dorsal slab fracture of the radial carpal bone. (b) Lag screw repair.

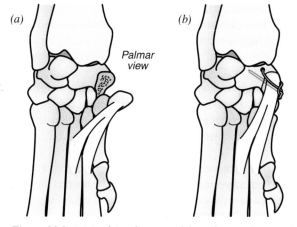

Figure 20.2: (a) Avulsion fracture of the palmar radiocarpal–metacarpal ligament origin. (b) Pin and tension band repair.

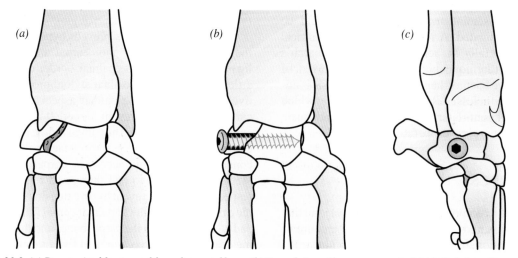

Figure 20.3: (a) Parasagittal fracture of the radiocarpal bone. (b) Dorsal view of lag screw repair. (c) Medial view of lag screw repair.

distomedially toward the second carpal bone. They are generally complete but occasionally hairline fractures may not involve the distal articular surface.

> **WARNING**
> **A sesamoid in the tendon of the abductor pollicis longus muscle is located medial to the radial carpal bone and should not be misdiagnosed as a fracture.**

Incomplete fractures are easy to miss and may present with subtle soft tissue swelling, slight pain on carpal flexion and a mild reduction in range of joint movement. Complete fractures present with more obvious swelling, pain on carpal flexion and possibly crepitus. Occasionally, dogs may present with a chronic lameness, a thickened carpus and considerably reduced range of joint flexion but no known history of trauma.

Lag screw fixation of acute fractures should be performed. The screw should be started extra-articularly from the palmaromedial aspect to avoid the joint space between the radial carpal and ulnar carpal bones. A 2.0 or 2.7 mm screw is used in small dogs; in large dogs a 3.5 or 4.0 mm screw is used (Figure 20.3).

> **PRACTICAL TIP**
> **The glide hole should be started at the insertion of the oblique component of the radial collateral ligament to ensure it is started sufficiently palmarly. There is no need to countersink the screw head.**

Chronic fractures may heal if compressed with a lag screw but owners should be warned that the non-union may persist. A pancarpal arthrodesis can be performed as the definitive treatment for these chronic cases, or it may be performed if lag screw fixation is unsuccessful.

Fracture–luxation of the radiocarpal bone
Luxation of the radial carpal bone is uncommon (Punzet, 1974; Miller *et al.*, 1990). Rupture of the radial collateral and other dorsal and intercarpal ligaments allows the radial carpal bone to rotate caudal to the radius. The palmar ligaments are unaffected and hyperextension is usually not present. In some instances, the luxation is accompanied by a parasagittal fracture of the radial carpal bone.

Treatment involves open reduction of the luxation, repair of the fracture (see parasagittal fracture above) and repair of the ruptured radial collateral ligament by either primary suture or synthetic reconstruction. The repaired ligament can be protected using a figure-of-eight loop of 0.8 to 1.0 mm stainless steel wire anchored around screws and washers in the radial styloid process and radial carpal bone. Alternatively, non-absorbable suture material can be threaded through bone tunnels in the radius and radial carpal bone. The joint is cast in 20° flexion for 6 weeks followed by 3

weeks in a support bandage.

Some degree of loss of carpal flexion should be anticipated. The wire and screws may be removed 6–8 weeks following surgery to minimize joint stiffness.

Fractures of the ulnar carpal bone
These are rare, and should be managed using the same principles as for the radial carpal bone.

Fractures of the distal carpal bones
These are generally small dorsal chips, although rarely a slab fracture occurs. Small fragments should be excised in the athletic dog. In the pet dog, the joint may be cast for 4 weeks, but if lameness persists the fragments should be removed.

A dorsal surgical approach is employed (Operative Technique 20.1), with dissection of the synovium from the surface of the affected bone.

> **PRACTICAL TIP**
> **It is often necessary to split the tendon of extensor carpi radialis if access to the third carpal bone is required.**

Proximal metacarpal bone fractures
These are discussed in Chapter 16.

Accessory carpal bone fractures
This injury is commonly seen in the racing Greyhound but it also occurs in similar dogs such as Whippets and Lurchers. In the racing dog, the fracture usually occurs in the right carpus as a sprain- or strain-avulsion injury caused by carpal hyperextension.

Five types of accessory carpal bone fracture have been described (Johnson, 1987; Johnson *et al.*, 1988) (Figure 20.4). Type I and II fractures are strain-avulsion fractures of the ligaments that connect the accessory

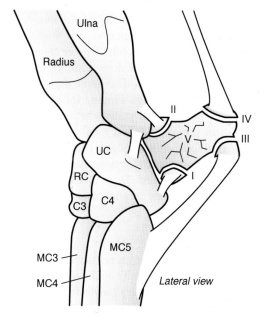

Figure 20.4: *Classification of accessory carpal bone fractures.*

carpal bone to the ulnar carpal bone and to the distal ulna and radius, respectively. Type III fractures are strain-avulsion fractures of the origin of the accessoro-meta-carpal ligaments, while type IV fractures represent sprain-avulsions of the insertion of the flexor carpi ulnaris muscle. Type V fractures are comminuted.

Types I and II are articular fractures. Thus, either can cause disruption of the accessoro-ulnar carpal joint and produce secondary osteoarthritis. Types II and III are often accompanied by a type I fracture.

The racing dog usually comes off the track lame, but clinical signs may not be evident until the next day. These signs will depend upon the type of fracture and the length of time between the injury and the examination. The intra-articular fractures are initially associated with a reduced range of carpal flexion, pain on joint flexion and mild joint swelling. The extra-articular fractures are more likely to show greater swelling and pain on joint extension.

Joint swelling and lameness often resolve with rest and anti-inflammatory management, and affected dogs may remain sound in light work. However, lameness recurs when they return to racing. The usual clinical signs at this time are palmar swelling or thickening around the base of the affected accessory carpal bone, pain on joint flexion and discomfort on direct palpation of the bone.

Fracture types I to IV are best treated surgically, unless the dog is to be retired from racing. Type I fractures should be repaired with a 2.0 mm positional screw via a palmarolateral approach (Operative Technique 20.3). Excision of type I fragments is an alternative to screw fixation. A similar surgical approach is employed.

Type II, III and IV fractures are generally managed by excision of small fragments. Larger fragments should be repaired either with screws or with a tension-band. Type V fractures are best managed conservatively by casting the carpus in 20° of flexion.

Johnson *et al.* (1989) reported a 45% chance of recovery to winning form, while Brinker *et al.* (1990) reported fewer than 50% of dogs winning following excision of the fragments. The latter authors report approximately 90% of dogs winning following screw fixation, but they do not state whether these dogs returned to the same grade of race. All dogs tend to lose carpal flexion following accessory carpal bone repair, and it is important to practise good case selection if the best outcome is required. Dogs that have minimal damage to the rest of the carpus tend to have the most favourable outcome.

Shearing injuries

Shearing injuries of the carpus result in a variable loss of soft tissue and bone, usually on the medial aspect of the joint. The degree of injury ranges from minor skin defects to loss of collateral ligaments and part of the styloid process and carpal bones.

The principles of treatment are similar to any other open fracture (Houlton, 1996) (Chapter 10). All foreign material must be removed, the wound debrided and lavaged, and the joint stabilized. An external skeletal fixator is recommended as this facilitates open wound management while providing support both for the soft tissues and for the joint. A technique of pin insertion into a block of wood incorporated in a cast applied around the metacarpus and digits – the 'fixator boot' – allows pins of reasonable size to be used distally without the risk of fracturing the small meta-carpal bones (Chapter 9).

THE HOCK

The hock is a compound joint comprising seven tarsal bones, the distal tibia and fibula, and the proximal metatarsals. The proximal row of tarsal bones comprises the calcaneus and talus. Distally there are two bone layers medially: the central tarsal bone and tarsal bones 1, 2 and 3. Laterally, there is only one bone: the fourth tarsal bone (T4).

The talocrural joint is a trochlear joint between the tibia and fibula and the talus. The proximal intertarsal joint has two parts: the talocalcaneocentral joint medially, and the calcaneoquartal joint laterally. The centrodistal joint is positioned between the central tarsal bone and T 1–3. The tarsometatarsal joint lies between the numbered tarsal bones and the metatarsal bones.

The talocalcaneal joint comprises three pairs of articular facets. The integrity of the joint is maintained by two strong ligaments which cross the tarsal sinus between the bones.

The plantar ligaments arise from the sustentaculum tali, the body, and the distolateral aspect of the cal-caneus, and insert on the distal tarsal bones and the metatarsal bones. They prevent hyperflexion of the joint during weight-bearing.

The common calcaneal tendon inserts on the tuber calcanei. The superficial digital flexor tendon (SDFT) passes distally over this point, protected by a synovial bursa.

The talocrural joint is supported medially and laterally by the collateral ligaments, each ligament being functionally composed of a long and short component. The long component of the medial ligament originates on the base of the medial malleolus of the tibia and inserts on the talus, the central and first tarsal bones and the first and second metatarsal bones. The tibiocentral part has its origin more craniodistal on the mallelus. It inserts on the talus and central and first tarsal bones. The origin of the short component arises deep to the tibiocentral ligament, while its insertion is on the medial trochlear ridge of the talus.

The long part of the lateral ligament runs from the base of the lateral malleolus to the calcaneus, the fourth

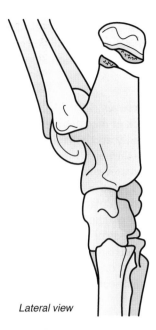

Figure 20.5: Type I Salter–Harris fracture of the proximal calcaneal physis.

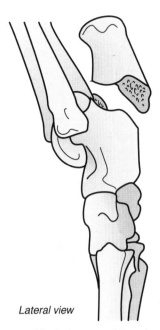

Figure 20.6: Mid-body fracture of the calcaneus.

tarsal bone and the fifth metatarsal bone. The short part of the ligament is composed of the calcaneofibular and talofibular ligaments.

The long and short components of the collateral ligaments stabilize the talocrural joint in extension and flexion, respectively.

Malleolar fractures of the distal tibia and fibula

These are discussed in Chapter 19.

Fractures of the calcaneus

Fracture/separation of the proximal calcaneal physis (Figure 20.5)

This is a type I Salter–Harris fracture which occurs, uncommonly, as an avulsion injury in the skeletally immature dog. The fracture is repaired using K-wires and figure-of-eight tension-band wire (Operative Technique 20.4).

Mid-body fractures (Figure 20.6)

Fractures of the right calcaneus are common in the racing Greyhound. Tension in the gastrocnemius tendon causes considerable displacement of the fragments and loss of the extensor mechanism results in a plantigrade stance. Repair is by pin and tension band (Operative Technique 20.4).

There are two biomechanical explanations for calcaneal fracture in the racing Greyhound. Most fractures are associated with a fracture of the central tarsal bone and subsequent distal migration of the talus. As a result, the calcaneus tilts dorsally and medially and is suddenly subjected to unexpected forces. In this situation, fractures tend to occur in the mid-body or are strain-avulsion fractures, such as dorsomedial or

lateral sagittal slab fractures (see below).

Those fractures not associated with central tarsal bone fracture are caused by excessive tension on the plantar aspect of the hock. Fracture of the plantar distal process or base of the calcaneus occurs, with subsequent subluxation of the proximal intertarsal joint.

Slab fractures

Slab fractures of the dorsomedial and distolateral calcaneus are best repaired with lag screws (Figure 20.7). Comminuted shaft fractures can generally be repaired with a combination of lag screws +/- K-wires combined with a pin and tension-band technique, as described above. Lateral buttress plate fixation is an alternative but is rarely required. A plantarolateral approach is used as described in Operative Technique 20.4.

Fractures of the base

These avulsion fractures of the origin of the plantar ligament are accompanied by plantar instability, subluxation of the proximal intertarsal joint and a plantigrade stance. They are treated by arthrodesis of the proximal intertarsal joint.

The prognosis is generally good for calcaneal fractures. However, racing dogs that have undergone proximal intertarsal arthrodesis do not successfully return to the track.

Fractures of the talus

Fractures of the talus are not common (Dee, 1988) and are generally classified as articular fractures of the body, or non-articular fractures of the head or neck.

Articular fractures (Figure 20.8)

Osteochondral fragments of the trochlear ridges may be associated with avulsion of the insertion of the short

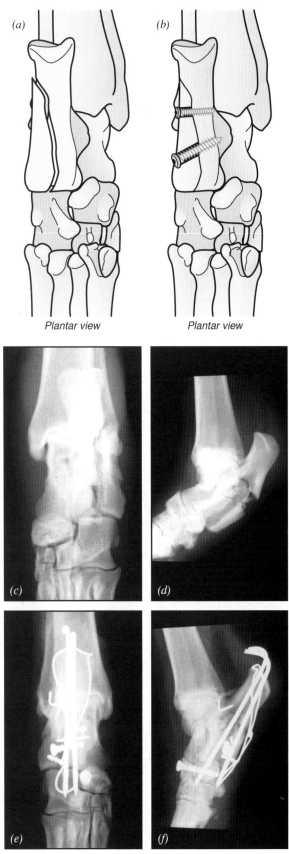

Figure 20.7: (a) Slab fracture of the distolateral calcaneus. (b) Fracture shown in (a) repaired with two lag screws. (c) and (d) Craniocaudal and lateral radiographs of a combined central tarsal bone fracture and comminuted calcaneal shaft fracture in a racing Greyhound. (e) and (f) Post-operative radiograph showing repair.

collateral ligaments. Small fragments should be removed via a talocrural arthrotomy. Larger fragments are managed by internal fixation (Operative Technique 20.5).

Non-articular fractures

Fractures of the neck of the talus are more common in the cat and are usually accompanied by a luxation of the body and base of the bone (Figure 20.9a). To reduce the bone, it is necessary to dorsiflex the proximal intertarsal joint and put the foot in a valgus position. The reduction is held in place with vulsellum forceps placed dorsally and plantarly. A positional screw is placed between the body of the talus and the calcaneus across the tarsal sinus (Figure 20.9b). The repair should be protected by a cast or splint for 4–6 weeks. Minimally displaced talar neck fractures may be managed by coaptation.

The prognosis for talar intra-articular fractures is variable and is influenced by the degree of articular congruency. Non-articular fractures of the talus carry a good prognosis.

Central tarsal bone fractures

Central tarsal bone fracture in the non-athletic dog is rare and generally involves avulsion fracture of the plantar process. Due to the small size of the fragment, the fracture should be managed by a mediolateral positional screw placed across the tarsal sinus into the fourth tarsal bone.

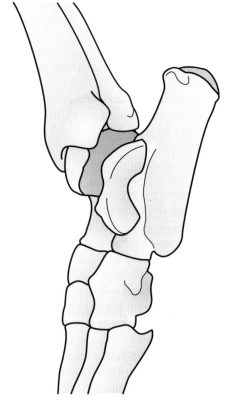

Figure 20.8: Fracture of the lateral ridge of the talus producing a large osteochondral fragment.

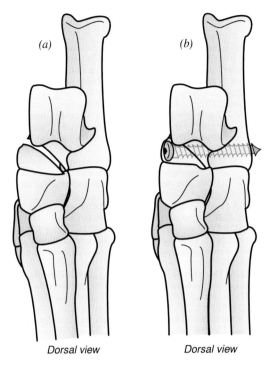

(a)   *(b)*

Dorsal view   Dorsal view

Figure 20.9: *(a) Fracture of the neck of the talus. (b) Repair using a mediolateral positional screw seated in the calcaneus.*

Central tarsal bone fractures commonly occur in the racing Greyhound, generally in the right hock due to racing anti-clockwise. Point pain and crepitus are evident on palpation, with variable soft tissue swelling. The degree of lameness may be mild and dogs can run on to finish races. With severe fracture, tarsal varus and plantar convexity may be apparent.

Central tarsal bone fractures have been classified by Boudrieau *et al.* (1984a) (Figure 20.10) as follows:

- **Type I**: dorsal slab with no displacement
- **Type II**: dorsal slab with displacement
- **Type III**: sagittal fracture with displacement of the medial fragment
- **Type IV**: both dorsal and medial slab fractures, with displacement
- **Type V**: severe comminution and displacement.

Central tarsal bone fractures in the Greyhound are frequently accompanied by other fractures – the two usual combinations being a compression fracture of T4, and a T4 fracture with avulsion of the lateral base of metatarsal V.

Internal fixation of central tarsal bone fractures using interfragmentary screws is the treatment of choice for the dog that hopes to return to the track (Boudrieau *et al.*, 1984b) (Operative Technique 20.6). However, coaptation fixation of type I and II fractures offers a fair prognosis for dogs that are to be retired or used for breeding. Type V fractures are usually not candidates for reconstruction and should be managed conservatively.

The prognosis for return to racing is very good for types I and II, good for types III and IV, and very poor for type V fractures (Boudrieau *et al.*, 1984b).

T2, T3 and T4 fractures

Fractures of the numbered tarsal bones are almost invariably associated with central tarsal bone fracture in the racing Greyhound. Compression fracture of T4 is most commonly observed. Placement of the mediolateral screw during central tarsal bone fixation is frequently the only repair required. If additional support is required, a second mediolateral screw can be placed through T2 and T3 into T4 (Dee, 1988).

Dorsal slab fractures of T3 can occur in isolation (Dee, 1988). Dorsoplantar lag screw fixation is the treatment of choice. The post-operative care is as for central tarsal bone fracture.

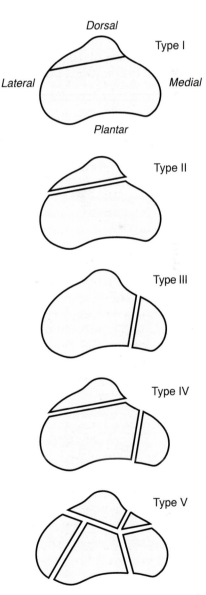

Dorsal

Lateral   Medial

Plantar

Type I

Type II

Type III

Type IV

Type V

Figure 20.10: *Schematic view of the proximal articular surface of the central tarsal bone to illustrate the fracture types (see text for details).*

Reduction of T2 and T3 fracture–luxation can be achieved by mediolateral transfixion screw.

Proximal metatarsal bone fractures

These are discussed in Chapter 21.

Shearing injury

A shearing injury of the hock is a frequent complication of road traffic accidents. The injury occurs as the limb is abraded along the road surface, causing loss of skin, underlying soft tissue and bone. The subcutaneous prominences of the medial (most commonly) and lateral malleoli are vulnerable to such injury. Medial malleolar shear is the more severe injury due to the normal valgus configuration of the pes. Although there may be extensive soft tissue loss, severe hock instability and intra-articular contamination, the prognosis is generally good. The management of open fractures is discussed in Chapter 10. The extent of malleolar shear which precludes joint salvage has not been specifically documented; however, if the axial part of the talar trochlear ridge is involved, or joint stability cannot be achieved, talocrural or pantarsal arthrodesis should be considered from the outset.

REFERENCES AND FURTHER READING

Boudrieau RJ, Dee JF and Dee LG (1984a) Central tarsal bone fractures in the racing greyhound: a review of 114 cases. *Journal of the American Veterinary Medical Association* **184**, 1486.

Boudrieau RJ, Dee JF and Dee LG (1984b) Treatment of central tarsal bone fractures in the racing greyhound. *Journal of the American Veterinary Medical Association* **184**, 1492.

Brinker WO, Piermattei DL and Flo GL (1990) Fractures of the carpus, metacarpus and phalanges. In: *Handbook of Small Animal Orthopaedics and Fracture Treatment*. WB Saunders Co., Philadelphia, 216.

Dee JF (1988) In: *Decision Making in Small Animal Orthopaedic Surgery*, ed. G Sumner-Smith. BC Decker Inc., Philadelphia.

Houlton JEF (1996) The management of open fractures. *Veterinary Annual* **36**, 173.

Johnson KA (1987) Accessory carpal bone fractures in the racing greyhound: classification and pathology. *Veterinary Surgery* **16**(1), 60.

Johnson KA, Piermattei DL, Davis PE and Bellenger CR (1988) Characteristics of the accessory carpal bone in 50 racing greyhounds. *Veterinary Comparative Orthopaedics and Traumatology* **1**, 104.

Johnson KA, Dee JF and Piermattei DL (1989) Screw fixation of accessory carpal bone fractures in racing greyhounds: 12 cases (1981–6). *Journal of the American Veterinary Medical Association* **194** (11) 1618.

Miller A, Carmichael S, Anderson TJ and Brown I (1990) Luxation of the radial carpal bone in four dogs. *Journal of Small Animal Practice* **31**, 148.

Punzet G (1974) Luxation of the os carpi radiale in the dog pathogenesis, symptoms and treatment. *Journal of Small Animal Practice* **15** (12), 751.

OPERATIVE TECHNIQUE 20.1
Dorsal approach to the carpus

Positioning
The dog may either be placed on its back with the affected limb drawn caudally to lie alongside its chest, or be placed in sternal recumbency with its limb drawn forwards. An extension arm added to the table is particularly useful if the latter approach is employed in large dogs.

Assistant
Optional.

Tray Extras
Gelpi retractors; small Hohmann retractor.

Surgical Approach
The skin incision is made on the mid-dorsal surface of the joint, curving laterally at its distal end parallel with the cephalic vein, allowing the latter to be retracted medially (Figure 20.11). The incision is continued between the tendons of the common digital extensor and the extensor carpi radialis and through the periosteum of the distal radius. This is elevated on either side of the incision so that the tendons can be elevated without disturbing their sheaths. The tendons are retracted laterally and medially, respectively, with Gelpi retractors. The joint capsule can be incised either parallel to the tendons or, if greater visualization is required, transversely. The synovium attached to the dorsal surface of the carpal bones must be incised around the bone in question in order to expose them.

> **PRACTICAL TIP**
> **Exposure is improved by flexing the carpus and readjusting the Gelpi retractors.**

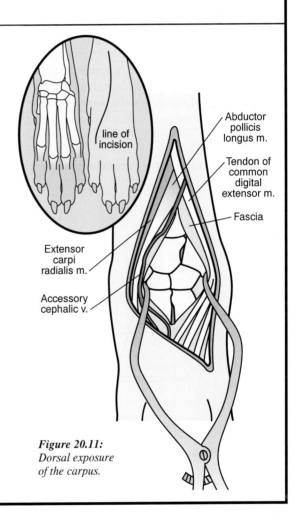

Figure 20.11:
Dorsal exposure
of the carpus.

line of incision

Abductor pollicis longus m.

Tendon of common digital extensor m.

Fascia

Extensor carpi radialis m.

Accessory cephalic v.

OPERATIVE TECHNIQUE 20.2
Palmaromedial approach to the radial carpal bone

Positioning
Dorsal recumbency with the affected limb drawn cranially so that the palmar surface of the foot is uppermost.

Assistant
Useful.

Tray Extras
Gelpi retractors; small Hohmann retractor. Rake-type retractors may be useful.

Surgical Approach
A skin incision is made equidistant between the radial styloid process and the carpal pad. The underlying cephalic vein is ligated and transected (Figure 20.12). The flexor retinaculum is incised in a similar direction to expose the tendons of the flexor carpi radialis and the digital flexor muscles. The antebrachiocarpal joint space is identified with a 21 g needle and the deep fascia and joint capsule are incised at this level. There is a daunting number of vessels and nerves, but most can be retracted if care is taken. The median artery and nerve, the ulnar nerve, and the deep palmar arch and palmar metacarpal arteries are the most important and must be preserved

WARNING
This approach is not recommended for inexperienced surgeons.

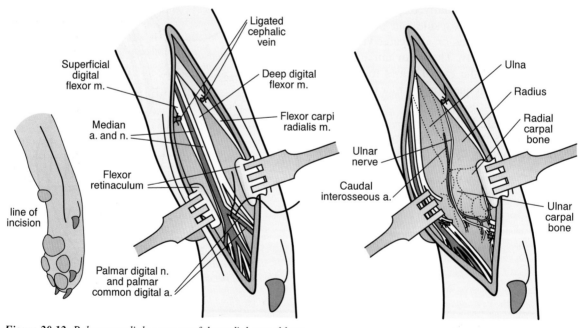

Figure 20.12: Palmaromedial exposure of the radial carpal bone.

OPERATIVE TECHNIQUE 20.3

Screw fixation of type I and II accessory carpal bone fractures

Positioning
Dorsal recumbency with the affected limb pulled cranially so that the palmar aspect of the foot is uppermost.

Assistant
Useful.

Tray Extras
Gelpi retractors; small Hohmann retractor; 1.5/2.0 mm screw sets; drill (ideally, mini air drill); small periosteal elevator; small pointed reduction forceps; Number 11 or 15 scalpel blade.

Surgical Approach
A palmarolateral approach is made. The skin incision is started at the caudomedial border of the distal ulna, taken around the accessory carpal bone, and ended distally over metacarpal V (Figure 20.13). The subcutaneous tissues are incised along the same line. The lateral flexor retinaculum is sharply incised with a scalpel, and a pair of Gelpi retractors is placed to retract the two accessoro-metacarpal ligaments medially. If further visualization of the distal border of the bone is required, sharp dissection of the origin of the abductor digiti quinti muscle is performed.

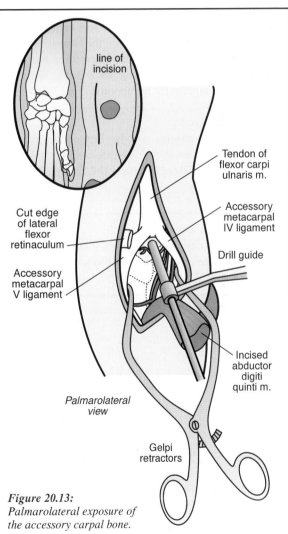

Figure 20.13:
Palmarolateral exposure of the accessory carpal bone.

→

OPERATIVE TECHNIQUE 20.3 (CONTINUED)

Screw fixation of type I and II accessory carpal bone fractures

Reduction and Fixation

The carpus should be extended and the slab pushed forwards with a small periosteal elevator so as to line up the palmar fracture line. Once reduced, the fragment should be clamped with a pair of small reduction forceps placed as close to the articular surface of the bone as possible. A 1.5 mm drill hole is started in the centre of the fragment. The hole should be drilled parallel to the metacarpal bones. The 2.0 mm screw is inserted and the screw tightened before removing the forceps. Overtightening of the screw will cause its head to shear, but the screw threads are likely to retain sufficient purchase in the bone fragment to maintain the reduction (Figure 20.14).

> **WARNING**
> **The screw should not be lagged, nor should its head be countersunk, to reduce the risk of splitting the thin slab of bone.**

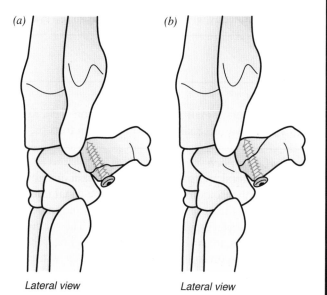

(a) Lateral view   *(b)* Lateral view

Figure 20.14: *Screw fixation of (a) type I and (b) type II articular fractures of the accessory carpal bone.*

Post-operative Care

The carpus is cast in flexion for a total of 6–8 weeks. Each second or third week the cast should be replaced and the joint re-cast in a less flexed position. At the end of this period, the carpus will have a restricted range of movement which will improve with a gradual increase in exercise level.

OPERATIVE TECHNIQUE 20.4
Pin and tension-band fixation of calcaneal fractures

Positioning
Dorsal recumbency with the affected limb drawn forwards or lateral recumbency.

Assistant
Optional.

Tray Extras
Gelpi retractors; K-wires; wire for tension-band; small chuck; pin/wire cutters; pliers/wire twisters; pointed reduction forceps; drill bits.

Surgical Approach
A plantarolateral approach (Figure 20.15) is made to the calcaneus to avoid the point of the tuber calcis. The skin incision begins on the lateral aspect of the calcaneal/achilles tendon and curves distally. The deep fascia is incised lateral to and parallel with the superficial digital flexor tendon. Medial retraction of the superficial digital flexor tendon from the gastrocnemius tendon completes the exposure.

> **WARNING**
> It is unwise to use an Esmarchs bandage and tourniquet when repairing calcaneal fractures, as the tourniquet will apply tension to the Achilles tendon and hinder fracture reduction.

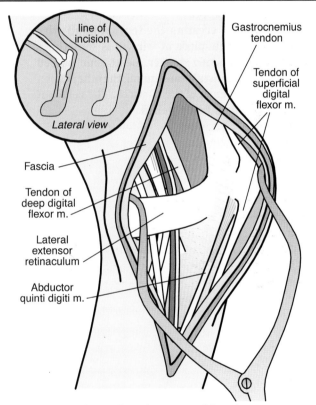

Figure 20.15: *Plantarolateral exposure of the calcaneus.*

Reduction and Fixation

> **PRACTICAL TIP**
> Extension of the hock will assist fracture reduction.

The transverse hole for the tension-band wire should be drilled first so that there is no danger of hitting the pins. Retraction of the superficial digital flexor tendon medially with a small pointed Hohmann retractor will enable the end of the wire to be grasped when it is threaded through the bone tunnel.

When managing physeal separation in puppies, the K-wires should be driven side by side as far laterally and medially as possible. The tension-band wire is then completed, making sure that it is adjacent to the bone and under the tendon of the superficial digital flexor. The ends of the K-wires must be bent over as close to the surface of the bone as possible, to minimize soft tissue irritation (Figure 20.16).

→

OPERATIVE TECHNIQUE 20.4 (CONTINUED)
Pin and tension-band fixation of calcaneal fractures

In adults with mid-body fractures, countersunk pins can be used as these interfere less with superficial digital flexor tendon function and create fewer soft tissue problems. A single pin is adequate and the tension-band is taken through two transverse tunnels: one proximal to and one distal to the fracture (Figure 20.17). Pre-drilling the calcaneus with a slightly smaller drill bit than the final pin is strongly advised as this is a very dense bone.

PRACTICAL TIP
Rather than creating the tension-band wire out of a single piece of wire, it is sometimes easier to use two shorter pieces, one passed through the distal bone tunnel, the other taken around the ends of the K-wires. The relevant ends can then be tightened.

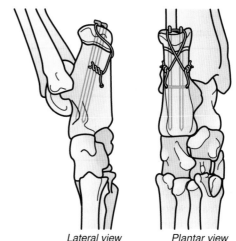

Lateral view   Plantar view

Figure 20.16: Pin and tension-band repair of a Salter–Harris type I fracture of the proximal calcaneal physis.

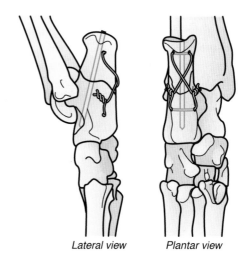

Lateral view   Plantar view

Figure 20.17: Pin and tension-band repair of a mid-body fracture of the calcaneus.

Post-operative Care
The hock is supported in slight extension for 6–8 weeks using a light cast or a short lateral splint and padded bandage. Greyhounds with calcaneal fractures are often retired from racing. If an attempt is made to return them to racing, then implants should be removed.

OPERATIVE TECHNIQUE 20.5

Internal fixation of articular fractures of the talus

Positioning
Medial or lateral recumbency, depending on which region of the talar surface is being exposed.

Assistant
Useful.

Tray Extras
Gelpi retractors; small Hohmann retractor; osteotome and mallet; small chuck; K-wires; pointed reduction forceps. Possibly 1.5/2.0 mm screw set. Rake-type retractors may be useful.

Surgical Approach
The exposure is as for the relevant malleolus described in Chapter 19, with an additional incision into the joint capsule. Adequate exposure of larger fragments may not be possible without a malleolar osteotomy. To expose the medial condyle, the medial collateral ligament is isolated by incising either side of it and removing the malleolus with an osteotome (Figure 20.18). This is not an easy osteotomy since it should be deep enough to include most of the origin of the malleolus, but not so deep as to involve the weight-bearing articular surface. To expose the lateral condyle, the distal fibula is isolated by a transverse osteotomy (Figure 20.19a).

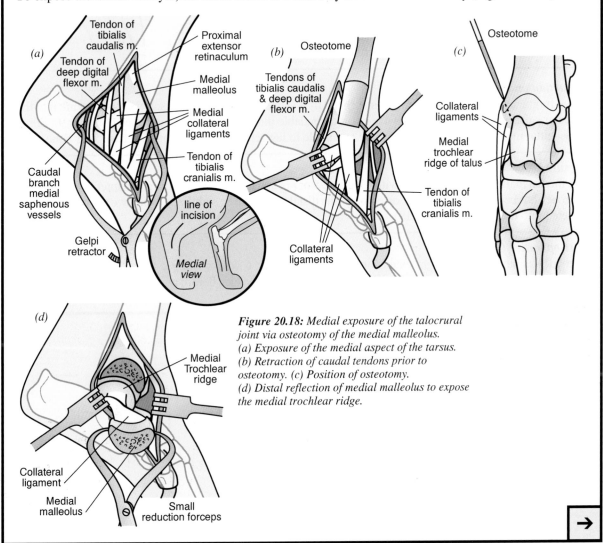

Figure 20.18: *Medial exposure of the talocrural joint via osteotomy of the medial malleolus. (a) Exposure of the medial aspect of the tarsus. (b) Retraction of caudal tendons prior to osteotomy. (c) Position of osteotomy. (d) Distal reflection of medial malleolus to expose the medial trochlear ridge.*

→

OPERATIVE TECHNIQUE 20.5 (CONTINUED)

Internal fixation of articular fractures of the talus

PRACTICAL TIP
Drill the fixation
screw/K-wire holes
before performing the
osteotomy.

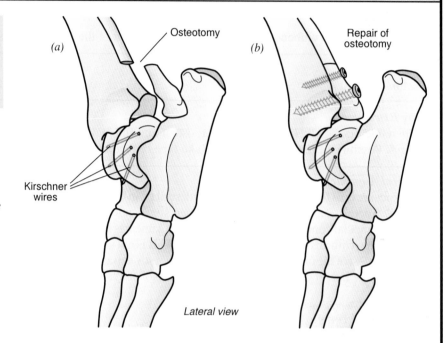

Figure 20.19: (a) Repair of the articular fracture shown in Figure 20.8 using countersunk K-wires. The fracture is exposed via osteotomy of the distal fibula and lateral reflection of the malleolus. (b) The fibular osteotomy is repaired using two positional screws into the distal tibia.

Reduction and Fixation

Large fragments should be reduced and stabilized by K-wires or 1.5 or 2.0 mm screws countersunk into the articular surface (Figure 20.19). The use of biodegradable pins has also been suggested (Chapter 9). Some parasagittal intertrochlear fractures may be amenable to lag screw fixation through subarticular bone.

Closure

The medial malleolus is re-attached with a lag screw or pin and tension-band wiring (Chapter 19). If a lateral approach has been used with fibular osteotomy, the distal fibula can be stabilized using two positional screws directed into the tibia (Figure 20.19).

Post-operative Care

The hock is supported in slight extension for approximately 6 weeks using a light cast. Following cast removal, activity is restricted to lead-walking for a further 2–4 weeks, before gradually increasing the dog's exercise.

OPERATIVE TECHNIQUE 20.6
Internal fixation of central tarsal bone fractures

Positioning
Dorsal recumbency with the affected leg extended caudally.

> **PRACTICAL TIP**
> When positioning the dog, it is helpful to extend the limb so that the hock and pes are parallel to the ground. This aids accurate drilling in a dorsoplantar direction.

Assistant
Helpful during exposure of fracture.

Tray Extras
Appropriate size bone screw set, drill bits, etc.; drill; Gelpi retractors; small Hohmann retractor; Vulsellum forceps.

Surgical Approach
The surgical approach is dorsomedial (Figure 20.20). A skin incision is made from the medial malleolus to metatarsal II between the saphenous and medial saphenous vein, lateral to the tendon of insertion of the cranial tibialis muscle. A small Hohmann retractor is used to retract the tendon medially and expose the dorsal surface of the central tarsal bone.

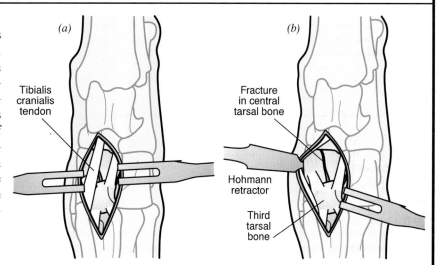

Figure 20.20: Dorsomedial exposure of the central tarsal bone. (a) Incision through skin and subdermal fascia. (b) Retraction of the tibialis cranialis tendon exposes the fracture.

Reduction and Fixation
Type I and II fractures are repaired using a dorsoplantar 2.7 mm lag screw (Figure 20.21). The fracture is reduced by extending the hock and lining up the articular surfaces. The reduction is maintained with Vulsellum forceps. Care should be taken to start the drill bit in the centre of the bone – too proximally and it will enter the talocalcaneocentral joint. If the hock is parallel with the floor and the drill bit directed vertically, the screw will be in the correct dorsoplantar direction.

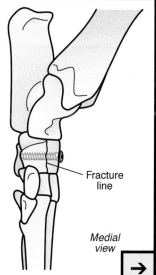

Figure 20.21: Repair of a type I/II central tarsal bone fracture using a dorsoplantar lag screw.

→

OPERATIVE TECHNIQUE 20.6 (CONTINUED)
Internal fixation of central tarsal bone fractures

Type IV fractures are repaired using a mediolateral 4.0 mm partially threaded cancellous bone screw to transfix the medial slab and a 2.7 mm lag screw through the dorsal slab. The use of a cancellous mediolateral screw helps to stabilize compression fractures in T4, and the non-threaded portion within the central tarsal bone allows easier placement of the dorsoplantar screw (Figure 20.22). Screw placement is critical if both screws are to avoid the talocalcaneocentral and centrodistal joint spaces. The mediolateral screw should be placed first, starting at the junction of the middle and distal third of the slab. The dorsoplantar screw is started at the junction of the proximal and middle third of the bone.

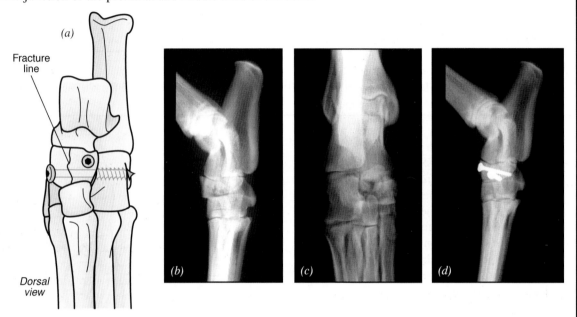

Figure 20.22: (a) Schematic to show screw position in the repair of a type IV central tarsal bone fracture. A mediolateral partially threaded cancellous screw is used to fix the medial slab. This allows more space for the insertion of the dorsoplantar lag screw to fix the cranial slab as shown in Figure 20.21. (b), (c) Pre-operative radiographs of a type IV central tarsal bone fracture in a racing Greyhound. (d) Post-operative radiographs showing lag screw repair.

Post-operative Care
The hock is supported in slight extension for 6 weeks using a light cast. Following cast removal, activity is restricted to lead exercise for the next 6 weeks. Training may generally resume at 12 weeks.

CHAPTER TWENTY ONE

The Distal Limb

Jonathan Dyce

This chapter reviews the management of fractures distal to the carpometacarpal and tarsometatarsal joints. In order to avoid repetition, anatomical terms relating to the forelimb only will be used. The text is equally applicable to the corresponding bones of the hindlimb, unless stated. High performance dogs are particularly vulnerable to distal limb injury and consequently this chapter is weighted towards the Greyhound. Where there are differences in management between the pet and the athlete, these are stated in the text.

ANATOMICAL CONSIDERATIONS

For detailed descriptions of regional anatomy in the dog and cat, refer to Evans (1993) and Hudson and Hamilton (1993).

The four main metacarpal bones are arranged in a diverging dorsally convex arcade. The base of a metacarpal bone is the proximal part, contributing to the carpometacarpal joint and providing insertion for carpal ligaments. The body has a greater dorsopalmar than mediolateral dimension, and extends distally to the neck (the site of the metacarpal growth plate). The head articulates distally with the first phalanx (P1) (Figure 21.1) and the paired palmar proximal sesamoid bones, which lie at either side of the sagittal condylar ridge. Sesamoids are numbered from medial to lateral, 1 to 8. The vestigial metacarpal I of the dew claw articulates with a single phalanx and unnumbered

sesamoid. A variable vestige of the first metatarsal bone is present in the hindlimb.

The anatomy of the proximal palmar sesamoid bones is of particular interest (Davis *et al.*, 1969; Robins and Read, 1993). The bones lie within the insertion of the interosseous muscles; they have a triangular cross-section and, with the intersesamoidean ligament, form a sulcus for the overlying digital flexor tendons. The sesamoids (3–6) of the axial digits form symmetrical pairs and are consequently loaded evenly as tension develops in the flexor tendons (Figure 21.2a). Due to the conformation of the metacarpus, the sesamoids of the abaxial digits are loaded eccentrically, with sesamoids 2 and 7 subjected to greater loading than sesamoids 1 and 8. In addition, sesamoids 2 and 7 are unusual in presenting a flat palmar surface to the flexor tendons (Figure 21.2b). Consequently,

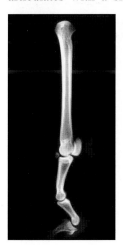

Figure 21.1: Lateral radiograph of an isolated canine left fore digit III.

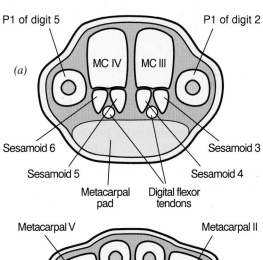

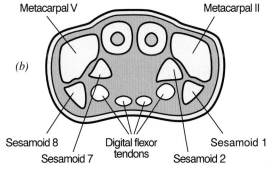

Figure 21.2: (a) Cross-section of the metacarpus at the level of the axial sesamoid bones. (b) Cross-section of the metacarpus at the level of the abaxial sesamoid bones. (Redrawn from Davis et al., 1969.)

pathology is most commonly seen in these bones.

Small single dorsal sesamoid bones lie within the digital extensor tendons at the level of the carpometacarpal and proximal interphalangeal joint. These sesamoids are very rarely of clinical importance (Brinker *et al.*, 1990).

GENERAL SURGICAL CONSIDERATIONS IN DISTAL LIMB SURGERY

Routine orthopaedic surgical asepsis is practised but the proximity of the nails and pads implies likely contamination of the surgical site. Nails should be scrubbed and should be isolated from the surgical site if possible. The use of sterile plastic foot bags or adhesive drapes should therefore be considered. The routine use of perioperative antibiosis is advised for surgery of the foot.

Surgical incisions overlie the region of interest. The bones of the foot are essentially subcutaneous and therefore easily exposed. To conserve delicate digital tendons and their accompanying vasculature, and thereby reduce the risk of adhesion formation, precise dissection is required. A bloodless surgical field can be created by exsanguination of the distal limb using an Esmarch bandage and subsequent application of a tourniquet. This is strongly recommended for procedures about the palmar foot, such as sesamoidectomy. If a tourniquet is used, a compression bandage should be applied on tourniquet removal and changed 24 hours later to allow inspection of the soft tissues.

Fracture repairs are generally coapted for 4–6 weeks. Adequate padding should be placed between the toes and all bandages should be monitored diligently. Ready-made or individually moulded thermoplastic metasplints are often more appropriate than full cylinder casts, which permit weight bearing on the digital pads. No foot should be cast before significant soft tissue swelling has resolved.

> **WARNING**
> **Improperly applied and maintained coaptation is the most significant cause of patient morbidity following distal limb surgery.**

METACARPAL/METATARSAL FRACTURES

Proximal avulsion
Oblique fractures of the bases of metacarpals II and V (Figure 21.3) are commonly associated with avulsion of the flexor carpi radialis and palmar radial carpal-metacarpal ligament, or ulnaris lateralis and palmar accessory carpal-metacarpal ligament, respectively. Collateral stress will demonstrate any resultant carpal valgus or

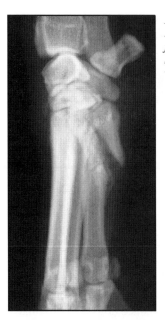

Figure 21.3: Chronic metacarpal V oblique fracture in an Old English Sheepdog (unstressed view).

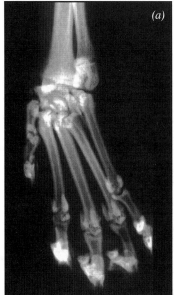

(a)

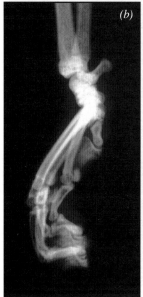

(b)

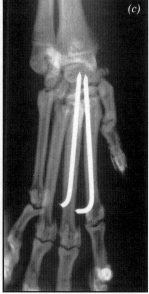

(c)

Figure 21.4: Acute carpometacarpal hyperextension and valgus displacement in a cat with proximal metacarpal V fracture/ luxation:
(a) dorsopalmar view;
(b) lateral view.
(c) Partial carpal arthrodesis stabilized with K-wires inserted proximally through the dorsal cortex of metacarpal II and III.

varus displacement. Such fractures are unlikely to be the sole significant pathology and should alert the surgeon to the probability of carpal hyperextension injury.

> **WARNING**
> **Metacarpal base fractures are likely to be associated with carpal hyperextension.**

The distractive forces may be neutralized by K-wire and figure-of-eight tension-band wire in cases of metacarpal II avulsion fractures, which tend to produce a smaller fragment than metacarpal V avulsion fractures (Dee, 1988a). Lag screw fixation may be more suitable for such metacarpal V fractures.

Carpal stability should be checked post-operatively and significant concomitant injuries treated. If there is severe carpometacarpal disruption (Figure 21.4a,b), or in cases that have been managed inappropriately by coaptation, partial (Figure 21.4c) or pancarpal arthrodesis (Figure 21.5) is indicated.

The lateral base of metatarsal V provides the insertion for fibularis brevis, abductor digiti quinti and lateral collateral ligament. Avulsion fracture of the lateral base is seen exclusively in the racing Greyhound following fracture of the central tarsal bone. The resultant dorsomedial collapse of the tarsus generates increased tension in the soft tissues inserting on the lateral base. Lateral subluxation of a compressed fourth tarsal bone further predisposes to lateral base fracture (Dee, 1993). This small fracture is managed conservatively and does not affect the prognosis for central tarsal fracture repair (Boudrieau *et al.*, 1984).

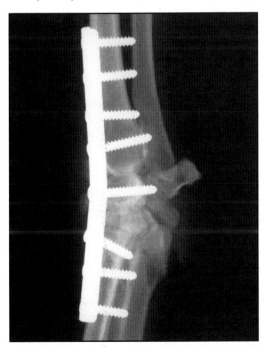

Figure 21.5: *Pancarpal arthrodesis stabilized with a 3.5 mm DCP, in an Old English Sheepdog with chronic middle carpal hyperextension following coaptation of an oblique proximal metacarpal V fracture.*

Stress fractures

Metacarpal/metatarsal stress fractures are seen in the racing Greyhound in training, or early in the racing career, with a peak incidence at 16–22 months of age (Gannon, 1972; Bellenger *et al.*, 1981). Dogs race anticlockwise and such injuries are seen much more commonly in the side of the foot nearer to the inner rail. There is no history of external trauma. Left metacarpal V fracture is significantly more common than right metacarpal II fracture. There is a lower prevalence of metatarsal stress fractures, with right metatarsal III most frequently affected.

The adaptation of bone to increasing repetitive deformation, as occurs during training, is a normal phenomenon and is manifest radiographically by increasing cortical width. However, if bone is overloaded and reparative remodelling is inadequate, then stress fractures become likely.

Combined bending and compressive forces produce a consistent fracture configuration, with a transverse palmar cortical fracture overlain by a dorsal butterfly fragment (Figure 21.6), at the junction of the proximal third and distal two-thirds of the bone. The distal fragment may displace in a palmar direction.

For displaced fractures, internal fixation is indicated (Operative Technique 21.1). The best management for non-displaced stress fractures is less well defined. Internal fixation, as described below, will yield excellent results. For reviews of non-surgical management of stress fractures, see Boemo (1989) or Blythe *et al.* (1994).

If internal fixation is not performed, the foot should be coapted with a palmar splint for 4 weeks, to prevent fracture displacement. If radiographic reassessment then confirms ongoing fracture repair, a gradually increasing plane of exercise is recommended. Training may re-

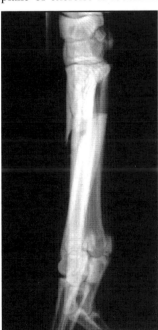

Figure 21.6: *Displaced metatarsal III stress fracture in a racing Greyhound.*

commence after 8-12 weeks, but initial trials should avoid cornering. Cast management may be inappropriate as Ness (1993) describes a high incidence of metatarsal III non-union with such coaptation.

If radiographic reassessment at 3-4 weeks shows no evidence of fracture healing in conservatively managed cases, consider internal fixation.

> **WARNING**
> **Acute proximal metacarpal pain in the racing Greyhound may be associated with radiographically covert stress fracture.**

It should be recognized that many stress fractures are initially undiagnosed and are only revealed retrospectively by radiographic disclosure of chronic cortical remodelling, medullary obliteration and periosteal reaction. Chronically remodelled but symptomatic stress fractures may benefit from forage or debridement of exuberant callus.

Other fractures

If the metacarpus is not completely disrupted, metacarpal fractures can be successfully managed in a splinted bandage. Coaptation of total metacarpal fracture is likely to result in a degree of malunion, with palmar bowing of the metacarpus, unless the splint is accurately contoured (Brinker *et al.*, 1990).

Internal fixation should be considered for single metacarpal fractures in the Greyhound as this normally offers an improved prognosis for return to racing (Operative Technique 21.1). In other dogs and cats, internal fixation is generally reserved for cases with more than two metacarpal fractures. If the longer axial metacarpal bones are stabilized, this generally permits the abaxial fractures to be managed simply by coaptation. Transverse fractures may be treated by intramedullary pin or plate fixation (Operative Technique 21.1). Repair with intramedullary pins is an example of adaptation osteosynthesis, with small pins used for ease of insertion and preservation of the medullary blood supply.

Fractures of the neck, including physeal separation, are managed by K-wire insertion using a Rush-pin method, entering the abaxial cortex just proximal to the metacarpophalangeal joint (Dee, 1988a). Lag screw fixation is most appropriate for long oblique fractures and intra-articular fractures of the metacarpal head. Intramedullary pin and cerclage wire fixation is most suitable for the abaxial metacarpals, due to difficulties in passing proximal wires about metacarpals III and IV.

Shearing injury

The general principles of open fracture management are described in Chapter 10. Following shearing injury, if two or more metacarpal bones remain, or can be reconstructed, restoration of foot function should be possible, given favourable soft tissue conditions.

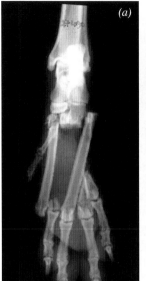
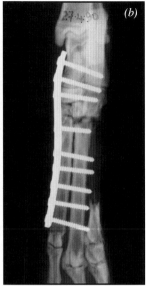
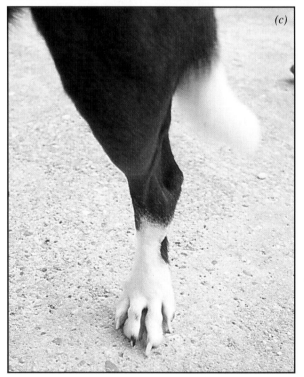

Figure 21.7: (a) Severe lateral metatarsal shearing injury, tarsometatarsal fracture/luxation, and metatarsophalangeal luxation, in a Collie. (b) Tarsometatarsal arthrodesis stabilized using a medial 2.7 mm DCP. Delayed full thickness open mesh autogenous skin grafting was also performed. (c) Foot posture 2 years post-operatively. Implants had been removed previously.

Pancarpal or tarsometatarsal (Figure 21.7) arthrodesis may be appropriate for cases with unstable proximal metapodal fracture, or carpometacarpal/tarsometatarsal subluxation, respectively. In cases of severe shearing injury of the distal limb including metacarpal trauma, which are managed with external skeletal fixation, consider extending a padded U-shaped 'walking bar' distally from a bilateral frame. This allows metacarpal pin placement, and also protects the foot from disruptive weight bearing.

SESAMOID FRACTURE

Transverse or polar avulsion fractures of the palmar proximal sesamoid bones are not uncommon in the racing Greyhound (Bateman, 1959; Davis *et al.*, 1969). Metacarpophalangeal hyperextension is a more likely aetiology than direct trauma. Sesamoids 2 and 7 are most frequently affected (see above).

Acute sesamoid fracture should be distinguished from bipartite/tripartite sesamoids and sesamoid disease, which also affect sesamoids 2 and 7 primarily but are likely to be incidental findings. In a survey of 100 racing Greyhounds, 27% were found to have asymptomatic sesamoid pathology (Eaton-Wells, 1989). Similarly, a 44% occurrence of incidental sesamoid disease has been documented in the Rottweiler (Vaughan and France, 1986).

> **WARNING**
> **Radiography frequently discloses asymptomatic sesamoid pathology. Correlation with specific clinical signs of sesamoid pathology is essential for diagnosis of significance.**

Acute sesamoid fractures are characterized radiographically by sharp demarcation of the fracture plane, whereas chronically fractured or bipartite sesamoids have non-complementary apposed surfaces (Figure 21.8). Sesamoid disease encompasses a variety of changes, from single small ectopic calcified bodies to grossly enlarged multipartite sesamoid bones.

Clinically significant sesamoid fractures are associated with pain and possible crepitus on direct palpation and metacarpophalangeal manipulation; metacarpophalangeal effusion; and significant response to an excitatory flexion test, or local anaesthetic infiltration. The degree of lameness is variable.

Sesamoidectomy is the treatment of choice for clinically significant acutely fractured sesamoid bones and offers a good prognosis for return to racing (Blythe *et al.*, 1994). Partial sesamoidectomy may be appropriate for small polar avulsions; however, total sesamoidectomy is most frequently performed (Operative Technique 21.2).

PHALANGEAL FRACTURES

Phalangeal fractures are commonly shaft fractures or collateral avulsions. Coaptation is the treatment of choice for most shaft fractures. Mini-plate fixation of unstable P1/P2 fractures or lag screw fixation of oblique fractures may be favoured in the racing Greyhound (Dee, 1988b) (Figure 21.9). Large proximal and distal interphalangeal collateral avulsions can be managed by lag screw fixation (Figure 21.10). If fixation of the avulsed fragment(s) is not practical, then fragment removal and prosthetic ligament repair are indicated (Eaton-Wells, 1994). Arthrotomy is mandatory in cases of interphalangeal luxation managed by open reduction, in order to remove any intra-articular osteochondral debris.

Irreparable intra-articular phalangeal fractures are rarely candidates for interphalangeal arthrodesis, which would be stabilized with angled miniplate or pin and tension-band wire. Amputation offers a more reliable prognosis in cases of comminuted intra-articular and compound phalangeal fractures.

Avulsion of the SDFT from the proximal palmar surface of P2 will result in a 'dropped toe'. This is unlikely to have more than cosmetic significance. In the acute case, if the fragment is large enough, it is possible to reattach this using a wire mattress suture placed through two dorsopalmar transosseous tunnels (Dee, 1988b).

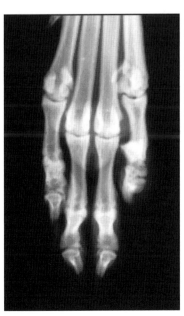

Figure 21.8: *Bipartite sesamoid 2, tripartite sesamoid 7 in a racing Greyhound. The significant pathology in this case is proximal interphalangeal luxation in digit V.*

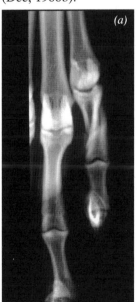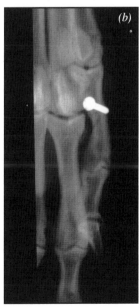

Figure 21.9: *(a) Oblique P1 fracture in a racing Greyhound. (b) Fracture fixation using a 1.5 mm lag screw.*

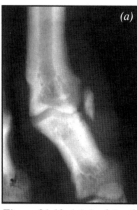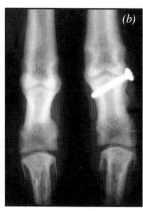

Figure 21.10: *(a) Avulsion fracture of the insertion of the medial proximal interphalangeal collateral ligament, in a racing Greyhound. (b) Repair using a 1.5 mm lag screw.*

Avulsion of the DDFT from the palmar protruberence of P3 will result in overextension of P3 – a 'knocked up' toe. Again, this is rarely of clinical significance. Other fractures of P3 that are not simple fractures of the ungual process are most effectively managed by distal P2 amputation.

Amputation of the digit

Amputation is a possible management for any injury of the digit but it is currently difficult to make objective specific recommendations regarding the relative merits of amputation and reconstruction. The advantages of digital amputation are that it is a single definitive procedure with a lower complication rate and that there is more rapid recovery without the requirement for prolonged coaptation. The disadvantage is that there will be increased loading of the other digits of the same foot, which may predispose to new pathology or exacerbate previously subclinical pathology. Although the majority of digital amputations are performed in Greyhounds, the effect of the procedure on performance and longevity of racing career has yet to be quantified.

Digital amputation is strongly recommended for:

* metacarpophalangeal luxation
* irreparable intra-articular fracture
* compound fracture or luxation.

Amputation may also be used to revise failed primary repair.

The surgical approach is via a dorsal or abaxial inverted Y-shaped incision. Amputation is performed for fractures of P1, 2 and 3 by osteotomy at the level of distal metacarpus, distal P1 and distal P2, respectively. Disarticulation is a less satisfactory procedure. The severed digital flexor and extensor tendons may be sutured over the cut bone surface to cushion the stump. The palmar proximal sesamoid bones should be re-moved during distal metacarpal amputation. It is possible to conserve the digital pad usefully with amputation up to the level of distal P1.

In the Greyhound consideration should be given to the racing surface, with more abrasive surfaces perhaps indicating a relatively higher amputation for a given injury (Dee *et al.*, 1990). Dogs should be able to resume training 3–4 weeks after amputation.

REFERENCES

Bateman JK (1959) Fractured sesamoids in the greyhound. *Veterinary Record* **71**, 101.

Bellenger CR, Johnson KA, Davis PE and Ilkiw JE (1981) Fixation of metacarpal and metatarsal fractures in greyhounds. *Australian Veterinary Journal* **57**, 205.

Blythe LL, Gannon JR and Craig AM (1994) Breaking-in or schooling. In: *Care of the Racing Greyhound*, ed. LL Blythe, JR Gannon and AM Craig. American Greyhound Council Inc.

Boemo CM (1989) Metacarpal injury. In: *Greyhound Medicine and Surgery*. Proc. **122** Post Graduate Committee in Veterinary Science, University of Sydney.

Boudrieau RJ, Dee JF and Dee LG (1984) Treatment of central tarsal bone fractures in the racing greyhound. *Journal of the American Veterinary Medical Association* **184**, 1492.

Brinker WO, Piermattei DL and Flo GL (1990) Fractures of the carpus, metacarpus and phalanges. In: *Handbook of Small Animal Orthopaedics and Fracture Treatment*, eds WO Brinker, DL Piermattei and GL Flo. WB Saunders, Philadelphia.

Bruse S, Dee JF and Prieur WD (1989) Internal fixation with a veterinary cuttable plate in small animals. *Veterinary and Comparative Orthopaedics and Traumatology* **1**, 40.

Davis PE, Bellenger CR and Turner DM (1969) Fractures of the sesamoid bones in the greyhound. *Australian Veterinary Journal* **45**, 15.

Dee, JF (1988a) Metacarpal (metatarsal) fracture. In: *Decision Making in Small Animal Orthopaedic Surgery*, ed. G Sumner-Smith. BC Decker Inc., Philadelphia.

Dee JF (1988b) Phalangeal fracture. In: *Decision Making in Small Animal Orthopaedic Surgery*, ed. G Sumner-Smith, BC Decker Inc., Philadelphia.

Dee JF (1993) Fractures in racing greyhounds. In: *Disease Mechanisms in Small Animal Surgery*, 2nd edn, ed. MJ Bojrab. Lea & Febiger, Philadelphia.

Dee JF, Dee LG and Eaton-Wells RD (1990) Injuries of high performance dogs. In: *Canine Orthopaedics*, 2nd edn, ed. WG Whittick. Lea & Febiger, Philadelphia.

Denny HR (1990) Pectoral limb fractures. In: *Canine Orthopaedics*, 2nd edn, ed. WG Whittick. Lea & Febiger, Philadelphia.

Eaton-Wells RD (1989) Prognosis for return to racing following surgical repair of musculoskeletal injury. In: *Greyhound Medicine and Surgery*. Proc. 122 Post Graduate Committee in Veterinary Science, University of Sydney.

Eaton-Wells RD (1994) The digits. In: *Manual of Small Animal Arthrology*, ed. JEF Houlton. BSAVA, Cheltenham.

Evans HE (1993) In: *Millers Anatomy of the Dog*, 3rd edn. WB Saunders, Philadelphia.

Gannon JR (1972) Stress fractures in the greyhound. *Australian Veterinary Journal* **48**, 244.

Gentry SJ, Taylor RA and Dee JF (1993) The use of veterinary cuttable plates: 21 cases. *Journal of the American Animal Hospital Association* **29**, 455.

Hudson LC and Hamilton WP (1993) *Atlas of Feline Anatomy for Veterinarians*. WB Saunders, Philadelphia.

Ness MG (1993) Metatarsal III fractures in the racing greyhound. *Journal of Small Animal Practice* **34**, 85.

Robins GM and Read RA (1993) Diseases of the sesamoid bones. In: *Disease Mechanisms in Small Animal Surgery*, 2nd edn, ed. MJ Bojrab Lea & Febiger, Philadelphia.

Vaughan LC and France C (1986) Abnormalities of the volar and plantar sesamoid bones in Rottweilers. *Journal of Small Animal Practice* **27**, 551.

OPERATIVE TECHNIQUE 21.1

Fractures of the metacarpus

Positioning
Dorsal recumbency with the affected limb extended caudally. Also see General Considerations section.

Assistant
Optional.

Tray Extras
Gelpi self-retaining retractor ± Kilner hand-held retractor; small Hohmann retractor; small pointed reduction forceps; appropriate pins, chuck, pliers and pincutters if pinning; 1.5/2.0 mm plate and screw sets, drill bits, etc., if plating.

Surgical Approach
Where a single metacarpal bone is fractured in the Greyhound, a longitudinal incision directly over the fractured bone can be used. In cases of total metacarpal fracture, all affected bones may be exposed by a dorsal approach through an elongated X-shaped incision (Denny, 1990) (Figure 21.11).

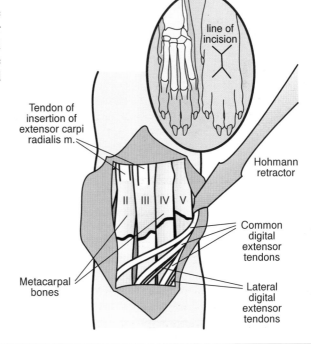

Figure 21.11 Dorsal approach to the left metacarpus.

Fixation
For plating, a veterinary cuttable plate 1 mm thick (Synthes), which accommodates 1.5 and 2.0 mm screws, is the implant of choice (Bruse *et al.*, 1989, Gentry *et al.*, 1993). It is applied as a neutralization plate with lag screw transfixion of the dorsal butterfly fragment (Figure 21.12).

Plates are applied to the medial surface of metacarpal II and the lateral surface of metacarpal V to reduce interference with the digital tendons. Conformation of the metacarpus dictates dorsal plate position on metacarpals III and IV.

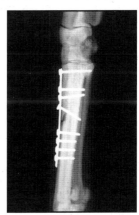

Figure 21.12: Repair of the fracture shown in Figure 21.6, using a veterinary cuttable plate and 2 mm screws. The dorsal butterfly fragment has been lagged through the plate.

→

OPERATIVE TECHNIQUE 21.1 (CONTINUED)
Fractures of the metacarpus

If intramedullary pinning is used, the pins are inserted orthograde. This is best accomplished via slots burred in the dorsal cortex of the distal fragment, in order to avoid penetration of the metacarpophalangeal joint (Dee, 1988a) (Figure 21.13).

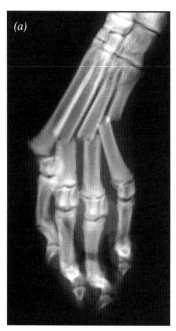 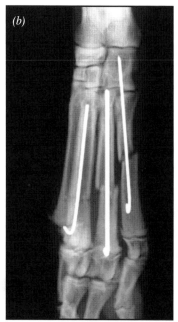 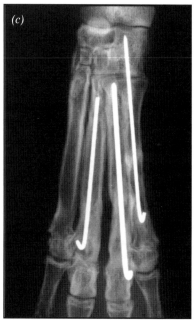

Figure 21.13: (a) Metatarsal II–V fracture in a 4-month-old Labrador Retriever. (b) Post-operative radiograph after repair using K-wires inserted proximally through the dorsal cortex of metatarsal III–V. (c) Five weeks post-operatively: wires were removed at this stage. The splinting of the repaired metatarsal bones and external coaptation allowed the metatarsal II physeal fracture to be managed conservatively.

Closure
The subcutaneous layers are closed with synthetic absorbable suture material used in a continuous or interrupted pattern. Skin closure is routine.

Post-operative Care
Implants are not removed routinely. In the Greyhound, the prognosis for a return to racing is very good following plate fixation.

OPERATIVE TECHNIQUE 21.2
Sesamoidectomy

Positioning
Forelimb: dorsal recumbency with affected limb extended cranially. Hindlimb: sternal recumbency with the affected limb extended caudally. Also see General Considerations section.

Assistant
Useful for retraction.

Tray Extras
Kilner hand-held retractors.

Surgical Approach
A palmar surgical approach is made over the affected sesamoid, avoiding the metacarpal pad (Figure 21.14). The annular ligament is transected, and the underlying digital flexor tendons are displaced to expose the palmar surface of the sesamoid. Using a No.11 blade against the bone, the fragments are dissected from the interosseous tendon proximally, and sesamoidean ligaments. The joint is lavaged, the flexor tendons are replaced, and the annular ligament is reapposed.

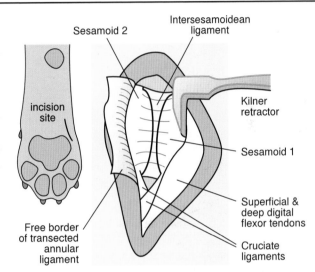

Figure 21.14: Surgical approach to left fore sesamoid 2.

Closure
The subcutaneous layers are closed with synthetic absorbable suture material used in a continuous or interrupted pattern. Skin closure is routine. The nail should be cut short to decrease metacarpophalangeal loading during convalescence.

Post-operative Care
The foot is bandaged for 3 days and exercise restricted for 6 weeks.

CHAPTER TWENTY TWO

Patella and Fabellae

Ralph H. Abercromby

INTRODUCTION

Fractures of the patella or fabellae are infrequently encountered. Care should be taken not to misdiagnose the more common, and generally clinically insignificant, bi- or poly-partite sesamoids as fractures.

PATELLA

The patella confers a mechanical advantage on the quadriceps muscle complex and is therefore a major component of the extensor apparatus of the stifle. The patella is an ossification or sesamoid bone in the tendon of insertion of the quadriceps muscle group. The quadriceps muscles converge distally as the quadriceps tendon, fibres of which pass over the patella and merge with the patellar ligament. Fibrocartilages are present on either side of the patella. In humans, resection of part or all of the patella results in quadriceps muscle atrophy and decreased strength of the extensor mechanism (Sutton *et al.*, 1976).

Fracture incidence is low, at a reported frequency of between 0.1% and 0.26% of all bone fractures (Leonard, 1960; Harari *et al.*, 1990). Any breed or age and either sex may be affected.

Fractures may occur as a consequence of intense forces generated on contraction of the quadriceps muscles — for example, when jumping or landing — but most commonly occur due to direct trauma, such as the patella being struck when the animal attempts to jump an obstacle.

Fracture classification
Fractures of the patella can be classified as either displaced or undisplaced and as transverse, longitudinal, polar or comminuted (Figure 22.1).

Clinical presentation
Non-weight-bearing lameness will be noted in many animals. Others may be surprisingly sound, especially those with undisplaced longitudinal fractures. In those caused by direct trauma, a wound or haemorrhage may be evident and may extend into the joint (open intra-articular fracture). The affected patella will be less well defined than the unaffected one due to swelling and bruising, though bilateral fractures are possible. Crepitus and pain may be evident on stifle manipulation, especially if pressure is applied to the patella. The patient may be unable, as opposed to unwilling, to bear weight on the affected limb if there is marked distraction of fragments and disruption of soft tissues. Severe disruption of the extensor apparatus is confirmed by an ability to flex the stifle with the hip concurrently extended.

Clinical signs may be suggestive of patellar fracture but confirmation requires radiography.

Radiography
Good quality caudocranial and flexed mediolateral radiographs are most useful. Fractures are usually displaced and obvious on such radiographs. Should uncertainty persist, additional projections including

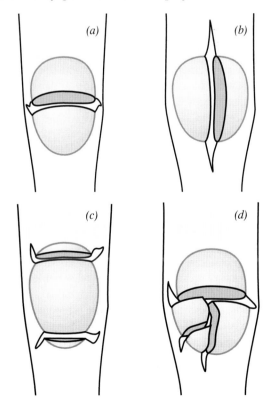

Figure 22.1: Fractures of the patella: (a) transverse; (b) longitudinal; (c) polar; (d) comminuted.

tangential/skyline, oblique, or flexed and extended views may be of some assistance.

The tangential or skyline radiographic projection permits a transverse view of the patella and can be useful for identifying undisplaced longitudinal fractures. The X-ray beam is centred between the femoral condyles and directed parallel with the trochlea and the long axis of the patella.

Surgical versus non-surgical management

Treatment aims to preserve a functional extensor apparatus and to limit degenerative joint disease. Large forces will act across any repair technique until bone union has occurred; and patellar fractures almost invariably affect the articular surface. Therefore, accurate reduction and stable fixation are usually required. External support alone is rarely indicated.

Undisplaced fractures, except perhaps where the fracture is longitudinal, are rarely encountered because of the distractive effect of the quadriceps. Such fractures may be managed conservatively by restricting physical activity and supporting the limb in moderate extension for 4 to 6 weeks. Regular radiographic monitoring is required to ensure that fragment displacement is not occurring. Rather than risk such deterioration and joint stiffness it is more usual to perform surgical repair.

Surgical management of patellar fractures

Despite earlier reports to the contrary, Howard *et al.* (1986) demonstrated that the canine patellar afferent blood supply enters at multiple sites on the medial, lateral, apical, basal and cranial surfaces and has extensive anastomoses within. Reduction and rigid fixation should result in successful bone union. The surgical options include:

- Internal fixation
- Excision of small fragments
- Patellectomy - partial or total.

Transverse fractures
Transverse fractures (Figure 22.1a) are the most commonly encountered patellar fractures. Where only two fragments are present and each is of reasonable size, it is possible to perform open reduction and fixation.

A pin and tension-band technique is recommended (Weber *et al.*, 1980) (Operative Technique 22.1). Simple wiring techniques have been shown to fail.

Longitudinal fractures
Longitudinal fractures of the patella (Figure 22.1b) are uncommon and result from direct trauma. The patella is split from proximal to distal. Should patellar tendon,

ligament and adjacent soft tissues be relatively undamaged the fracture will remain essentially undisplaced and lameness will be minimal. If soft tissue damage is extensive and displacement occurs, lameness may be marked (Operative Technique 22.2).

Polar fractures
Fractures of either patellar pole (proximal = base, distal = apex) (Figure 22.1c) are unlikely to be avulsion fractures because they are relatively unattached to patellar ligament or tendon. Where size allows they may be fixed in position by K-wire, pin and tension-band or small orthopaedic screw. Their small size and limited contribution to femoropatellar articulation means they may be safely discarded or treated conservatively. A radiographic non-union of a polar fracture does not appear to cause lameness as long as the extensor apparatus is functional.

Comminuted fractures
Repair techniques applied to comminuted patellar fractures (Figure 22.1d) depend on degree of comminution and fragment size (Operative Technique 22.3).

Patellectomy
Removal of the patella consistently alters biomechanics and has been demonstrated in clinical human and experimental animal cases (De Palma and Flynn, 1958) to result in degenerative stifle lesions and to increase the force required for knee extension. It is therefore preferable to preserve the patella wherever possible or, if not, to preserve a fragment large enough to contribute to the extensor mechanism (partial patellectomy). Carb (1975) reported a limited series including two canine patellar fractures successfully treated by partial patellectomy in which DJD resulted in only one case and was considered clinically insignificant. He proposed partial patellectomy as a first choice treatment of transverse patellar fractures.

In cases where fibrous non-union has occurred, such as following fracture of a patella weakened by disease or congenital malformation and not diagnosed or treated early, partial patellectomy has provided, for some, more satisfactory results than has late primary repair (White, 1977). Arnbjerg and Bindseil (1994) reported good function without patellectomy in cats with non-union of either transverse or polar type fractures which had occurred despite or without reparative surgery. It would appear, especially in the cat, that if partial patellectomy is considered, surgery may be temporarily delayed in order to assess whether conservative management is likely to be successful (Operative Technique 22.4).

General post-operative care of patellar surgery cases

Accurate reduction and internal fixation should allow early joint motion and weight bearing. Controlled early joint use will reduce development of DJD and fracture disease.

A soft dressing will limit but not prevent stifle motion. Care should be taken as a Robert Jones dressing that slips may actually increase the load on the repair, by restricting hock but not stifle motion. An unbandaged limb, on which the animal initially bears little weight because of the effects of injury or surgery, and an owner who understands the reasons and methods for restricted and controlled activity may be better. Exercise should be controlled for at least 4 to 6 weeks.

Where stifle movement is to be severely restricted, such as for a reconstructed comminuted patellar fracture or following patellectomy, a spica splint or Schroeder Thomas splint is to be recommended, perhaps to be replaced by a softer dressing after 2 weeks.

Should stifle motion be restricted by desire or otherwise, it will be useful to instigate a degree of passive physiotherapy at an appropriate time. Lead walking when the limb has begun to bear weight is an effective form of active physiotherapy.

Implant failure is likely to be the result of poor surgical choice but may also reflect the inability of the surgeon and owner to control activity adequately (the patient does not know any better).

Implants used in successful fracture fixation rarely break but may require removal following bone union should their subcutaneous position cause discomfort or skin problems. This is especially so for thin-skinned dogs such as Greyhound or Lurcher.

Wire passed around the patella and tibial crest to neutralize quadriceps forces on the patella is likely to fracture and may require removal. A planned removal may be performed 4 to 6 weeks post surgery or if/when a problem occurs.

Prognosis

For all but the worst comminuted fractures, the prognosis is good. Where the fracture is considered irreparable there is always the option of patellectomy or arthrodesis for salvage, the latter being a last resort when other surgical options have been tried and failed.

FABELLAE AND POPLITEAL SESAMOIDS

The fabellae and popliteal sesamoid bones are situated within the tendons of origin of the gastrocnemius and popliteus muscles, respectively. As a consequence, fracture results in displacement of the distal fragment. Fracture is rare; it may be caused by direct trauma and is often mistaken for the more common and benign bi-/poly-partite sesamoid condition. Lameness is expected and exquisite pain may be localized on deep palpation. Radiography confirms the diagnosis.

If untreated, non-union results and it may or may not cause pain (McCurnin, 1977). Internal reduction and fixation are not usually practical because of size. Where conservative management has failed or surgery is considered applicable, the proximal fragment, and others if size dictate, is removed and a suture (monofilament steel or non-absorbable synthetic) passed around the distal fragment and/or through the tendon of origin and through a femoral bone tunnel or strong soft tissues adjacent to the tendon of origin. Early surgery is generally indicated to limit the distractive effect of muscle contraction.

REFERENCES AND FURTHER READING

Alvarenga J (1973) Patellar fracture in the dog. *Modern Veterinary Practice* **54**, 43.

Arnbjerg J and Bindseil E (1994) Patella fracture in cats. *Feline Practice* **22**, 31.

Arnoczky SP and Tarvin GB (1980) Surgery of the stifle — the patella. *Compendium on Continuing Education* **2**, 200.

Betts CW and Walker M (1975) Lag screw fixation of a patellar fracture. *Journal of Small Animal Practice* **16**, 21.

Brinker WO, Piermattei, DL and Flo GL (eds) (1990) *Handbook of Small Animal Orthopaedics and Fracture Treatment.* WB Saunders, Philadelphia.

Brinker WO, Hohn RB and Prieur WD (eds) (1984) Fractures of the patella. In: *Manual of Internal Fixation in Small Animals*, 1st edn. p. 176., Springer-Verlag, Berlin.

Brunnberg L, Durr E and Knospe C (1991) Zu den Verletzungen der Patella und des Ligamentum Patellae bei Hund und Katze. 1. Patellafraktur. *Kleintierpraxis* **36**, 547.

Carb A (1975) A partial patellectomy procedure for transverse patellar fractures in the dog and cat. *Journal of the American Animal Hospital Association* **11**, 649.

De Angelis M (1981) Fractures of the appendicular and heterotopic skeleton. In: *Pathophysiology in Small Animal Surgery*, ed. MJ Bojrab, pp. 632, 787. Lea and Febiger, Philadelphia.

DePalma AF and Flynn JJ (1958) Joint changes following experimental partial and total patellectomy. *Journal of Bone and Joint Surgery* **40A**, 395.

Harari JS, Person M and Berardi C (1990) Fractures of the patella in dogs and cats. *Compendium on Continuing Education. Small Animal Practice* **12**, 1557.

Howard PE, Wilson JW, Robbins TA and Ribble GA (1986) Normal blood supply of the canine patella. *American Journal of Veterinary Research* **47**, 401.

Kaufer H and Arbor A (1971) Mechanical function of the patella. *Journal of Bone and Joint Surgery* **53A**, 1551.

Leonard EP (ed.) (1960) *Orthopaedic Surgery of the Dog and Cat.* WB Saunders Co., Philadelphia.

McCurnin DM (1977) Separation of the canine fabella. *Veterinary Medicine (Small Animal Clinician)* **72**, 1438.

Sutton FS, Thompson CH, Lipke J and Kettelkamp DB (1976) The effect of patellectomy on knee function. *Journal of Bone and Joint Surgery* **58A**, 537.

Weber MJ, Janecki CD, McLeod P. *et al.* (1980) Efficacy of various forms of fixation of transverse fractures of the patella. *Journal of Bone and Joint Surgery* **62A**, 215.

White RAS (1977) Bilateral patellar fracture in a dog. *Journal of Small Animal Practice* **18**, 261.

OPERATIVE TECHNIQUE 22.1
Patella: transverse fractures

Positioning
Dorsal recumbency.

Assistant
Optional.

Tray Extras
K-wires; wire for tension-band; chuck; pin/wire cutters; pliers/wire twisters; pointed reduction forceps; wide-bore hypodermic needle; ± 2.0 mm and 1.5 mm screw sets; drill and bits.

Surgical Approach
A cranial skin incision is made over the patella. Intra-articular structures should be examined. In many instances of direct trauma there is considerable damage to peripatellar soft tissues. In some cases one may choose to perform intra-articular examination through the laceration which can function as a transverse arthrotomy, rather than inflict further tissue trauma with a standard parapatellar arthrotomy. Blood and debris are lavaged from the joint.

Reduction and Fixation
The stifle is extended to ensure that fragments can be accurately reduced. Reduction may be assisted with reduction forceps applied to each pole of the patella. Alternatively, apply and tighten orthopaedic wire around either the circumference of the patella or immediately above the proximal fragment and through the tibial crest.

> **PRACTICAL TIP**
> **Extend stifle during repair to assist fragment reduction.**

The K-wire may be inserted through the reduced fragments in a normograde manner from one pole to the other. Alternatively it may be inserted in retrograde fashion (Figure 22.2a) from the centre of one fracture surface to the pole of that fragment, the fragment accurately reduced and the K-wire advanced to exit near the opposite pole (Figure 22.2b).

> **PRACTICAL TIP**
> **Pre-drill the hole in the first fragment with a power drill as it can be difficult to control the direction of a K-wire with a hand chuck.**

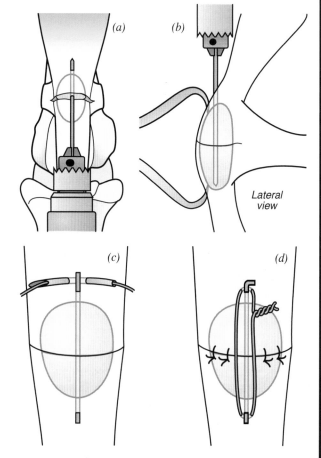

Figure 22.2: *Application of a pin and tension-band for transverse patellar fracture. (a) Retrograde placement of pin in the proximal fragment. A pilot hole can be made first with a suitable drill bit. (b) Fracture held in reduction using small pointed reduction forceps. The pin is advanced through the distal fragment. (c) Wire passed through the patellar tendon and behind the K-wire at each pole via the lumen of a pre-placed hypodermic needle. The needle can be bent into a gentle curve to facilitate placement. (d) Tension-band wire tightened and soft tissues closed.*

→

OPERATIVE TECHNIQUE 22.1 (CONTINUED)
Patella: transverse fractures

The use of two parallel wires may improve rotational stability and reduce the likelihood of breakage of the tension-band wire but is usually neither necessary nor practical, except in large dogs.

Articular surfaces should be observed if possible during reduction and fixation.

Orthopaedic wire is placed around the K-wire to function as a tension-band (Figure 22.2c,d). It is imperative that the orthopaedic wire is applied correctly and is of sufficient gauge (0.5 mm or 0.8 mm, cat and small dog; 1.0 mm, medium-sized dog; 1.25 mm, large dog).

> ### PRACTICAL TIPS
> **Orthopaedic monofilament wire is used, not suture material.**
> **Use a large hypodermic needle as a wire passer to allow correct positioning of the horizontal arms of the tension-band.**

The horizontal arms of the wire should pass immediately caudal to the K-wire and the patellar attachments of the quadriceps tendon and ligament. The vertical arms must lie on the cranial surface of the patella. Wire placed on the cranial surface will prevent the force of the quadriceps mechanism distracting the fracture (Figure 22.3).

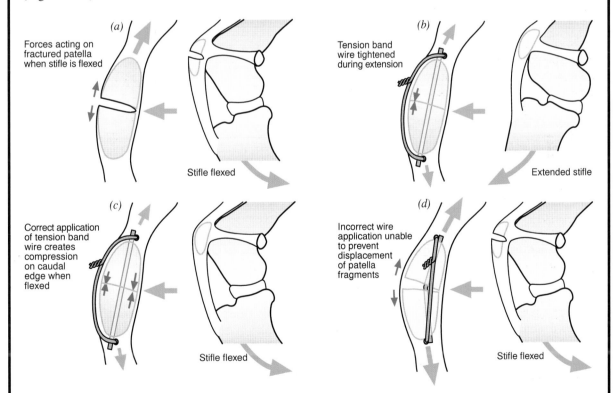

Figure 22.3: Importance of correct positioning of tension band wire in repair of transverse patellar fractures. (a) Forces acting at the site of patellar fracture during stifle flexion. (b) Tension-band wire tightened on cranial surface of the patella. The wire is tightened with stifle in extension, as in this position the polar distractive forces and caudal bending force are relatively small. (c) When the stifle is now flexed, a cranially placed wire opposes distractive and bending forces and converts them into compression at the fracture site. (d) If the wire is incorrectly placed, the caudal compressive force from the femur opens the fracture site cranially and the pin is exposed to large bending forces, leading to premature implant failure.

→

OPERATIVE TECHNIQUE 22.1 (CONTINUED)
Patella: transverse fractures

WARNING
Incorrect placement of the wire will allow distraction of the cranial aspect of the fracture on weightbearing.

The repair technique bears considerable load until bone union has occurred. To protect this to some degree and therefore lessen the risk of implant failure, or where there is concurrent damage to the patellar ligament, orthopaedic wire may be passed immediately proximal to the patella and through the tibial crest and tightened. This second wire functions as a prosthetic patellar ligament (Figure 22.4) and transfers forces directly between the insertion of the patellar tendon on the patella and the insertion of the patellar ligament on the tibial crest, thereby bypassing the fracture site.

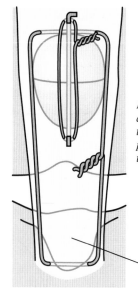

Figure 22.4: Wire placed around proximal patella and through the tibial tuberosity to protect the repair of a transverse patellar fracture.

Tibial crest

Wound Closure
Routine. Periosteum and deep fascia can be closed as one layer.

Post-operative Care
See main text.

Alternative Technique
Successful treatment of transverse fractures by partial patellectomy is reported (Carb, 1975) but results are often poorer than successful reconstruction and fixation. Conservative management of transverse patellar fractures has been reported to have failed in the dog (Alvarenga, 1973), but to have succeeded in the cat (Arnbjerg and Bindseil, 1994).

WARNING
Until a large series of canine patellar fractures treated by conservative management is reported it is probably better to treat them surgically.

OPERATIVE TECHNIQUE 22.2
Patella: longitudinal fractures

Positioning
Dorsal recumbency.

Assistant
Optional.

Tray Extras
As for Operative Technique 22.1.

Surgical Approach
As for Operative Technique 22.1.

Management
The author prefers a pin and wire technique similar to that used in transverse patellar fractures except rotated 180°, i.e. pin and wire directed in a lateromedial direction (Figure 22.5). An interfragmentary screw can be used (Betts and Walker, 1975) but fragment size often makes this more difficult than using pin and wire, and implant failure is more likely.

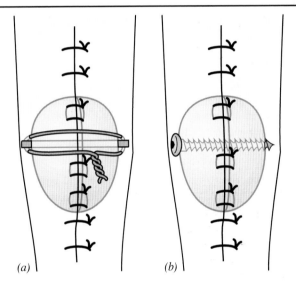

(a) (b)

Figure 22.5: *Methods of repairing longitudinal patellar fractures: (a) pin and tension-band wire; (b) lag screw.*

OPERATIVE TECHNIQUE 22.3
Patella: comminuted fractures

Positioning
Dorsal recumbency.

Assistant
Optional.

Tray Extras
As for Operative Technique 22.1

Surgical Approach
As for Operative Technique 22.1

Management
Where practical, the articular surface is reconstructed and stabilized with internal fixation. This often involves a combination of techniques including pin and tension-band, transfixion pins, orthopaedic wire and lag or positional screws (Figure 22.6a,b). Small fragments that cannot be accurately and rigidly reduced should be discarded (Figure 22.6c).

> **PRACTICAL TIP**
> If fragment size and type or surgical equipment and skills preclude fixation, consider patellectomy – either partial or total.

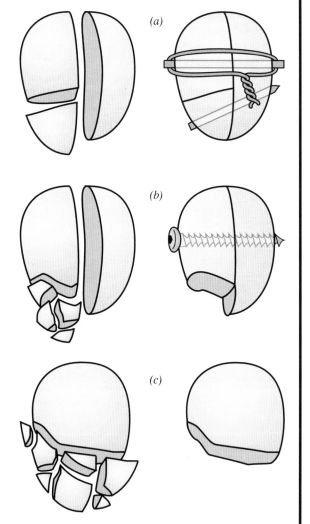

Figure 22.6: *Possible treatments of comminuted patellar fractures. (a) Reconstruction – K-wires and tension-band. (b) Partial reconstruction – screw (or pin and tension band) and smaller fragments discarded. (c) Partial patellectomy.*

OPERATIVE TECHNIQUE 22.4
Patellectomy

Positioning
Dorsal recumbency.

Assistant
Optional. Can be useful for everting the patella as the fragments are excised.

Tray Extras
As for Operative Technique 22.1, plus hand-held or self-retaining retractors; periosteal elevator; rongeurs.

Surgical Approach
The patella is approached via a standard parapatellar arthrotomy and is everted.

Technique
Fragments to be discarded are carefully excised with a scalpel or removed with rongeurs, avoiding where possible additional damage to the soft tissues (Figure 22.7). The extensor apparatus is obviously weakened in this area and will probably lengthen or fail if not protected. The area of patellectomy is 'snugged up' with Bunnell type or mattress sutures (Figure 22.7b). Where the most proximal fragment is preserved the soft tissues can be protected with a temporary wire prosthetic ligament as described for Operative Technique 22.1. Further support may be provided by a strip of fascia lata which remains attached proximal to the previous position of the patella, is reflected distally and is sutured to the peripatellar soft tissues and tibial crest.

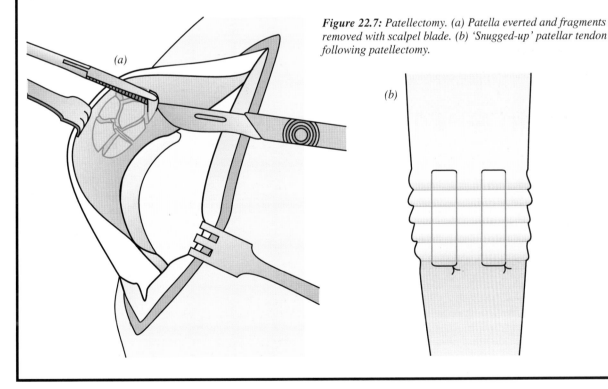

Figure 22.7: Patellectomy. (a) Patella everted and fragments removed with scalpel blade. (b) 'Snugged-up' patellar tendon following patellectomy.

PART FOUR

Complications of Fracture Management

CHAPTER TWENTY THREE

Fracture Disease

John F. Ferguson

INTRODUCTION

Fracture disease is the term used to describe the complication where a limb remains with no function, or suboptimal function, after treatment of fractures. The phrase was used by Muller (1963) to describe the syndrome of muscle atrophy or contracture, joint stiffness and osteoporosis resulting from prolonged immobilization of a limb. Functional disability may persist long after the fracture has healed.

Complications arising as a consequence of prolonged periods of limb immobilization stimulated the formation of the AO/ASIF group. This group developed instruments and implants to facilitate accurate fracture reduction and stabilization, which ensures early limb use so that controlled ambulation can be encouraged in the early post-operative period, reducing the chance of fracture disease occurring.

AETIOLOGY

Immobilization of a limb can lead to many structural, biomechanical, biochemical and metabolic changes in the affected tissues. It is well known that bone in an immobilized limb undergoes atrophy. The fact that other limb tissues – including muscles, ligaments, articular cartilage and synovium – atrophy as well has probably received less recognition. This is an important consideration as changes in articular cartilage and joint capsule may be irreversible and progressive (Akeson *et al.*, 1987).

Fracture disease usually occurs in association with surgical treatments and immobilization methods that do not provide optimal stability or that limit or prevent early active movement and limb use (Figure 23.1a,b). Non-union, delayed union, osteomyelitis and improper treatment of articular fractures all predispose to fracture disease (Figures 23.2a,b and 23.3). Fractures close to joints cause reduced range of joint movement due to the healing response and the development of adhesions in periarticular connective tissues. Fibrous adhesions between joint capsule, muscle, tendon and bone limit the normal sliding between these structures. Effects of muscle trauma seem to play a limited role in the development of joint stiffness. Immobilization of the stifle joint for three weeks with and without concurrent muscle trauma in growing dogs did not lead to a permanent reduction in range of joint motion (Shires *et al.*, 1982). However, immobilization of distal femoral fractures treated by external splintage resulted in a stiff stifle joint after a period of 3–7 weeks.

The elbow and stifle joints appear most susceptible to post-traumatic stiffness. The number of joints that a muscle group crosses affects its tendency to atrophy by virtue of the extent of immobilization the muscle group experiences. With elbow immobilization, for

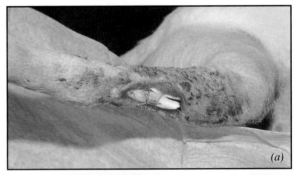

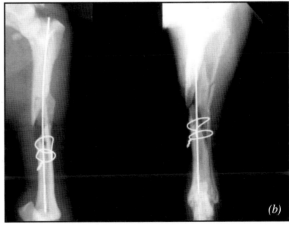

Figure 23.1: (a) A 2-year-old Jack Russell terrier, 2 weeks after surgical treatment of a closed comminuted diaphyseal tibial fracture. Note the loss of soft tissue around the fracture site. Two cerclage wires are visible. (b) Mediolateral and craniocaudal radiographs of the tibia of the same dog. Gross instability at the fracture site has resulted from the inappropriate use of implants. A Robert Jones dressing had been applied post-operatively to help to 'stabilize' the fracture.

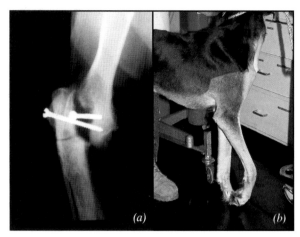

Figure 23.2: *(a) Craniocaudal radiograph of a Saluki-cross with a lateral humeral condylar fracture 8 weeks post-operatively. A non-union has resulted due to failure to reduce the fracture and gain rigid stability. (b) The same dog, showing signs of 'fracture disease' of the right forelimb. Note the presence of severe muscle atrophy.*

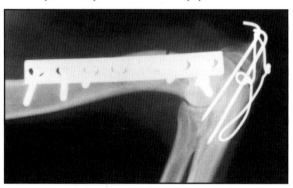

Figure 23.3: *Post-operative lateral radiograph of the right elbow of a 5 year-old Springer Spaniel. One of the K-wires used to re-attach the olecranon is placed intra-articularly. The dog did not use the limb until the K-wire was removed 3 weeks post-operatively.*

in joint range of motion may be evident. Manipulation of the joints may elicit pain. Ligamentous laxity after prolonged support is common, especially in immature animals. Joint hyperextension at the time of cast removal in young dogs results in abnormal joint posture (Figure 23.4a). This usually resolves as muscle tone returns following limb use and exercise. Animals with fracture disease after intra- or peri-articular fractures may have a severe or non-weightbearing lameness, marked muscle atrophy and decreased or loss of joint range of motion. Radiography may reveal osteoporosis (Figure 23.4b). Animals with severe quadriceps muscle contracture show characteristic signs and this condition will be discussed later in the chapter.

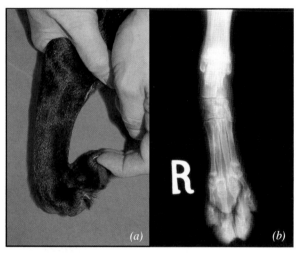

Figure 23.4: *(a) A 12-week-old Labrador's hindlimb after being in a cast for 3 weeks to treat a tibial fracture. Note the severe hyperextension of the digits due to laxity of the associated soft tissues. The signs resolved 4 weeks later. (b) Dorsopalmar radiograph of the foot of the same dog, showing osteoporosis of the bones in the distal limb.*

example, the effect on the triceps brachii muscle is greater than that on the elbow flexors because the triceps is closer to being a 'one joint' muscle than the elbow flexors (Anderson, 1991). Immobilization of the limbs of animals during their rapid growth phase may have especially dramatic consequences on the entire limb. Fracture disease in the young animal may result in disturbances in the growth of bones, joint subluxation, bone hypoplasia and limb shortening (Bardet and Hohn, 1984).

The atrophy of muscles, ligaments, articular cartilage and synovium is not caused by decreased blood flow. Richards and Schemitsh (1989) showed that blood flow to the affected limb actually increases during fracture healing and limb immobilization.

CLINICAL SIGNS

The clinical signs of fracture disease depend on the duration and severity of the condition. Immediately after cast removal, mild muscle atrophy and reduction

PATHOPHYSIOLOGY

The effects of experimental immobilization on limb tissue has been studied in various species, including the dog and cat. Changes in bones, muscles, articular cartilage, synovium, ligaments and other peri-articular structures have been demonstrated.

Muscle atrophy
Elimination of normal weightbearing forces and muscle activity leads to flaccidity and atrophy of skeletal muscles within 3–5 days of immobilization. This decrease in muscle size results in decreased muscle strength. Braund *et al.* (1986) found muscles composed of type I fibres ('slow' fibres) atrophy to a greater extent than muscles composed of type II fibres ('fast' fibres). Half of the total muscle mass lost during long-term immobilization occurs in the first 9 days (Booth, 1987). Anti-gravity muscles atrophy to a greater extent than their antagonists. Disuse muscle atrophy is generally reversible: unlike disuse osteoporosis, it appears that atrophic muscle maintains its regenerative

capacity even after long periods of immobilization. However, the recovery period varies between two and four times the duration of the immobilization.

Disuse osteoporosis

Disuse osteoporosis is characterized by decreased bone mass resulting from muscular inactivity and reduction in weight bearing. Osteoporosis after immobilization can be divided into phases. Uhthoff and Jaworski (1978) examined limbs of Beagles that had been immobilized and found the bone mass responded in three stages: it declined rapidly for the first 6 weeks but returned almost to control values during the following 8-12 weeks of immobilization; a second phase of slower but longer-lasting bone loss ended 24-32 weeks after immobilization; the third stage was characterized by maintenance of the bone mass by some 30-50% of original values. The distal limb bones lost more bone than the proximal limb bones.

The initiating cause of disuse osteoporosis is not well understood. Lack of muscular activity, increased vascular supply to the affected limb and absence of weightbearing, which decreases the piezoelectric action of crystals on bone cells, are important factors in inducing bone atrophy. The production of new bone after immobilization occurs 10 times more slowly than bone removal. Also, there is evidence that osteoporosis in young dogs and in limbs immobilized longer than 12 weeks may not be totally reversible (Bardet, 1987).

Articular and periarticular changes

Cartilage and menisci depend on synovial fluid for their nourishment and lubrication. Motion is important in producing circulation of synovial fluid and thus the flow of nutrients throughout the joint. Articular changes can occur within a few days of immobilization and are more pronounced in joints that are not subject to intermittent loadbearing (Jurvelin, 1986; Bardet, 1995). Substantial reduction in cartilage proteoglycan synthesis and content with subsequent cartilage softening occurs. Intra-articular fibro-fatty connective tissue forms within a month of immobilization, and between 1 and 2 months adhesions can occur between this tissue and the underlying cartilage. With time, major cartilage alterations occur including fibrillation, deep erosion and cleft formation. Fibrous and sometimes cartilaginous or bony ankylosis between adjacent joint surfaces may take place. Biochemical and morphological changes are rarely irreversible before 4 weeks of immobilization, but after 7 weeks changes in articular cartilage may be permanent and even become progressive despite remobilization (Akeson *et al.*, 1987). Mechanical restriction in motion leads to periarticular tissue contractures, the severity of which is related to the duration of immobilization.

The position in which the joint is immobilized appears to be significant. When rabbit stifles were immobilized in flexion, the incidence of osteoarthritis was less than when immobilized in extension (Ouzounian 1986). Thickening of the joint capsule occurs, due to fibrous hyperplasia, and type B synoviocytes proliferate in the synovial lining. Stress deprivation weakens articular ligaments due to alterations in the glycosaminoglycan and collagen fibre relationship. Bone reabsorbtion in the cortex immediately beneath the ligament attachment site may lead to avulsion fractures (Noyes, 1977).

Growth disturbances

Immobilization of limbs of growing animals may lead to severe growth disturbances in the entire limb. Immobilization of the stifle in dogs younger than 3 months of age can lead to hip subluxation, bone hypoplasia and increased femoral torsion. Hip subluxation is seen consistently after 8 weeks of cast application with the stifle fixed in an extended position (Bardet, 1987). Lack of weightbearing leads to reduction in osteoblast activity and a resultant decreased physeal growth.

QUADRICEPS CONTRACTURE

Quadriceps muscle contracture is a common complication of distal femoral fractures and is probably the commonest manifestation of fracture disease in the dog. Fractures treated by internal fixation, supplemented by extension splints, are more prone to developing this complication. The initiating factor appears to be fibrous adhesions tying down the vastus intermedius to the distal end of the femur with incorporation of the muscle into the organizing callus. This occurs most often and is likely to be most severe in young growing dogs.

Clinical signs

There is rigid hyperextension of the affected limb with reduced flexion of both the hock and stifle joints. The quadriceps muscles are firm and atrophied (Figure 23.5). Stifle hyperextension may be present to such a degree that it is bent backward, termed genu recurvatum

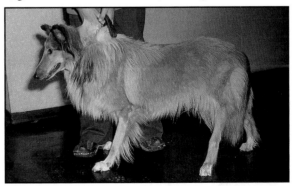

Figure 23.5: A 1-year-old Shetland Sheepdog showing signs of severe quadriceps muscle contracture. Hyperextension of both the stifle and hock joints is present.
Supplied by Mr C Stead.

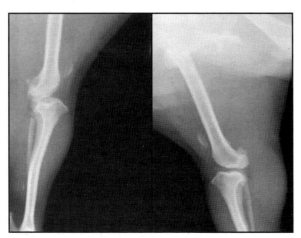

Figure 23.6: *Mediolateral radiograph of the left stifle joint of the dog in Figure 23.5. The joint is hyperextended and the patella is proximal to the trochlear groove.*
Supplied by Mr C Stead.

(Figure 23.6). The patella is pulled proximally in the trochlear groove and may be luxated medially. In young dogs, subluxation of the hip with reduced internal and external rotation and a positive Ortolani sign may be present.

Treatment

If the changes are mild then a conservative approach may be the best option. In moderate or severe cases surgery may be indicated. The aim of surgical treatment is to restore a functional range of motion to the stifle joint by freeing adhesions between muscle groups and the femur, breaking down the periarticular adhesions, lengthening the quadriceps muscle groups and regaining an angulation of the stifle joint to allow weightbearing. If the limb is severely short or if hip subluxation and severe disuse osteoporosis are present then surgical treatment is contraindicated.

Many surgical techniques have been described for the treatment of quadriceps contracture and include partial quadriceps myotomy (Leighton, 1981), Z-myoplasty (Bloomberg, 1993), freeing of adhesions and implantation of plastic sheeting between the quadriceps and distal femur (Wright, 1981), sliding myoplasty and quadriceps insertion relocation (Bloomberg, 1993). Excision of the vastus intermedius appears to be the single procedure most likely to be successful – but only in the early stages of the condition, before development of irreversible joint changes. Bardet (1987) gives a full account of the operative technique. Regardless of the surgery performed, it is important to maintain the stifle in flexion with either a figure-of-eight dressing or external pin splintage for 4–7 days.

Passive flexion and extension is performed when the supports are removed. The use of a dynamic apparatus for the prevention of recurrence of quadriceps contracture has been described (Wilkens *et al.*, 1993).

Prognosis

The prognosis for a full return to limb function is extremely poor and is guarded even for a return to reasonable function. Residual lameness is to be expected. Stifle arthrodesis or limb amputation may be necessary if there are advanced changes in the stifle or if severe hip subluxation or limb shortening is present.

CLINICAL CONSIDERATIONS IN AVOIDING FRACTURE DISEASE

The basic guideline of providing stable fixation when treating fractures to facilitate early return to limb function is critical to a satisfactory outcome and avoidance of fracture disease. In some circumstances immobilization of the limb in a cast is the treatment of choice, although the clinician should remember that fracture disease is a potential complication with this method. The duration of immobilization should be only as long as necessary to achieve bony union, and the limb should be placed in a flexed position to enable the animal to walk on the immobilized leg.

When internal fixation is used, devices that lead to rapid return of limb function should be chosen. For example, dogs with transverse mid-diaphyseal fractures of the femur stabilized with bone plates benefited from full function of the limb in an average of 3.5 weeks, compared with 7.5 weeks in dogs treated with intramedullary pins and half Kirschner splints. When intramedullary pins were used alone the time taken for normal limb function to be restored was 9.2 weeks (Braden and Brinker, 1973). Any delay in return of limb function will increase the chance of fracture disease developing. The application of Schroeder–Thomas splints (Figure 23.7) has a high incidence of developing serious complications, including non-unions, malunion and fracture disease. In the author's opinion, there is no place for the use of these devices in modern small animal veterinary practice.

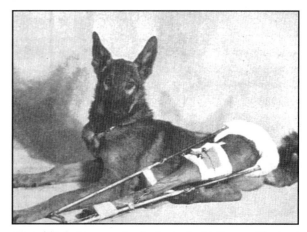

Figure 23.7: *Photograph of a 6-month-old German Shepherd Dog with a Shroeder—Thomas extension splint applied to the hindlimb for the treatment of a distal femoral fracture.*

When periarticular contractures occur, active exercise and physical therapy may be beneficial. In a study by Olson (1987), 12 dogs had their carpi immobilized in a cast for 6 weeks. In the ensuing 4 weeks, after cast removal, half the dogs received daily passive physiotherapy while the others did not. The dogs were allowed to ambulate freely in their cages during this period. Dogs that had received physiotherapy had a statistically greater range of carpal joint motion than dogs that had not received physiotherapy. However, the mean range of motion difference between the two groups was small (an average of 2°). These results would suggest that physiotherapy may only have a small effect on joint stiffness and little effect over and above the mobilizing effect of ambulation.

Swimming provides an excellent form of active, weight-supported exercise in the early rehabilitation period (Figure 23.8). Goniometry (Figure 23.9) is important if objective assessments for response to treatment are to be made.

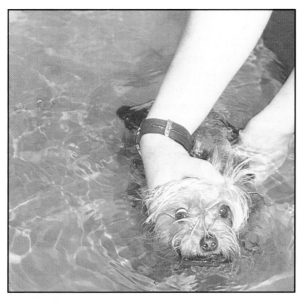

Figure 23.8: Swimming in a bath tub provides excellent weight-supported exercise and physiotherapy in the early post-operative period.

Manipulation of chronic stiff joints under anaesthesia can sometimes be used to restore normal motion by tearing adhesions and other soft tissues. Generally, however, this technique is discouraged by most physiotherapists and in fact forceful stretching techniques that cause tearing of tissues can promote further scar formation and increase joint stiffness (Herbert, 1993). Furthermore, manual stretching of adhesions is often contra-indicated because this technique usually exacerbates the severity of the mature contracture. A stretch reflex may be stimulated which is painful, causes further muscle contraction and has few long-term beneficial effects.

An alternative, more useful technique when dealing with contractures is activation or strengthening of the weak opponent muscle. In veterinary medicine,

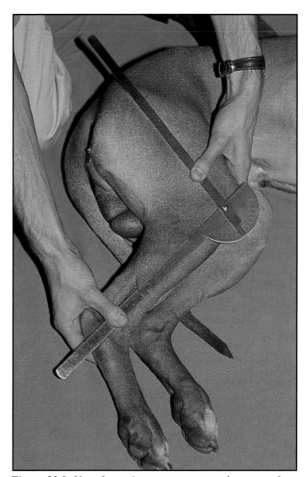

Figure 23.9: Use of a goniometer to measure the range of movement of the stifle joint after treatment of a supracondylar femoral fracture.

this can only realistically be achieved by active exercise – either weightbearing or swimming. Cooling by applying ice locally to decrease nerve conduction velocity and thus myotactic reflex activity may increase inhibition of the contracted muscle immediately before exercise periods. Passive lengthening using splints is used in humans to produce increasing but gentle prolonged stretch of contracted muscles and induces less reflex stimulation than periods of rapid muscle stretching. Non-steroidal anti-inflammatory drugs (NSAIDs) appear to have little effect on post-traumatic joint stiffness but have been shown to reduce joint swelling after trauma (More *et al.*, 1989). The analgesic effect of NSAIDs has an important role in encouraging return to weightbearing and limb function in the early post-operative period.

Experimentally, joints immobilized for 4 weeks and then treated with four weekly intra-articular hyaluronic acid injections showed reduced cartilage proteoglycan loss and reduced joint stiffness, and superficial cartilage damage was prevented (Keller *et al.*, 1994). Dexamethasone (1 mg/kg) has been shown to decrease joint stiffness after trauma although no statistically significant effect on joint swelling was seen (Grauer *et al.*, 1989). The corticosteroid effect of reducing inflammatory mediators and decreasing collagen production and cross-linking is likely to be responsible. The use of hyaluronic acid and corticosteroids has not been fully evaluated in canine fracture disease and so is not currently advocated for use in clinical practice

SUMMARY

Fracture disease is most commonly encountered with external coaptation of a limb by using a cast. However, the changes occur to a lesser extent with other means of fixation. The clinician should adhere to the principles of fracture repair and make every attempt to avoid fracture disease, since no satisfactory treatment exists. Stable fixation of fractures that allows the limb the most rapid return to functional weightbearing without immobilization should be employed. If a cast is used, the limb should be fixed in a walking position. Severe manifestations of fracture disease can be avoided with proper fracture management.

REFERENCES

Akeson D, Amiel D and Abel MF (1987) Effects of immobilization on joints. *Clinical Orthopaedics and Related Research* **219**, 28–37.

Anderson GI (1991) Fracture disease and related contractures. *Veterinary Clinics of North America* **21**, 845–858.

Bardet JF (1987) Quadriceps contracture and fracture disease. *Veterinary Clinics of North America* **17**, 957–993.

Bardet JF (1995) Fracture disease. In: *Small Animal Orthopaedics*, ed. M Olmstead, pp. 319–329. Mosby-Year Book Inc., Missouri.

Bardet JF and Hohn RB (1984) Subluxation of the hip joint and bone hypoplasia associated with quadriceps contracture in young dogs. *Journal of American Veterinary Medical Association* **20**, 421–428.

Bloomberg M (1993) Muscles and tendons. In: *Textbook of Small Animal Surgery* 2nd edn, ed. S Slatter, pp. 2010–2011. WB Saunders & Co., Philadelphia.

Booth FW (1987) Physiologic and biochemical effects of immobilization on muscle. *Clinical Orthopaedics and Related Research* **219**, 15–20.

Braden TD and Brinker WO (1973) Effect of certain fixation devices on functional limb usage in dogs. *Journal of the American Veterinary Medical Association* **162**, 642–646.

Braund KJ, Shires PK and Mikeal RL (1986) Type I fibre atrophy in the vastus lateralis in dogs with femoral fractures treated by hyperextension. *Veterinary Pathology* **17**, 166–177.

Grauer JD, Kabo JM, Dorey FJ and Meals RA (1989) The effects of dexamethasone on periarticular swelling and joint stiffness following fracture in a rabbit model. *Clinical Orthopaedics and Related Research* **242**, 277–284.

Herbert R (1993) Preventing and treating stiff joints. In: *Key Issues in Musculoskeletal Physiotherapy*, ed. J Crosbie and J MacConnel, pp. 114–141. Butterworth-Heinmann, Oxford.

Jurvelin J (1986) Softening of canine articular cartilage after immobilization of the knee joint. *Clinical Orthopaedics and Related Research* **207**, 246–250.

Keller GW, Aron DA, Rowland GN, Odend'hal S and Brown J (1994) The effect of trans-stifle external skeletal fixation and hyaluronic acid therapy on articular cartilage in the dog. *Veterinary Surgery* **23**, 119–128.

Leighton RL (1981) Muscle contractures in the limbs of dogs and cats. *Veterinary Surgery* **10**, 132.

More RC, Kody MH, Kabo JM, Dorey FJ and Meals RA (1989) The effects of two non-steroidal anti-inflammatory drugs on limb swelling, joint stiffness, and bone torsional strength following fracture in a rabbit model. *Clinical Orthopaedics and Related Research* **247**, 306–311.

Muller ME (1963) Internal fixation for fresh fractures and for non-union. *Proceedings of the Royal Society of Medicine* **56**, 455–460.

Noyes FR (1977) Functional properties of knee ligaments and alterations induced by immobilization. *Clinical Orthopaedics and Related Research* **123**, 210–42.

Olson VL (1987) Evaluation of joint mobilization treatments. *Physical Therapy* **67**, 351–356.

Ouzounian TJ (1986) The effect of pressurisation on fracture swelling and joint stiffness in the rabbit hind limb. *Clinical Orthopaedics and Related Research* **210**, 252–257.

Richards RR and Schemitsh EH (1989) The effect of flap coverage on bone and soft tissue on blood flow following devascularisation of a segment of tibia. An experimental investigation in the dog. *Journal of Orthopaedic Research* **7**, 550–558.

Shires PK, Braund KG, Milton JL and Lui W (1982) Effect of localised trauma and temporary splinting on immature skeletal muscle and mobility of the femorotibial joint in the dog. *American Journal of Veterinary Research* **3**, 454–60.

Uhthoff HK and Jaworski ZFG (1978) Bone loss in response to long term immobilization. *Journal of Bone and Joint Surgery* **60B**, 420–429.

Wilkens BE, McDonald DE and Hulse DA (1993) Utilization of a dynamic stifle flexion apparatus in preventing recurrence of quadriceps contracture: a clinical report. *Veterinary Comparative Orthopaedics and Traumatology* **6**, 219–223.

Wright RJ (1980) Correction of quadriceps contractures. *California Veterinarian* **1**, 7–10.

CHAPTER TWENTY FOUR

Implant Failure

Malcolm G. Ness

Most failures in orthopaedics can be placed at the feet of the surgeon

D.L. Piermattei

If a bone is subjected to moderately increased stress — be it from increased activity, patient weight gain, biomechanical alterations or other reasons — the bone will undergo reactive hyperplasia. This process is described by Wolff's Law. Following fracture surgery the metal implants used in fracture repair must bear all or part of the load usually carried by the bone. Without bone's capacity for reactive hyperplasia, overloaded metal implants may fatigue and fail.

Is occasional implant failure an inevitable complication of fracture surgery or can it be avoided? The purpose of this chapter is to look more closely at how and why implants fail in the hope that an increased understanding of the relevant biological, biomechanical, mechanical and metallurgic phenomena can be usefully applied to the benefit of patients. Fracture repair by open reduction and internal fixation has been described as a race between bone healing and implant failure. Whilst such biomechanical brinkmanship cannot be condoned two points are well made: metallic implants cannot be expected to function indefinitely and biological factors such as patient age, disease status, surgical technique, etc. can greatly influence the rate of bone healing.

This review of implant failure in small animal fracture surgery will be divided into three subsections:

1. The properties of 316L stainless steel — the material from which almost all veterinary orthopaedic implants are made (Chapter 8).
2. Mechanics of material failure with reference to 316L stainless steel.
3. Modes of failure of metallic orthopaedic implants *in vivo*.

316L STAINLESS STEEL

Almost all implants currently used in small animal fracture are manufactured from 316L stainless steel (316L). Although titanium alloy plates and screws are widely used in human orthopaedics, they perform only marginally better, yet are significantly more expensive, than 316L stainless steel implants and so they have not found favour in veterinary orthopaedics.

316L is an alloy of iron (55—60%), chromium (17—20%), nickel (10—14%), molybdenum (2—4%) and traces of other elements, notably carbon. Carbon content is kept below 0.03% — the 'L' of 316L stands for 'low carbon'. This particular alloy has been developed from earlier materials — the addition of molybdenum and chromium to the recipe has enhanced the corrosion resistance of today's implants when compared with those in use in the 1920s.

Despite these improvements, 316L, when perfectly clean, is remarkably reactive and therefore prone to corrosion. In practice this reactivity is beneficial, as it leads to the formation of a tightly bound oxide film which covers the entire surface of the metal, and provides significant protection against further corrosion of the implant *in vivo*. However, corrosion resistance of 316L stainless implants remains marginal and some corrosion is inevitable in most fractures where a plate and screws are used. The amount of corrosion will not usually be enough in itself to be obviously significant, but may act in concert with stress concentration and metal fatigue phenomena to cause ultimate failure of implants.

316L is a relatively strong material, being able to withstand forces in the region of 7×10^8 Newtons/m^2 in compression and the same under tension. This compares with cortical bone, which can withstand forces of about 1.5×10^8 Newtons/m^2 in compression but rather less under tension — bone, unlike 316L, is anisotropic. A fuller description of the material properties of bone can be found in Chapter 3. Many of the mechanical principles governing the way in which bone fractures can equally be applied to fracture of 316L, though obviously the forces required and amounts of energy involved are very much greater.

This inherent strength of 316L allows plates, pins, etc. to be made sufficiently small to allow implantation, while remaining strong enough to resist the biomechanical forces acting through the implant—bone composite during fracture healing.

The mechanical properties and corrosion resistance of 316L can vary greatly, depending on how an implant is made from the stock metal. For example, 316L implants made by casting rather than forging have poor corrosion resistance and are relatively weak, being only marginally stronger than cortical bone. This observation need not trouble the surgeon, because almost all implants used in veterinary fracture surgery are forged.

In conclusion, 316L can be forged and worked to form a variety of useful orthopaedic implants. It is non-toxic, biochemically inert, and strong enough and stiff enough to resist the stresses normally encountered in small animal orthopaedics although, like many metals, it is prone to fatigue failure and its corrosion resistance is only just adequate.

IMPLANT MATERIAL FAILURE

A detailed account of the mechanics of 316L is beyond the scope of this chapter, but it is interesting to compare the acute material failure occasionally seen in implants with the material failure of cortical bone during fracture, a process that has been described in some detail in Chapter 3. Similarly, the concepts of stress concentration and fatigue failure are important to the understanding of how and why an implant might fail and will be discussed in some detail.

Early acute material failure of a metal implant is analogous to the material failure seen in bone as it fractures and is extremely uncommon in small animal orthopaedics. Such sudden and catastrophic failure of a metal implies the development and propagation of a crack in the material. When compared with fracturing bone, massive amounts of energy are required to propagate a crack in metal as strong as 316L stainless steel; consequently this type of failure is rarely seen in small animal orthopaedics, where the necessary energy and force cannot be generated. Contrast this with the failures sometimes seen in equine long bone fracture repair, when plates fracture as the patient attempts to rise following surgery. The considerable stresses generated in the plate by the uncoordinated efforts of the horse to stand are sufficient to initiate a crack in the implant, and the availability of large amounts of energy related to muscle strength and body mass allows propagation of the crack and causes acute material failure of the implant.

In small animal orthopaedics, implant failure typically occurs some weeks after an apparently successful fracture repair. The concepts of metal fatigue and fatigue failure help to explain these cases.

Stresses well below those needed to fracture an implant have the potential to alter the implant material permanently. It has been shown experimentally that cyclical stresses applied to a metal, whilst not enough to fracture the material, will cause microscopic cracks which will be advanced, perhaps by only a fraction of a micron, each time the stress is re-applied. These experimentally applied cyclical stresses are not dissimilar to those applied to an orthopaedic implant during normal weightbearing activity.

The fatigue characteristics for a metal can be determined experimentally and described graphically (Figure 24.1). From this, we can see that larger stresses will lead to earlier fatigue failure and also that there is a level of stress below which fatigue failure will not occur — the fatigue limit.

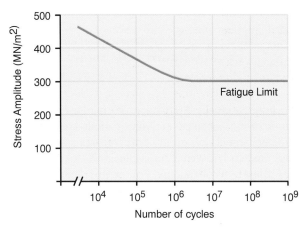

Figure 24.1: *Curve for stress versus number of cycles, determined experimentally for 1045 carbon steel. The fatigue limit is a level of stress that will never cause material failure, no matter how often the stress is applied. The curve also shows that even quite modest increases in stress amplitude can greatly reduce the number of cycles to failure: a 50% increase in stress might reduce the life of the material by a factor of 10 or more. Much larger stresses — higher than those recorded on this curve — will lead to permanent (plastic) deformation or even fracture of the material. (Redrawn from Radin et al., 1992.)*

In practice, this raises the possibility of an implant with infinite life expectancy, though in reality such an implant might be unacceptably large and unwieldy. Similarly, an implant subjected to sufficiently large cyclical stresses will have a reduced life expectancy, and as the stress is increased the life span of the implant will be shortened. This information can be used by the surgeon to select suitably strong implants which will not be prone to fatigue failure before bony union is achieved. Equally the surgeon can consider restricting the patient's activity in an attempt to maximize implant longevity. In practice, the extent to which we can vary implant size or levels of patient activity are limited and will have a relatively small effect on implant stress levels and implant longevity. Of more significance in this respect is the effect of stress concentration, which has the potential to increase local stresses by several orders of magnitude, significantly reducing the time (number of cycles) to failure.

If a tensile force is applied to a metal bar, the stresses will be spread equally across the bar (Figure 24.2). If a hole or notch is cut into the bar, the same stresses will be distributed less evenly and areas of stress concentration will arise (Figure 24.3). Areas where stress concentration occurs are known as stress risers.

The similarities between these hypothetical models and some of our implants are obvious and the importance of this stress concentration effect should not be underestimated: sharp, deep defects in a metal bar can result in local stresses being increased 1000 times or more. Most plates and wires in small animal orthopaedics are placed on the tension aspect of long bones and are therefore subjected mainly to tensile stresses. Similarly, repeated bending stresses, which are a frequent precursor to implant failure, can be considered as cyclical tensile stresses applied to the convex surface of the implant, with the largest tensile stresses being recorded at the abaxial surface of the implant. Applying this information to the example of a bone plate on the lateral (tension) surface of a dog's femur, we can appreciate that the tensile stresses on the outer aspect of the plate will be exaggerated and that the screw holes will further enhance the stress concentration. Consequently, some of the metal making up the plate will be subjected to stresses many times greater than could be expected if only the patient's weight and the cross-sectional area of the plate were taken into consideration.

The concept of stress concentration is essential to the understanding of why implants of seemingly reasonable size can fail.

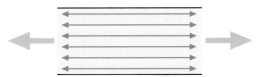

Figure 24.2: *When a metal bar is placed under tension, the stress (shown here by lines of force) is spread evenly across the bar.*

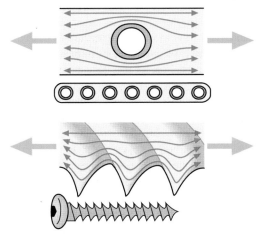

Figure 24.3: *With the bar under tension, the number of lines of force at any cross-section must remain constant. Cutting a hole or notch into the bar will lead to concentrations of stress around the hole or at the extremity of the notch. The similarities between these hypothetical models and our bone plates and screws are obvious.*

MODES OF FAILURE OF METALLIC IMPLANTS

Having considered in some detail, but in isolation, the failure of a metal subjected to simple mechanical forces (material failure), we must now relate this to the clinical situation (implant failure). Two major differences exist between the hypothetical models of material failure previously discussed and the failed implants encountered in small animal orthopaedic practice:

- All orthopaedic implants are fixed to bone and so, from a mechanical viewpoint, they are part of a bone—metal composite and the size and distribution of stresses through the implant will be enormously influenced by its relationship to the bone.
- Orthopaedic implants are continually bathed in extracellular fluid which, being ionic and oxygen rich, is potentially corrosive.

We can propose five distinct mechanisms that may cause, or at least contribute to, the failure of a metallic implant:

- Material failure due to metallurgic imperfections or manufacturing faults
- Acute overload
- Electrochemical corrosion
- Oxidation—reduction corrosion ('crevice corrosion')
- Fatigue failure.

It is not unusual for several of these processes to be acting concurrently, and there exists potential for a destructive synergism that can easily be exacerbated by technical errors, such as inadequate fracture reduction, damage and marking of implants, poor tissue handling causing delayed union, etc.

Failure due to metallurgic imperfections or manufacturing faults

316L is a relatively simple material to manufacture. The metal is extensively worked, forged and polished before being delivered as a finished implant and so the potential for an implant made from imperfect material getting as far as the surgeon is small. Implant failure due to metallurgic imperfection is correspondingly rare.

Acute overload of implant

Acute material failure of an implant (as distinct from fatigue failure) is not common in small animal orthopaedics. Such fracture implies the development and then (importantly) the rapid propagation of a crack in the implant material, a process that requires larger amounts of energy than are generally available in small animal fractures.

One example of acute implant failure which may be encountered is that of a screw head shearing off as the screw is overtightened. A screw is a simple machine that converts a small torque into a much larger axial force. During insertion, the screw head becomes restrained against cortex or bone plate. Further torque merely increases tensile force in the shaft of the screw. Applying knowledge of stress concentration phenomena we can predict a stress riser where the thread cuts into the screw shaft proximally, so that overtightening causes the screw head to snap off. Whilst this is certainly an example of acute material failure, the event is perhaps best viewed as technical error — it was not that the screw was too weak but that the surgeon was too strong.

Electrochemical corrosion

The principle of the electrical storage battery is familiar to anyone who has studied elementary science. The key chemical reaction is that of a more active metal displacing a less active metal from solution. For example, if we have two implants made of different alloys bathed in a solution (extracellular fluid) then we can expect the more reactive metals to displace the less reactive from solution. The net result of this chemistry is loss of substance, and therefore strength, from the implant — i.e. corrosion.

The orthopaedic surgeon must be aware that implants of differing composition should never be mixed. Because almost all small animal orthopaedic implants are made from 316L, electrochemical corrosion is an uncommon occurrence in our patients. However, inadvertent use of titanium plates with 316L screws or the use of non-standard drill bits which may snap and be left *in situ* are scenarios that may lead to electrochemical corrosion. Corrosion products cause pain, inflammation and bone necrosis and in practice the surgeon will recognize these cases primarily as painful delayed unions, before significant implant erosion or failure occurs.

Oxidation—reduction corrosion ('crevice corrosion')

The above description of electrochemical corrosion explained how metals of differing reactivity placed in solution give rise to an electric current at the expense of loss of the more reactive metal in solution. Similarly, identical metals in environments with differing oxidation—reduction (redox) potentials will display different levels of reactivity and consequently can become involved in electrochemical reactions comparable with those described above. The key chemical reaction is:

$$2Fe + 2H_2O + O_2 \rightleftharpoons 2Fe(OH)_2$$

The reaction is driven by the higher oxidation potential on the left side of the equation. The net result is loss of elemental iron into solution under conditions of low oxygen tension and is manifest as corrosion of the metallic implant.

In practice, this type of corrosion occurs quite frequently — usually between screw heads and plates or between a plate and cortical bone; hence the description 'crevice corrosion'. Although unlikely to result in extensive damage to implants, the importance of crevice corrosion is its action in potentiating other forms of implant degeneration. For example, crevice corrosion breaches the protective oxide film present on all 316L implants, exposing them to further corrosive attack. Additionally, the pits on the implant surface caused by crevice corrosion will act as stress risers, accelerating fatigue failure.

Fatigue failure

This is by far the most important mode of implant failure encountered in small animal orthopaedics. Typically, the patient will have shown an early return to function and will have seemed to be well until the implant 'suddenly' breaks some weeks after surgery. Fatigue failure occurs after an implant has been exposed to repeated cyclical stresses which, though not large enough to cause acute material failure, will cause a small, permanent alteration to the structure of the metal. The size of this microscopic defect will be proportional to the applied load and similarly the time to failure of the implant will be inversely proportional to the applied load.

> ### PRACTICAL TIP
> **Except in cases where an unusually small implant has been used in error, most instances of fatigue failure of implants encountered in small animal practice result from stress concentration effects (often with other mechanical phenomena) acting in an unstable or poorly reduced fracture.**

Recommendations to use complex rather than unilateral single bar external fixator frames in inherently unstable fractures, or to use larger implants when applying a plate as a buttress, represent a recognition that in some circumstances there is an increased risk of implant fatigue failure. Intuitively, we know that a plate over a poorly reduced fracture will be exposed to greater stresses than a plate over an anatomically reconstructed bone, but the full consequence in terms of the amount of increased stress may not be immediately obvious. Area moment of inertia (AMI), discussed in Chapter 3 in relation to the biomechanics of fracture repair, is an expression of a structure's ability to resist bending. AMI depends not only on the mass of material but also, and importantly in this context, on the distance of mass from the neutral axis of the structure. The neutral axis is that part of a structure under bending (or eccentric axial loading) which is exposed to neither tensile nor compressive force, and the importance of estimating the neutral axis (and AMI) of a proposed bone—implant composite during fracture repair has been described in Chapter 3.

Figure 24.4a shows an anatomically reduced fracture fixed with a plate applied to the lateral (tension) aspect of the femur. The neutral axis is displaced laterally but remains within the bone. In Figure 24.4b the neutral axis lies within the plate itself; consequently, the AMI in this example is low, not only because the bone does not contribute, but also because the mass of the plate is close to the neutral axis.

> **PRACTICAL TIP**
> **In essence, the presence of a mechanically competent cortex opposite a bone plate not only shares the load but also greatly enhances the mechanical environment by moving the neutral axis away from the plate.**

The low resistance to bending (low AMI) characterized in Figure 24.4b, which accelerates fatigue failure, will at the same time permit movement at the fracture. This may delay fracture healing, and therefore further increase the risk of implant failure. The possibility of implant failure in this situation is recognized by most orthopaedic surgeons, who will avoid leaving fracture gaps or an open opposite cortex. When unavoidable, the use of cancellous bone autografts will encourage prompt new bone formation, thus restoring mechani-

cal competence to the opposite cortex and easing the stress acting through the implant.

The broken plate shown in Figure 24.5 is a good example of fatigue failure resulting from stress concentration in an implant caused by the lack of a mechanically competent opposite cortex. It is tempting to think that the plate was just too small. While a larger implant might have delayed failure, it probably would not have prevented it as the plate (no matter how large) remains mechanically exposed. Had the cranial cortex been reconstructed, the AMI would have been increased and the stress levels in the plate consequently decreased. An alternative solution would have been the application of a second plate. This would have been beneficial because of load sharing and, more importantly, because of the effect of increasing the AMI of the repair.

In conclusion, it is clear that most implant failures can be avoided and that implant failure must not be considered an inevitable complication of fracture surgery. An awareness of material failure, stress concentration, fatigue failure, etc. will help the aspiring fracture surgeon to avoid the technical errors that culminate in implant failure.

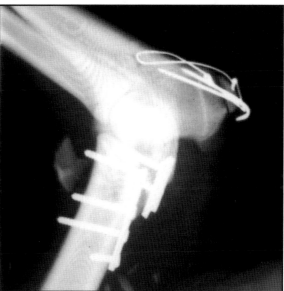

Figure 24.5: Lateral radiograph taken 4 weeks after open reduction and fixation of a comminuted intercondylar fracture of the distal humerus in a 25 kg dog. Early progress had been excellent and the patient was only slightly lame until the plate snapped the day before this radiograph was taken. Note the large cranial cortical fragment which was not reduced and fixed in the original repair.

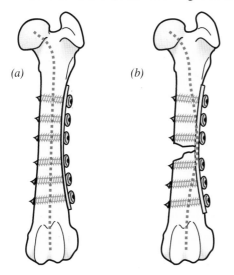

Figure 24.4: (a) Anatomically reduced mid-femoral fracture fixed with a plate and screws. The dashed line represents the estimated location of the neutral axis. Because there is a mass of material located some distance from the neutral axis (plate laterally and cortex medially) this bone and plate composite will have a high area of movement of inertia (high resistance to bending) and so will be inherently stable. (b) A similar fracture, but without benefit of a mechanically competent medial femoral cortex. Here, the neutral axis must lie within the plate itself and so the AMI is very much lower. Weightbearing in this limb will cause repeated bending stresses concentrated in the small part of the plate overlying the fracture — a recipe for fatigue failure.

REFERENCES AND FURTHER READING

Nordin M and Frankel VH (1989) *Basic Biomechanics of the Musculo-Skeletal System*, 2nd edn. Lea and Febiger, Philadelphia.

Perrens SM and Rahn BA (1978) Biomechanics of fracture healing, *Orthopaedic Survey* 2(2) 108—143.

Radin EL, Rose RM, Blaha JD and Litsky AS (1992) *Practical Biomechanics for the Orthopedic Surgeon*, 2nd edn. Churchill Livingstone, New York.

Sumner-Smith G (ed.) (1982) *Bone in Clinical Orthopedics*. WB Saunders, Philadelphia.

CHAPTER TWENTY FIVE

Osteomyelitis

Angus A. Anderson

INTRODUCTION

Osteomyelitis is defined as inflammation of the bone cortex and marrow. Osteitis, myelitis and periostitis refer to inflammation involving the bone cortex, marrow and periosteum, respectively. Although most commonly caused by bacteria, other infectious agents (fungi, viruses) may cause the disease, and corrosion of metallic implants may also initiate inflammatory responses in bone.

Osteomyelitis is often classified as being haematogenous or post-traumatic in origin. Post-traumatic osteomyelitis develops following the direct inoculation of bacteria into a fracture site either at the time the fracture occurs, or after contamination of the fracture site during internal fixation, or by extension of infection from adjacent soft tissues (e.g. following bite wounds). Haematogenous osteomyelitis results from blood-borne bacteria localizing to bones, but the source of these bacteria is frequently unknown. Although there is no very satisfactory definition that distinguishes acute from chronic forms of the disease, chronic osteomyelitis is usually characterized by the presence of avascular cortical bone and requires surgical intervention for the disease to resolve. Some bacteria (e.g. *Mycobacteria* spp.) and some fungi give rise to a disease that is chronic in nature.

PATHOGENESIS

Normal bone is relatively resistant to infection and studies of animal models of osteomyelitis have shown that chronic disease can only be generated if a number of factors are present. These include:

- An inoculum of sufficient numbers of pathogenic bacteria
- Avascular cortical bone
- Favourable environment for bacterial colonization and multiplication (metallic implants, haematomata, necrotic soft tissue).

Chronic osteomyelitis is unlikely to develop if these three factors are not present (Braden *et al.*, 1987).

Unfortunately, the commonest reason for the development of osteomyelitis in small animals is the open reduction of fractures. During surgery, bacteria from the animal's skin, the atmosphere or the surgeon frequently contaminate the exposed tissues and may colonize the surface of metallic implants (Smith *et al.*, 1989). Some bacteria possess mechanisms that ensure their persistence at fracture sites. These include the production of slime that consists of extracellular polysaccharides, ions and nutrients (Gristina *et al.*, 1985), phenotypic transformation to more virulent strains, and adherence to components of extracellular matrix (e.g. fibronectin, laminin) via specific receptors (Vercelotti *et al.*, 1985). Bacterial slime combines with host-derived substances to form biofilm, which surrounds bacterial colonies and protects them from host defences (phagocytosis, antibodies and complement) and the actions of some antibiotics (Figure 25.1).

Despite the high incidence of contamination during surgery, osteomyelitis only develops in a small proportion of cases (Smith *et al.*, 1989). Factors that increase the likelihood of the development of infection include excessive trauma to soft tissues, periosteal stripping resulting in devascularization of cortical bone, fracture instability, and the presence of individual host factors that may alter local defences (e.g. malignancy, diabetes mellitus).

If infection becomes established, inflammatory exudate may be forced along the Haversian and Volkmann's canals of the cortex, under the periosteum (particularly in young animals where the periosteum is more loosely attached to underlying cortical bone) and into the medullary canal (Figure 25.1). Fragments of cortical bone that have lost their blood supply (sequestra) may become surrounded by exudate and act as persistent foci of infection. The periosteum and endosteum of cortical bone adjacent to a sequestrum may attempt to wall off this infected material by depositing new bone (involucrum) around it.

Fracture instability is an important mechanism potentiating infection. Lysis of cortical bone adjacent to implants, as a result of the infection, may lead to implant loosening and increased interfragmentary movement. This effect may be compounded by excessive movement at the fracture site caused by

Contaminated site following surgery

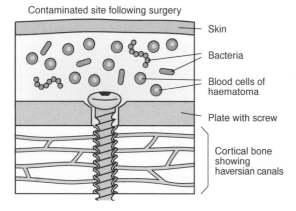

— Skin

— Bacteria

— Blood cells of
   haematoma

— Plate with screw

Cortical bone
showing
haversian canals

Host inflammatory response

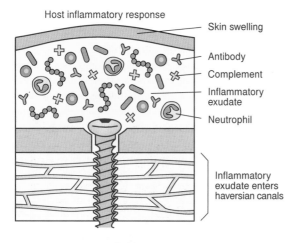

— Skin swelling

— Antibody

— Complement

— Inflammatory
   exudate

— Neutrophil

Inflammatory
exudate enters
haversian canals

Biofilm formation and bone death

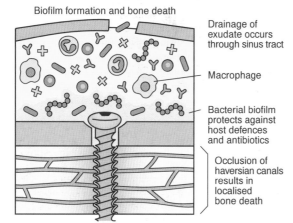

Drainage of
exudate occurs
through sinus tract

Macrophage

Bacterial biofilm
protects against
host defences
and antibiotics

Occlusion of
haversian canals
results in
localised
bone death

Bone lysis and plate loosening

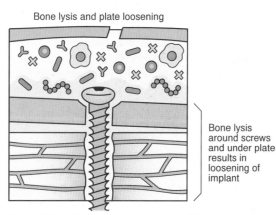

Bone lysis
around screws
and under plate
results in
loosening of
implant

Figure 25.1: Pathogenesis of osteomyelitis.

inadequate fracture fixation, or technical errors in implant application. The resulting triad of infection, cortical bone resorption and fracture instability usually leads to delayed fracture healing or non-union (Johnson, 1994).

DIAGNOSIS

A diagnosis of osteomyelitis is suggested from the history, clinical signs and radiographic findings. Confirmation requires bacteriological culture of the causative organism(s).

History

Because the majority of cases of osteomyelitis develop as a result of open reduction of fractures, there is usually a history of fracture repair. Where osteomyelitis develops as a result of extension of infection from an adjacent site, the commonest sources of infection include bite wounds, teeth, nailbeds and the middle ear (Caywood *et al.*, 1978; Muir and Johnson, 1992). In haematogenous osteomyelitis, clinical evidence of a septic focus elsewhere in the body may be present (e.g. prostate, uterus, lungs), although frequently the source of the infection remains unknown.

Clinical and laboratory findings

Clinical signs depend on the stage of the disease process and the bone(s) affected. During the acute stage of the disease the affected animal may show:

- Pain on palpation of the bone and associated soft tissues
- Swollen, inflamed soft tissues (Figure 25.2)
- Pyrexia, anorexia, lethargy
- (Discharge from sinus tracts).

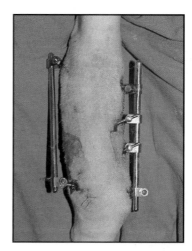

Figure 25.2: Acute osteomyelitis following application of a modified type II external skeletal fixator to stabilize an osteotomy of the distal radius and ulna. The limb is swollen, and purulent material is discharging through the skin incision on the lateral aspect of the limb.

Haematological examination may reveal a neutrophilia with a left shift. Differentiating acute osteomyelitis from deep wound infection may be very difficult because radiographic changes in bone will not appear immediately following infection. Needle aspiration from around the fracture site may reveal large numbers of neutrophils with bacteria suggestive of infection involving the bone.

During the more chronic stages of the disease process, systemic signs are usually absent and the main clinical findings are:

- Lameness
- Discharging sinus tracts
- Pain on palpation of the bone
- Disuse muscle atrophy
- Instability at the fracture site
- Intermittent soft tissue swelling.

Haematological examination is usually normal.

Radiography and other imaging modalities

The radiographic appearance of osteomyelitis is variable and depends on the stage of the disease process (see Chapter 5). During the acute stages, the only visible changes may be soft tissue swelling. More rarely, gas shadows may be present if the causative organism is a gas-producer (e.g. some *Clostridium* spp.) (Figure 25.3). It may take up to 2 weeks for radiographic changes to appear in the bone. As the disease becomes more chronic the following features may be evident (Figures 25.4, 25.5 and 25.6):

- Bone lysis (usually focal or adjacent to metallic implants)
- Periosteal new bone (smooth or irregular)
- Sclerosis
- Cortical thinning
- Involucrum (identified as an area of sclerotic bone surrounding a sequestrum)
- Delayed fracture healing or nonunion
- Sequestrum (identified as a radiodense fragment of cortical bone surrounded by a zone of radiolucency).

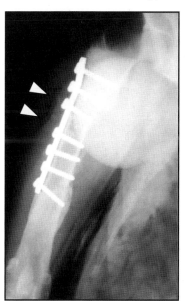

Figure 25.3: Mediolateral radiograph of a femur showing gas in the soft tissues (shown by arrows) overlying a fracture stabilized with a bone plate. Gas production was due to infection with Clostridium novyi.
Courtesy of AC Stead.

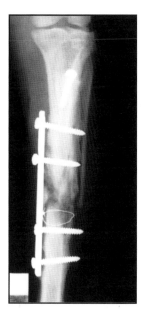

Figure 25.4: Craniocaudal radiograph of a tibia showing chronic osteomyelitis following application of a bone plate. There is lysis of bone under the plate and around the screws, fracture non-union, an irregular periosteal reaction and soft tissue swelling.

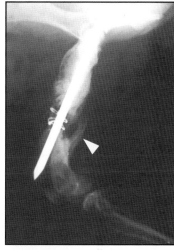

Figure 25.5: Mediolateral radiograph of a femur showing chronic osteomyelitis following fracture fixation with an intramedullary pin. There is extensive periosteal new bone on the proximal fragment, fracture non-union and large periosteal spurs on the distal fragment (arrow).

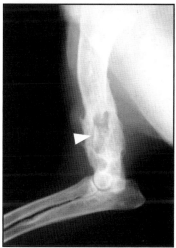

Figure 25.6: Mediolateral radiograph of a humerus showing chronic osteomyelitis. Although the fracture has healed, a large sequestrum is present (arrow) surrounded by an involucrum.

Sequestra are sometimes difficult to visualize and repeated radiographic examination may be necessary for their identification, together with oblique projections in addition to the standard views in two planes. They may vary in size from very small fragments to large segments of the diaphyseal cortex. Sequestra adjacent to external fixator pin tracts have been referred to as ring sequestra (Kantrowitz *et al.*, 1988) because of their characteristic radiographic appearance. They may be caused by excessive thermal necrosis at the time of pin insertion, movement of the pin and localized infection (Figure 25.7).

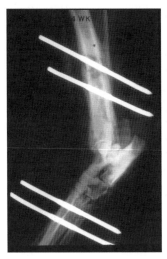

Figure 25.7: Mediolateral radiograph of a distal hindlimb showing a trans-articular external skeletal fixator used for immobilization of an unstable tibiotarsal joint. A sequestrum is visible surrounding the most proximal pin.
Courtesy of B Kirby.

Injection of water-soluble contrast media up discharging sinus tracts (sinography) may help to confirm the location of foreign bodies (e.g. surgical swabs) if these are the cause of the disease (Caywood, 1983), or to delineate sequestra.

Where osteomyelitis has developed as a result of infection spreading from adjacent tissues, the initial radiological manifestation is usually a periosteal reaction (Figure 25.8). It must be emphasized that the radiographic features of osteomyelitis are not peculiar to this disease, and have to be differentiated from normal bone healing and disease processes such as neoplasia, vascular infarction and trauma.

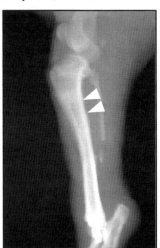

Figure 25.8: Mediolateral radiograph of a tibia showing chronic osteomyelitis following extensive soft tissue trauma to the limb. Arrows show an irregular periosteal response.

Bone scintigraphy using technetium 99m-methylene diphosphonate (^{99m}Tc-MDP) may facilitate the early diagnosis of osteomyelitis (Aliabadi and Nikpoor, 1994) and reveal foci of active inflammation in chronic disease (Lamb, 1987). Use of this technique may reveal areas of increased activity in affected bones within three days of infection (Lamb, 1987), consider-

ably in advance of radiographic changes. Although the sensitivity of ^{99m}Tc-MDP bone scanning is high (90%), its specificity is relatively low (60–70%). This specificity can be increased by using Gallium 67 or white blood cells labelled *in vitro* with Indium II oxide. In humans, computed tomography and magnetic resonance imaging have been found to be of value in the diagnosis of osteomyelitis and in the detection and localization of sequestra (Aliabadi and Nikpoor, 1994).

Bacteriology

Bacterial infections of bone may be mono- or polymicrobial. The majority of infections are reported to be monomicrobial (Caywood *et al.*, 1978; Hirsh and Smith, 1978) and the most commonly isolated organisms are shown in Table 25.1. The commonest organism to be isolated is *Staphylococcus intermedius*, the majority of which are ß-lactamase producers. Polymicrobial infections may involve Gram-negative and Gram-positive organisms, aerobes and anaerobes.

Aerobes	**Anaerobes**
Staphylococcus spp. *Streptococcus* spp. *Escherischia coli* *Pseudomonas aeruginosa* *Proteus* spp. *Klebsiella* spp. *Pasteurella* spp. *Nocardia* spp.	*Bacteroides* spp. *Fusobacterium* spp. *Actinomyces* spp. *Clostridium* spp. *Peptostreptococcus* spp.

Table 25.1: Bacteria isolated from dogs with osteomyelitis (from Hirsh and Smith, 1978; Stead, 1984; Muir and Johnson, 1992).

Tissue samples for culture should ideally be obtained from the affected bone, adjacent soft tissues or implants that are removed during debridement. In situations where debridement is not performed, a sample of bone may be obtained by a closed needle biopsy technique using a Jamshidi or similar bone marrow biopsy needle. However, studies in humans have shown that this is a less reliable method of obtaining the causative organism(s) than culture of tissues removed at open debridement (Perry *et al.*, 1991). Similarly, swabs taken from discharging sinuses may not isolate the causative organism(s), particularly where an infection is polymicrobial or where anaerobes are present (Perry *et al.*, 1991). Gram staining of smears made from swabs taken from the bone or discharging sinuses may give some indication of the causative bacteria, prior to obtaining the results of culture.

Anaerobic bacteria may be present in osteomyelitic bone alone or in combination with aerobic bacteria (Muir and Johnson, 1992). The presence of anaerobes may be suggested by the presence of fight wounds, malodorous discharge, gas shadows on the radiographs (indicating the presence of gas-forming organisms such as *Clostridium* spp.) and the failure to isolate bacteria by aerobic culture when they have been identified on Gram-stained smears. Tissue samples for anaerobic culture should be exposed to an anaerobic environment promptly because failure to do so will reduce the rate at which these organisms are isolated. Advice on the appropriate media should be sought from the laboratory where the sample is to be sent.

Histopathology

Histopathological examination of affected bone is rarely necessary to obtain a diagnosis of osteomyelitis following trauma. Where there is no history of trauma it is sometimes performed to help to differentiate infection from other disease processes such as neoplasia and metaphyseal osteopathy. The morphological identification of bacteria or neutrophils with engulfed bacteria is considered diagnostic (Braden *et al.*, 1989). Fungal hyphae may be identified if these agents are the cause of the disease.

TREATMENT OF POST-TRAUMATIC OSTEOMYELITIS

Successful management of post-traumatic osteomyelitis usually requires a combination of surgery and a prolonged course of antibiotics. There are several basic principles that apply to the treatment of the disease:

* Surgical debridement to remove all dead and necrotic soft tissue and bone
* Allow drainage and obliterate dead space
* Stabilize the fracture site if necessary
* Prolonged course of antibiotics based on the results of culture and sensitivity.

These basic guidelines should be tailored to each individual case. Essentially, the same principles are applied to the management of acute and chronic osteomyelitis. However, chronic osteomyelitis is usually characterized by the presence of avascular cortical bone that requires removal for resolution of the infection and is usually associated with delayed fracture healing or non-union.

Surgical debridement and drainage

In acute infections, early aggressive treatment is essential to limit the spread of infection within the bone, prevent widespread cortical necrosis and prevent the disease from becoming chronic. The fracture site should be exposed via the same surgical approach that was used to repair the fracture initially. All necrotic soft tissues from around the fracture site should be debrided and the fracture site assessed for stability.

Although usually identifiable on radiographs, problems may sometimes be encountered locating sequestra at the time of surgery. This may be facilitated by instilling 2% methylene blue up sinus tracts where these are present, 24 hours prior to surgery. Methylene blue should not be used intravenously because of the risk of inducing acute renal failure (Osuna *et al.*, 1990). Avascular tissue will not clear the dye within this period and hence will appear blue, allowing differentiation of viable from non-viable bone.

Sequestra are usually 'free-floating' and can be identified *in situ* by their characteristic appearance (initially ivory-like, later becoming discoloured and pitted) (Figure 25.9). Where a sequestrum is surrounded by an involucrum, some of this new bone may require removal (using rongeurs or a mechanical burr) to enable the sequestrum to be removed (Figure 25.10). This may significantly weaken the bone, predisposing it to fracture (Figure 25.11). Although it has been recommended that ring sequestra are surgically removed (Kantrowitz *et al.*, 1988), other authors have stated that they will resolve spontaneously following external fixator pin removal.

Where new bone deposition has obliterated the medullary canal, channels should be made through this bone with a reaming device or a large drill bit (Figure 25.12). This will facilitate the ingrowth of new blood vessels and hasten resolution of infection and fracture

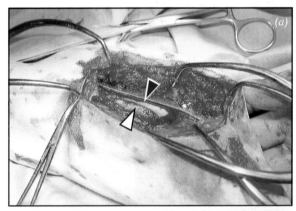

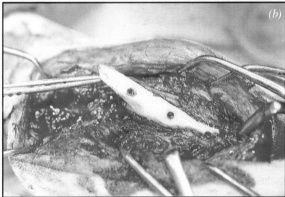

Figure 25.9 *Intra-operative appearance of chronic osteomyelitis of a femur following application of a bone plate for fracture stabilization. (a) Sequestered cortical bone is visible beneath the bone plate (black arrow); viable cortical bone is shown by the white arrow. (b) The sequestrum is more clearly visible following removal of the bone plate.*

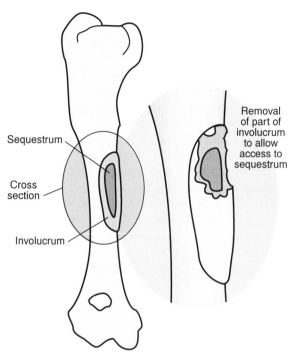

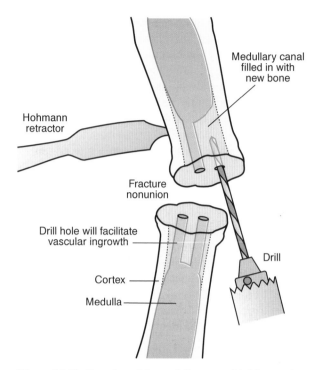

Figure 25.10: *Excision of part of an involucrum to allow removal of a sequestrum. The bone may require subsequent support with a fixation device if sequestrum removal has significantly weakened the bone (see Figures 25.11 and 25.16).*

Figure 25.12: *Reaming of the medullary canal (obliterated by new bone formation following infection) to facilitate vascular ingrowth and fracture healing.*

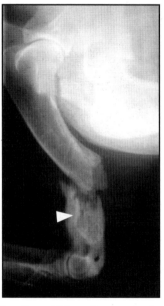

Figure 25.11: *Mediolateral radiograph of a humerus following an attempt to remove a sequestrum. The sequestrum was not found (shown by arrow) and the weakening of the bone resulted in its fracture.*

healing. Although some authors recommend debridement of sinus tracts, provided all the avascular, infected cortical bone is removed, discharge from these sinuses should quickly disappear.

The resulting wound can be managed in several ways, depending on the degree of discharge and the location of the affected bone. Where there is significant discharge the open wound can be packed with saline or povidone–iodine-soaked swabs and covered with a sterile dressing. The swabs and dressing should be changed daily (with the animal heavily sedated) until there is little evidence of suppuration, at which point the wound can be closed primarily or left to heal

by secondary intention. Packing the wound with swabs facilitates the removal of exudate and obliterates dead space. If there is little evidence of discharge the wound can be closed primarily, usually following the insertion of a drain which is removed after 24 to 48 hours. Closed suction or suction-irrigation drainage systems have been used although they probably confer little advantage over healing by secondary intention. Antibiotic therapy should be initiated immediately following the collection of samples for culture and modified according to the results.

Occasionally, in severe cases of osteomyelitis where there are serious joint or soft tissue complications, amputation may be the treatment of choice. Chronic infections of the metacarpal/metatarsal bones and digits where there is extensive involvement of adjacent soft tissues are best managed by amputation of the affected digit(s). Similarly, chronic infection of the sternebrae and mandible can be managed by *en bloc* resection of affected tissues (Fossum *et al.*, 1989) (Figure 25.13).

Fracture management

With infections where the fracture has not healed, the existing implants should not be removed if they are providing adequate stability. It is important to remember that fractures will heal in the presence of infection provided they are stable. If the fracture site is unstable the existing implants should be either supplemented or removed and replaced. External skeletal fixators are particularly useful in this respect because the pins can often be placed some distance

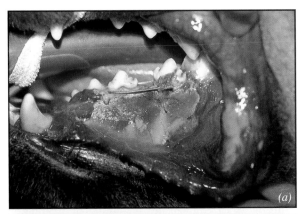

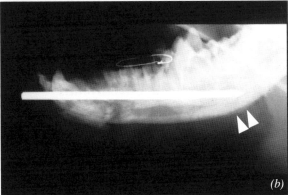

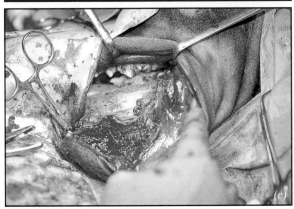

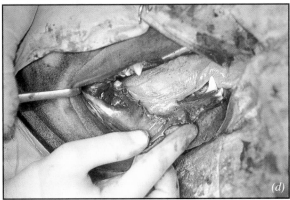

Figure 25.13: *(a) Chronic osteomyelitis with sequestration of a large segment of the mandible following the insertion of an intramedullary pin to stabilize a fracture. (b) Lateral radiograph of the mandible from the same dog showing an irregular periosteal response of the mandible adjacent to the distal end of the pin (shown by arrows). (c, d) Treatment for the dog involved rostral hemimandibulectomy to remove all dead, infected cortical bone.*

from the fracture site, limiting the amount of foreign material in the infected area, and their removal is quick and easy (Figure 25.14). Alternatively, bone plating provides excellent stability but requires more extensive surgery for their removal (Figure 25.15). Bone plates should be removed following fracture union, otherwise infection is likely to persist and clinical signs will recur. Intramedullary pins are best avoided because of the risk of disseminating infection throughout the medullary canal.

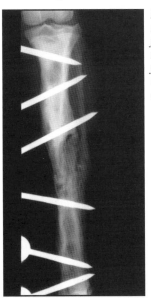

Figure 25.14 *Craniocaudal radiograph of a tibia following application of a type I external skeletal fixator to stabilize an infected fracture.*
Courtesy of J Ferguson.

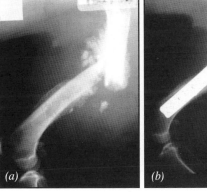

Figure 25.15: *(a) Mediolateral radiograph of a femur showing an infected non-union. (b) The fracture healed following stabilization with a bone plate.*

If the fracture has healed but following sequestrectomy and debridement the strength of the bone appears to be compromised, cancellous bone grafting and a period of supplemental support with an external skeletal fixator is advisable (Figure 25.16). In chronic low-grade infections where the fracture has healed, implant removal and a prolonged course of antibiotics may be all that is necessary for the infection to resolve (Figure 25.17).

Techniques employed in humans, including microvascular muscle and bone transplantation (Gordon and Chiu, 1988), have not been reported in the veterinary literature.

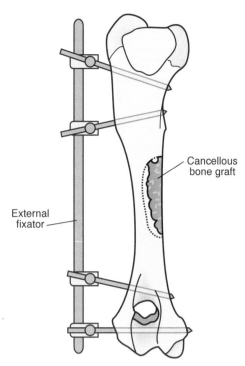

Figure 25.16 *Application of an external skeletal fixator to an infected bone to provide additional support following removal of a sequestrum. The defect has been packed with a cancellous bone graft.*

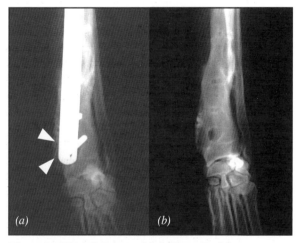

Figure 25.17 *(a) Craniocaudal radiograph of the antebrachium 2 years after the application of a bone plate to stabilize a fractured radius. The fracture has healed but there is evidence of low-grade osteomyelitis. An irregular periosteal response is present on the distal radius (shown with arrows). (b) Following removal of the   plate and a prolonged course of antibiotics, the infection resolved.*

Bone grafting

The value of cancellous bone grafting in the management of delayed and non-union fractures is well established. Cancellous bone grafting can be performed either immediately following debridement or as a delayed procedure up to 2 weeks later (Bardet *et al.*, 1983). These grafts will survive in the presence of infection, though their value is likely to be compromised in the presence of inflammatory exudate or where the local blood supply has been compromised.

Hence the procedure is sometimes delayed following initial surgical debridement. Where large cortical defects exist and large quantities of bone graft are needed to fill these areas, cancellous bone graft may need to be harvested from more than one donor site. Great care must be taken to ensure that infection is not transferred from the infected bone to the bone graft donor site. Following cancellous bone grafting it is best to close the soft tissues primarily over the grafted site rather than to allow healing by secondary intention.

Where large segmental cortical defects exist following debridement, an alternative to cancellous bone grafting is to employ the technique of distraction osteogenesis using either a modified type II or Ilizarov external fixator (Lesser, 1994). The use of cortical bone grafts in the presence of infection is contra-indicated.

Antibiotic therapy in osteomyelitis

At one time it was thought that bone possessed certain unique properties that prevented the penetration of some antibiotics, the so-called blood–bone barrier. Research has shown that most antibiotics can cross the capillary membranes of normal and infected bone but the effectiveness of these drugs depends upon the organisms(s) responsible for the infection and the surgical removal of dead, infected bone. Table 25.2 shows some of the antibiotics used more commonly in the treatment of osteomyelitis. The appropriate choice is based on the results of culture and sensitivity.

In acute osteomyelitis, samples for bacteriology should be obtained and treatment started immediately. Knowledge of the organisms most likely to be present dictates the initial choice of antibiotic. Because ß-lactamase-producing *Staphylococcus* spp. are the commonest cause of osteomyelitis, suitable first choices include cephalexin, clavulanate-potentiated amoxycillin or clindamycin. If the former two are used, the addition of metronidazole will broaden the spectrum to include the majority of anaerobes, including *Bacteroides* spp. This choice of antibiotic can be modified when the results of culture and sensitivity have been obtained.

In chronic osteomyelitis, antibiotic therapy should be started after samples have been obtained for culture during debridement. Initiating therapy intra-operatively will limit the effects of any 'bacteriological shower' during surgery and will ensure high levels of antibiotics in any haematomata that form. Where antibiotics have been administered prior to surgery, they should be stopped 2–3 days beforehand to increase the likelihood of isolating the causative organism(s). Therapy should continue for a minimum of 4–6 weeks.

Osteomyelitis caused by resistant organisms such as *Pseudomonas* spp. and some *Bacteroides* spp. poses certain problems. Although some drugs used in humans, such as carbenicillin, ticarcillin and second and third generation cephalosporins (e.g. ceftazidime), are

Drug	Dose (mg/kg)	Route	Frequency
Amoxycillin–clavulanate	12–25	oral	bid
Cephalexin	10–20	sc, im, oral	bid
Cephazolin[a]	20–25	iv	tid
Chloramphenicol	25–50	sc, oral	bid/tid
Clindamycin	5–11	oral	bid
Enrofloxacin	2.5	oral	bid
Gentamicin[b]	2	iv, im, sc	tid
Metronidazole	10–15	oral	bid

Table 25.2: *Antibiotics commonly used in the treatment of osteomyelitis.*

a   Cephazolin is not licensed for use in small animals. However, because it can be given intravenously it is commonly used prophylactically during orthopaedic surgery.

b   Gentamicin is nephrotoxic and should not be used for more than one week. Renal function should be monitored whilst it is being administered. Gentamicin is also available impregnated in polymethylmethacrylate beads though these are not licensed for use in animals.

frequently effective against these organisms, these are not currently licensed for use in small animals. Gentamicin and enrofloxacin are frequently effective against these organisms *in vitro*, but gentamicin is nephrotoxic and should not be used systemically for more than one week because of the risk of inducing acute renal failure. This serious side-effect can be overcome by local implantation of gentamicin-impregnated beads (Figure 25.18). Although fluoroquinolones such as ciprofloxacin have been used effectively in the treatment of osteomyelitis in man and experimental models of osteomyelitis, the efficacy of enrofloxacin in the treatment of osteomyelitis in dogs is not known. However, its low toxicity and oral dosing provide significant advantages over gentamicin and it

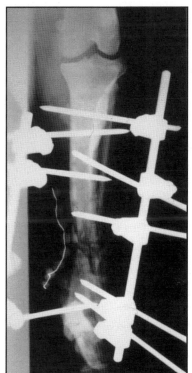

Figure 25.18: *Craniocaudal radiograph of an infected tibial fracture stabilized with an external skeletal fixator. Gentamicin-impregnated beads have been implanted at the fracture site.*
Courtesy of S Langley-Hobbs.

is probably the agent of choice – assuming the causative organism is susceptible.

HAEMATOGENOUS OSTEOMYELITIS

Osteomyelitis that arises other than following extension of infection from adjacent tissues, trauma or the migration of foreign bodies is presumed to be haematogenous in origin although the primary focus of infection is often not apparent. This is a rare condition in small animals and while it has been identified in adult dogs over 1 year of age (Caywood *et al.*, 1978), it is probably commoner in skeletally immature dogs (Nunamaker, 1985; Dunn *et al.*, 1992). It has also been reported in the cat (Dunn *et al.*, 1983).

Affected animals are usually presented with a history of lethargy, anorexia and lameness or stiffness. Pyrexia and pain localized to the affected areas of bone (usually the metaphyses of multiple long bones in skeletally immature dogs) are usually present and infection may spread into adjacent soft tissues or joints, resulting in a septic arthritis.

Radiographic findings include diffuse areas of bone lysis and periosteal reactions (Figure 25.19). Bacteriological culture of blood and aspirates from bone may fail to identify the causative organisms but they should be attempted. Treatment consists of broad spectrum antibiotics (Table 25.2) and exercise restriction for 6 weeks. If the infection extends into adjacent soft tissues the area should be drained and flushed. The prognosis is reported to be good.

Discospondylitis is an infection of the intervertebral disc space that extends into the adjacent vertebral bodies, although some dogs may show evidence of infection of the vertebral endplates in the apparent absence of infection in the intervertebral disc (Jimenez and O'Callaghan, 1995) (Figure 25.20). This disease is more common than the forms of haematogenous osteomyelitis described above. Treatment with a pro-

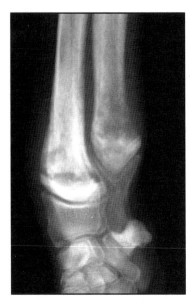

Figure 25.19:
Mediolateral radiograph of the distal radius and ulna from a dog with haematogenous osteomyelitis. Focal areas of lysis are present in the metaphyses of both bones.
Courtesy of J Houlton.

longed course of antibiotics (6–8 weeks) is usually successful but some animals may require curettage of the affected disc space or vertebral stabilization (Gage, 1975; Kornegay and Barber, 1980).

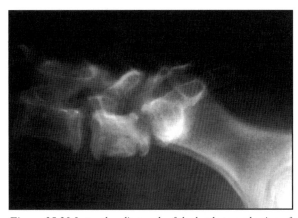

Figure 25.20 *Lateral radiograph of the lumbosacral spine of a 5-month-old dog with discospondylitis at the L7/S1 intervertebral disc space. There is widening of the affected disc space with lysis of the adjacent vertebral end-plates.*

FUNGAL OSTEOMYELITIS

Although not uncommon in some southern and western areas of the USA (Nunamaker, 1985), fungal osteomyelitis is very rare in the UK. In the USA the most commonly isolated causative agents are *Coccidioides immitis, Blastomyces dermatitidis, Histoplasma capsulatum* and *Cryptococcus neoformans* (Nunamaker, 1985). The main portal of entry is the respiratory tract, and in addition to respiratory signs affected animals may develop neural, ocular and skeletal lesions. Osteomyelitis caused by *C. neoformans* has been reported in the UK (Brearley and Jeffrey, 1992). Radiographic lesions resemble those previously described for chronic bacterial osteomyelitis (Figure 25.21). Diagnosis is based on the characteristic histo-

logical appearance of affected bone and isolation of the organism. Treatment with ketaconazole (10 mg/kg per day for 2 months, reducing to 5 mg/kg per day for a further 2 months) has been reported to be effective (Brearley and Jeffrey, 1992).

Osteomyelitis caused by *Aspergillus* spp. has also been reported from the USA and the UK (Butterworth *et al.*, 1995; Hotston Moore and Hanna, 1995). Although usually confined to the nasal cavity and paranasal sinuses, *Aspergillus* spp. can disseminate to other body systems, including the skeletal system. Female purebred German Shepherd Dogs are predisposed to this disease, with infection usually causing discospondylitis at multiple sites. The organism may be cultured from affected intervertebral discs and from urine sediment. Frequently, affected animals will not have serum antibodies to the organism (Watt *et al.*, 1995). Treatment with ketoconazole (10–15 mg/kg bid) or itraconazole (17 mg/kg sid) may control the infection in some dogs, but affected animals will need to be kept on medication permanently (Watt *et al.*, 1995). The prognosis is poor.

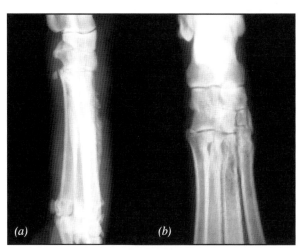

Figure 25.21: *(a) Mediolateral and (b) dorsoplantar radiographs of the metatarsus from a dog with osteomyelitis caused by* Cryptococcus neoformans. *There is an irregular periosteal response and areas of lysis of the third metatarsal bone.*
Courtesy of M Brearley.

REFERENCES

Aliabadi P and Nikpoor N (1994) Imaging osteomyelitis. *Arthritis and Rheumatism* **37**, 617.

Bardet JF, Hohn RB and Basinger R (1983) Open drainage and delayed autogenous bone grafting for treatment of chronic osteomyelitis in dogs and cats. *Journal of the American Veterinary Medical Association* **183**, 312.

Braden TD, Johnson CA, Gabel CL *et al.* (1987) Posologic evaluation of clindamycin, using a canine model of posttraumatic osteomyelitis. *American Journal of Veterinary Research* **48**, 1101.

Braden TD, Tvedten HW, Mostosky UV *et al.* (1989) The sensitivity and specificity of radiology and histopathology in the diagnosis of posttraumatic osteomyelitis. *Veterinary Comparative Orthopaedics and Traumatology* **3**, 98.

Brearley MJ and Jeffrey N (1992) Cryptococcal osteomyelitis in a dog. *Journal of Small Animal Practice* **33**, 601.

Butterworth SJ, Barr FJ, Pearson GR and Day MD (1995) Multiple discospondylitis associated with *Aspergillus* species infection in a dog. *Veterinary Record* **136**, 38.

Caywood DD, Wallace LJ and Braden TD (1978) Osteomyelitis in the dog. *Journal of the American Veterinary Medical Association* **172**, 943.

Caywood DD (1983) Osteomyelitis. *Veterinary Clinics of North America: Small Animal Practice* **13**, 43.

Dunn JK, Farrow CS and Doige CE (1983) Disseminated osteomyelitis caused by *Clostridrium novyi* in a cat. *Canadian Veterinary Journal* **24**, 312.

Dunn JK, Dennis R and Houlton JEF (1992) Successful treatment of metaphyseal osteomyelitis in the dog. *Journal of Small Animal Practice* **33**, 85.

Fossum TW, Hodges CC, Miller MW and Dupre GP (1989) Partial sternectomy for sternal osteomyelitis in the dog. *Journal of the American Animal Hospital Association* **25**, 435.

Gage ED (1975) Treatment of discospondylitis in the dog. *Journal of the American Veterinary Medical Association* **166**, 1164.

Gordon L and Chui EJ (1988) Treatment of infected non-unions and segmental defects of the tibia with staged microvascular muscle transplantation and bone grafting. *Journal of Bone and Joint Surgery* **70-A**, 377.

Gristina AG, Oga M, Webb LX and Hobgood CD (1985) Adherent bacterial colonisation in the pathogenesis of osteomyelitis. *Science* **228**, 990-993.

Hirsh DC and Smith TM (1978) Osteomyelitis in the dog: microorganisms and susceptibility to antimicrobial agents. *Journal of Small Animal Practice* **19**, 679.

Hotston Moore A and Hanna FY (1995) Mycotic osteomyelitis in a dog following nasal aspergillosis. *Veterinary Record* **137**, 349.

Jimenez MM and O'Callaghan MW (1995) Vertebral physitis: a radiographic diagnosis to be separated from discospondylitis. *Veterinary Radiology and Ultrasound* **36**, 188.

Johnson KA (1994) Osteomyelitis in dogs and cats. *Journal of the American Veterinary Medical Association* **205**, 1882.

Kantrowitz B, Smeak D and Vannini R (1988) Radiographic appearance of ring sequestrum with pin tract osteomyelitis in the dog. *Journal of the American Animal Hospital Association* **24**, 461.

Kornegay JN and Barber DL (1980) Discospondylitis in dogs. *Journal of the American Veterinary Medical Association* **177**, 337.

Lamb CR (1987) Bone scintigraphy in small animals. *Journal of the American Veterinary Medical Association* **191**, 1616.

Lesser AS (1994) Segmental bone transport for the treatment of bone deficits. *Journal of the American Animal Hospital Association* **30**, 322.

Muir P and Johnson KA (1992) Anaerobic bacteria isolated from osteomyelitis in dogs and cats. *Veterinary Surgery* **21**, 463.

Nunamaker DM (1985) Osteomyelitis. In: *Textbook of Small Animal Orthopaedics*, ed. CD Newton, DM Nunamaker. JB Lippincott Co., Philadelphia.

Osuna DJ, Armstrong PJ, Duncan DE and Breitschwerdt EB (1990) Acute renal failure after methylene blue infusion in a dog. *Journal of the American Animal Hospital Association* **26**, 410.

Perry CR, Pearson RL and Miller GA (1991) Accuracy of cultures of material from swabbing of the superficial aspect of the wound and needle biopsy in the preoperative assessment of osteomyelitis. *Journal of Bone and Joint Surgery* **73-A,** 745.

Smith MM, Vasseur PB and Saunders HM (1989) Bacterial growth associated with metallic implants in dogs. *Journal of the American Animal Hospital Association* **195**, 765.

Stead AC (1984) Osteomyelitis in the dog and cat. *Journal of Small Animal Practice.* **25**, 1.

Vercelotti GM, McCarthy JB, Lindholm P *et al.* (1985) Extracellular matrix proteins bind and aggregate bacteria. *American Journal of Pathology* **120**, 13.

Watt PR, Robins GM, Galloway AM and O'Boyle DA (1995) Disseminated opportunistic fungal disease in dogs: 10 cases (1982-1990). *Journal of the American Veterinary Medical Association* **207**, 67.

CHAPTER TWENTY SIX

Complications of Fracture Healing

David Bennett

INTRODUCTION

The objectives of the orthopaedic surgeon in fracture repair are to achieve a healed bone and normal limb function. However, complications will occasionally prevent these objectives from being achieved. Because of the many variables in each fracture case, very few are managed 'perfectly' from start to finish (Olmstead, 1991) and although fractures will heal in less than perfect conditions, we shall encounter problems if we ask too much of nature.

In fracture repair there are many causes of complications and one of the most important is the violation of orthopaedic or surgical principles. If we always obey the basic principles, complications will be minimal, but this is often a difficult goal to achieve. Sometimes it is a lack of owner compliance with the surgeon's instructions for convalescent care, or even a failure of communication between surgeon and owner. Occasionally the animal's personality and activity contribute to the complications. The patient's health status and general metabolism are sometimes factors. Very occasionally the implant is defective and produces complications.

Most complications, as stated, are due to failing to observe basic orthopaedic principles (Chapter 9), though it may be difficult for the surgeon to admit to this. Some principles are commonly ignored. A good orthopaedic surgeon realizes that all fractures can be adequately stabilized by several different methods; the surgeon must choose the fracture technique that has the greatest potential for success with the least risk to the patient. If a fracture is not stable at the end of the surgical procedure, the potential for complications is high (Sumner-Smith, 1991).

When complications do occur it is important that the surgeon attempts to find the cause since this will aid in establishing a treatment plan and also help to avoid recreating the problem in the future.

DEFINITIONS

Union

This term means that the fractured bone has healed. Although the exact definition varies between clinician,

radiologist and histologist, it is clinical union that is most relevant to the patient. Clinical union means that sufficient union has occurred to permit the patient to load the bone and ambulate without complications occurring. There is no movement or pain at the fracture site although the fracture line may still be evident on the radiographs.

Malunion

The fracture has healed but with poor alignment which, if severe enough, is not compatible with the normal function of that particular part of the skeleton.

Delayed union

This somewhat vague term is applied to a fracture that seems to be taking an excessive amount of time to heal – much longer than might be expected for that particular fracture (Figure 26.1). Certainly fracture healing time varies greatly and is influenced by the bone that has fractured, the site and type of fracture, the age of the patient, the method of fixation, general health of the patient and many other factors.

Non-union

This indicates that the fracture has not healed and is not likely to do so unless circumstances are altered by surgical or other intervention.

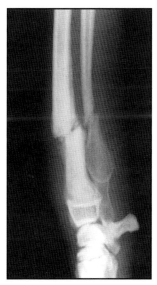

Figure 26.1: Lateral radiograph of the radius and ulna of a 9-month-old Collie, 4 weeks after an external support has been applied. The fracture is still unstable and radiographic union is not present. There is evidence of callus. This is an example of a delayed union; the cause was the use of an inappropriate external support. Clinical union would have been expected in a dog of this age by 4 weeks; the fracture will heal with further external support for a longer time.

Pseudarthrosis

This term indicates a non-union where there is considerable movement at the fracture site, such that a false joint has formed with a synovial cavity. The bone ends of most non-unions are joined by fibrous or cartilaginous tissue.

NON-UNION

Classification

Classification of non-unions is based on the fracture site (diaphyseal, metaphyseal or epiphyseal), displacement of fragments (displaced or in alignment), presence or absence of infection and the biological activity based on viability and osteogenic potential (which relates directly to the vascularity).

Non-union classification based on biological activity includes the viable and non-viable types. They are further classified as to the appearance of the fracture site (the Weber–Cech classification: Weber and Cech, 1976) (Figure 26.2) and the cellular response (Frost, 1989).

Viable

Viable non-union is usually the result of instability at the fracture site or a failure to reduce the fracture.

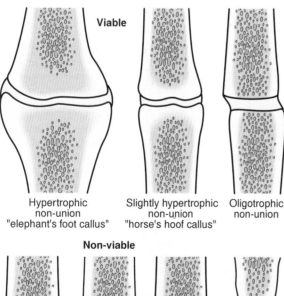

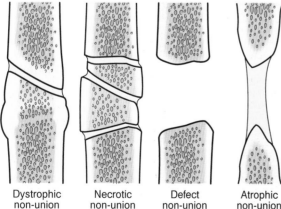

Figure 26.2: *The Weber–Cech classification of non-union fractures based on the radiographic appearance.*

Three types are recognized:

- Hypertrophic non-union ('elephant's foot callus') is characterized by abundant callus (Figures 26.3 and 26.4)
- Slightly hypertrophic non-union ('horse's hoof callus') is characterized by moderate callus production (Figures 26.5 and 26.6)
- Oligotrophic non-union is characterized by minimal callus production; the bone ends are joined by fibrous tissue (Figure 26.7 and 26.8).

Non-viable

The blood supply to the fracture site has been interrupted to such an extent that healing is greatly impaired. There is the presence of necrotic fragments or actual bone loss, which is not the case with viable non-unions. They are divided into four types:

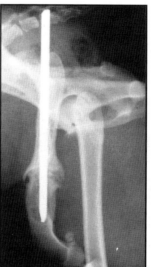

Figure 26.3: *Lateral radiograph showing a non-union fracture of the femur. This is an example of a hypertrophic viable non-union. The intramedullary pin has loosened; there is a radiolucent 'halo' around the distal end of the pin. It is likely that the pin did not have sufficient purchase in the distal fragment and rotation was present at the fracture site.*

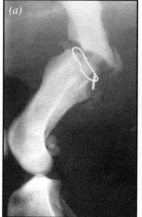

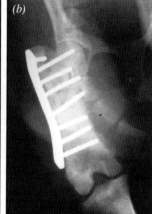

Figure 26.4: *(a) Lateral radiograph of the femur showing a hypertrophic viable non-union. The fracture had been treated with an intramedullary pin of too narrow a diameter and a single cerclage wire. The pin loosened and migrated proximally and was removed. Single cerclage wires have no place in the treatment of fractures. (b) This case was treated by removal of the cerclage wire, then osteotomy of the fracture ends to allow accurate reduction, and the application of a compression plate. Shortening of the femur resulted but fracture healing occurred.*

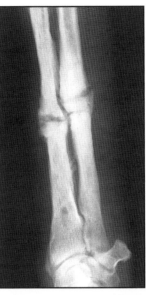

Figure 26.5: Lateral radiograph of a non-union fracture of the radius and ulna in a 7-year-old Rough Collie. This is an example of a slightly hypertrophic viable non-union. The fracture had been treated with an external fixator of insufficient rigidity.

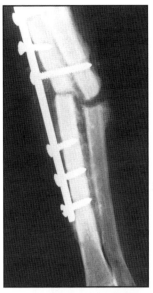

Figure 26.6: Lateral radiograph of the radius and ulna of a 6-year-old Border Collie. The implant has failed, resulting in movement of the fracture site. Radiolucent 'halos' are present around each of the screws. This is an example of a slightly hypertrophic viable non-union. A low-grade staphylococcal infection was also present, as suspected from the extensive periosteal reaction.

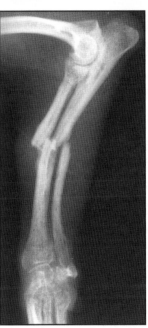

Figure 26.7: Lateral radiograph of a non-union fracture of the radius and ulna in a 4-year-old Spaniel cross. There is minimal callus and the fracture is very unstable. This is an example of an oligotrophic viable non-union. There is obvious disuse atrophy of the distal radius and ulna and of the carpal bones.

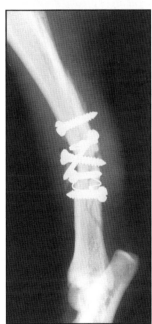

Figure 26.8: Lateral radiograph of the tibia of a 3-year-old Crossbred. A comminuted fracture of the tibia has been reconstructed with lag screws and cerclage wire, supplemented only with an external support. The implants have failed and angulation has occurred at the fracture. An oligotrophic non-union has resulted. Reconstruction of comminuted fractures with lag screws/cerclage wires must be accompanied by a plate and screws or by an external fixator to neutralize the forces at the fracture site. This non-union was treated by removal of the implants and stabilization of the fracture with a bilateral uniplanar external fixator.

- *Dystrophic non-union.* These are characterized by an intermediate fragment that has united with one main fragment but not the other. Vascularization of the intermediate fragment, which may be partially necrotic, takes place only from one side. Hypertrophic callus may be present on the vital side of the fragment but necrosis persists on the opposite side (Figure 26.9).
- *Necrotic non-union.* In these cases there is a major interruption to the blood supply of the fragments. There are two or more necrotic fragments and there is lack of callus and death of neighbouring bone. As a result, implants may loosen and fail (Figures 26.10 and 26.11).
- *Defect non-union.* In these cases there is a significant loss of bone at the fracture site. This may occur at the time of injury or may be an

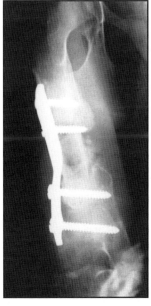

Figure 26.9: Craniocaudal radiograph of the femur of a 9-year-old Crossbred. A separated central cylinder of bone was left unsecured between the two main fragments, which were fixed with a plate and screws. Fixation is poor. The cylinder of bone has healed to the distal fragment but not the proximal. This is an example of a dystrophic non-viable non-union. The proximal end of the cylinder of bone was necrotic. Revision surgery involved removal of the implants, debridement of the bone ends, a cancellous bone graft and stabilization with a 7-hole 3.5 mm dynamic compression plate.

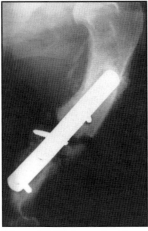
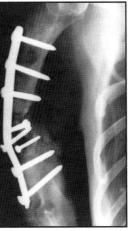

Figure 26.10: Lateral and craniocaudal views of the humerus, showing a necrotic non-union. This was a comminuted fracture where reconstruction was attempted using lag screws. There has been obvious bone loss at the fracture site. There are radiolucent areas around the plate and some of the screws, indicating loosening of the implants. The plate has bent at the fracture site. This case was treated by removal of the plate and screws, debridement at the fracture site, a cancellous bone graft and the application of a 3.5 mm dynamic compression plate.

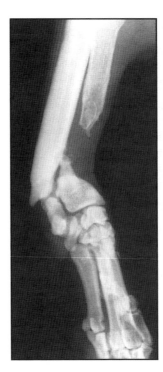

Figure 26.12: Craniocaudal radiograph of the radius and ulna of a 4-year-old crossbred dog showing a non-viable defect non-union of the radius. There is an oligotrophic non-union of the distal ulna. This non-union was of several months duration. Attempts at a repair using cancellous bone graft and plates and screws on both the radius and the ulna were unsuccessful.

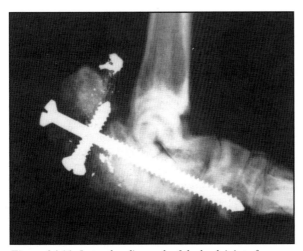

Figure 26.11: Lateral radiograph of the hock joint of a Collie showing a fibular tarsal bone fracture caused by gunshot. The fracture was repaired with two bone screws. The longer screw was of stainless steel and the shorter one of vitallium. Lead shot was also present. Severe bone loss has occurred and a necrotic non-union has resulted – the presence of dissimilar metals in close proximity has resulted in local bone necrosis.

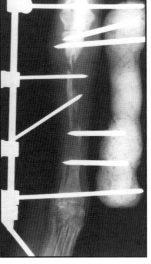

Figure 26.13: Craniocaudal radiograph of the radius and ulna of a 3-year-old Toy Poodle. The original mid-shaft fracture of the radius and ulna had been treated with an external fixator. An iatrogenic fracture of the proximal third of the radius then occurred through a fixation pin hole. The original external fixator was removed and a second external fixator was applied. Three weeks later an obvious non-viable atrophic non-union of both radius and ulna is present. Limb amputation was necessary in this case.

extension of the necrotic state, with subsequent separation and bone loss, or it may be iatrogenic as may occur with resection of a bony neoplasm (Figure 26.12).

- *Atrophic non-union.* These usually occur as a sequel to one of the three other types of non-viable non-unions. They are rare but are regularly seen in non-union fractures of the distal radius and ulna of the toy breeds (Figure 26.13).

Causes

The causes of non-unions are described in Table 26. 1.

Diagnosis

The diagnosis of non-union is based on clinical and radiographic evaluation and generally there will be several assessments over a period of weeks before a final diagnosis is made. Movement of the fracture site is a cardinal feature of non-union. This movement is often painful, certainly in the early stages; but pain is generally not a feature if a pseudarthrosis develops. Loss of function is present which, for the limb bones, shows as an obvious lameness. Depending on the type of non-union present, there may be obvious callus to palpate, or very little. Deformity of the fracture site is often a feature (e.g. shortening, angulation, rotation) and disuse atrophy of the musculature is prominent.

Radiography helps in confirming the diagnosis and deciding on treatment. The radiographic features vary according to the type of non-union present. A gap is

Inadequate immobilization of fracture
This is the commonest cause of non-union. When there is excessive movement at the fracture site neither the periosteal, intercortical nor endosteal callus is able to bridge the site effectively. The constant movement destroys the juvenile blood vessels that attempt to bridge the gap. The use of intramedullary pins of too small a diameter is one of the commonest mistakes leading to non-union.

Excessive gap at the fracture site
This may be caused by several different factors. The bone ends may be distracted by lack of immobilization or by the fixation technique used. There may be interposition of soft tissue which impedes callus formation, although callus can form and the soft tissue be organized into the callus. Loss of bone from the fracture site at the time of the trauma or removal of bone by the surgeon also creates gaps. Bone loss may also occur due to ischaemia and infection.

Loss of blood supply
Ischaemia of bone may result from the initial trauma to bone and soft tissue. In addition, loss of blood supply can be created by the surgeon due to excessive periosteal stripping, damage to the nutrient vessels and comminution or crushing of bone and soft tissue. Avascular necrosis is an extreme form of ischaemia in which an element of local bone or soft tissue becomes devoid of its blood supply and necroses, leaving a deficit.

Infection
Infection of bone involving the fracture ends or the neighbouring soft tissues delays healing. Infection lowers the normal pH, and this tends to put calcium into solution. In addition, infection interferes with the blood supply, occludes the Haversian systems, causes bone death and bone sclerosis, and interferes with nutrition of the callus. Implants loosen more readily in infected bone. Fractures can heal in the presence of infection but only if the fracture is rigid.

Hyperaemia
Hyperaemia is a normal feature of healing bone but it can become excessive (e.g. when infection is present) and prevent the laying down of collagen.

Compression
Although compression of the bone ends is often desirable in fracture repair, excessive compression can cause microfractures and necrosis of adjacent arteries.

Excessive quantities of implants
The presence of large amounts of metal work relative to the bone can seriously impede the blood supply to the area. Excessively large intramedullary pins may seriously damage the medullary blood flow. Plates and screws of an inappropriately large size can also create problems. Screws can obstruct the medullary blood supply and there may be insufficient blood reaching the cortex from the periosteum, especially if the latter has been damaged in the original accident or by the surgeon. The presence of a plate on the cortical surface may impede the centrifugal flow of blood from the medulla to the periosteal surface, causing the blood to divert laterally around the plate, and the flow to the cortex is accordingly diminished.

Severe comminution
Severely comminuted fractures are more likely to be associated with diminished blood supply between fragments, ischaemia, sequestration and instability.

Use of improper metals
The use of improper metals or combination of dissimilar metals produces an electrolytic reaction and consequent lysis of the local bone cells.

Inappropriate post-operative management
Modern techniques aim for early weightbearing and ambulation but this can sometimes be excessive. If too great a load is placed on the stabilizing device it may fail before the fracture has healed. Early weight-bearing is certainly desirable and will encourage fracture healing but this must be controlled in a sensible fashion.

General factors
Most of these do not themselves cause non-union but may predispose to it. Sufficient amounts of dietary calcium and phosphorus are important for correct mineralization of the callus. Metabolic disorders (e.g. liver failure, diabetes, hyperadrenocorticalism) may delay healing. Dogs receiving high doses of corticosteroids or cytotoxic drugs for other problems may be at risk of a non-union. Hyperparathyroidism (nutritional or renal) may also interfere with fracture healing. Geriatric patients are also at a greater risk of non-union.

Table 26.1: Causes of non-union.

evident at the fracture site. There are generally well defined fracture ends without an apparent healing activity, or at least no increased activity over a reasonable period of time. The bone ends may become sclerotic and the marrow cavity sealed off with endosteal callus at the fracture site. Callus, if present, does not bridge the fracture site. Deformity at the fracture site may be seen and osteopenia of the limb bones due to disuse atrophy may be apparent. The typical appearance of a pseudarthrosis may also be appreciated (Figure 26.3). Increased density of soft tissue surrounding the fracture site is often seen, and muscle atrophy may be evident.

Treatment

The creation of maximum stability and the encouragement of osteogenesis are of paramount importance in treating non-unions. This generally means compressing the fracture and using bone grafts. Treatment is influenced by the site of non-union, the presence or absence of infection, presence or absence of callus, the type of fracture, the experience of the surgeon and the availability of equipment.

Non-displaced non-union (non-infected)

Compression of the fracture together with a cancellous bone graft is often all that is required. Compression may be created with the dynamic compression plate, or the use of a compression device on the plate or by means of an external fixator. If non-union is the result of interference with blood supply then further damage to the blood supply should be avoided. The use of limited contact plates may help here or, even better, the use of an external fixator. A dynamic external fixator which generates specific amounts of micromovement at the fracture site has been used in successfully treating non-union fractures of the tibia (Kenwright and Goodship, 1989; Kenwright *et al.*, 1991). Micromovement in assisting fracture healing is, however, in dispute (Aro and Chao, 1993; Kershaw *et al.*, 1993; Noordeen *et al.*, 1995). Any callus that is present should be left intact. Healing can be assisted and accelerated by the use of a cancellous bone graft.

Displaced non-union (non-infected)

The fracture must be opened and reduced in these cases. Sufficient callus must be excised to permit reduction. This can be difficult if there is severe overriding and sometimes the use of a mechanical distractor can help. Sometimes shortening of the bone is necessary in order to achieve reduction. The medullary cavity should be opened to permit the growth of medullary blood vessels and allow the endosteum to contribute to healing. If the bone ends are rounded off at the fracture site, they must be resected to create transverse surfaces for apposition. Any bony callus removed during debridement can be grafted to the fracture site to help to stimulate osteogenesis. This may be supplemented with autogenous cancellous bone taken from one or more donor sites.

In cases where there are massive defects, the gap can be bridged with a corticocancellous graft such as a split rib, although large quantities of cancellous graft can be used. The application of microsurgical techniques now means that vascularized autogenous bone grafts (e.g. distal ulnar diaphysis) can be considered in treating non-union fractures. Such grafts bring about healing much more quickly than avascular cortical grafts (Szentimrey *et al.*, 1995).

An alternative approach to filling very large deficits is to use a 'bone transport' technique which utilizes the phenomenon of distraction osteogenesis (Reuter and Brutscher, 1988; Ilizarov, 1989). A corticotomy (or osteotomy) proximal to the non-union is carried out and generally a ring external fixator (Ilizarov fixator) is employed to move the diaphyseal segment distally (1 mm/day) to close the fracture gap. As the segment is moved, new bone is generated at the transection site. Once the non-union gap has been closed by the transplanted segment, the bone is left in the external fixator without further displacement until healing has occurred at the transection and non-union sites.

One reason for using cancellous bone grafts is because they contain bone morphogenetic proteins (BMPs), which are osteogenic growth factors; they induce transformation of undifferentiated mesenchymal cells into chondroblasts and osteoblasts in a dose-dependent manner (Kirker-Head, 1995). Recombinant DNA technology allows the production of these BMPs in large and highly purified quantities and their potential in stimulating bone healing is immense. They can be used to coat implants, or can be incorporated within bone matrix constituents, such as collagen, or into polymers, which can be used to fill very large bone defects. Implantation of skeletal stem cells with BMPs is also being assessed as a means of stimulating bone production. Other cytokines, such as transforming growth factor-ß and basic fibroblast growth factor, also stimulate bone growth and are being assessed for a possible clinical role (Iwasaki *et al.*, 1995; Sumner *et al.*, 1995). It is likely that recombinant BMPs will be available for clinical use within the next five years and will revolutionize the treatment of fractures. In addition, a gene therapy approach has already been studied in experimentral animals (Fang *et al.*, 1996)

The application of an electrical current to a non-union fracture has been used to stimulate repair in humans (Bassett *et al.*, 1982; Sharrard *et al.*, 1982) and in experimental animals but has not been established in clinical small animal orthopaedic surgery (Nunamaker *et al.*, 1985).

Metaphyseal and epiphyseal non-union

Treatment of these poses particular problems because of the effects on joint function. An arthrotomy must be performed and the joint thoroughly assessed. Any thickened synovium must be resected and any fragments of soft tissue and bone and hypertrophic callus removed. The fracture surfaces must be meticulously aligned and any defects may need reconstructing with cancellous bone or methylmethacrylate bone cement. The fracture must be adequately immobilized using lag screws and T-plates or possibly an external fixator. Early ambulation is essential if fracture disease is to be avoided. Appropriate physiotherapy should be given to prevent 'tie down' of the local retinaculum and musculature and in the early stages this will involve manipulation under general anaesthesia.

Infected non-unions

The treatment of osteomyelitis is described in Chapter 25. The non-union should be rigorously explored surgically and debrided. Any sinus tract should be explored and excised as well as all necrotic material, chronic fibrous tissue and granulation tissue. The exploration of sinus tracts can be facilitated by the installation of 1% methylene blue solution (approximately 5–10 ml). Any dead bone is removed. Implants can be left *in situ* if they are supporting the fracture and are not loosening. However, the implants must be removed if they are not supporting the fracture.

The use of the pulsating water jet has been advocated (Sumner-Smith, 1990). Water pressure between 50 and 70 psi is effective in removing necrotic tissue and debriding the wound without affecting the healthy tissue. Antibiotics can be added to the irrigation solution. Aerobic and anaerobic bacteriology cultures are taken from the fracture site and used to select the antimicrobial agent. If the original implant is left *in situ* a cancellous bone graft can be packed at the fracture site, even though its survival is seriously reduced by infection. If the original implant is removed, the fracture can initially be left unsupported or preferably an external fixator applied with transfixing pins inserted into the bone stock away from the infected fracture site. The wound can be left open to drain or, alternatively, closed and drainage tubes can be inserted and left in place for 5–7 days. Systemic antibiotics must be used for 6–8 weeks. The use of local gentamicin can be achieved by the insertion of gentamicin-impregnated methylmethacrylate beads at the fracture site (Brown and Bennett, 1989) for 3–4 weeks. Further stabilization of the fracture with plates and screws, for example, if indicated, should be delayed for at least 2 weeks. Alternatively, stabilization with an external fixator is acceptable; in this instance, a very rigid frame should be used which can be staged down throughout the healing process. Plates and screws should also be removed if the fracture has healed.

DELAYED UNION

The causes of delayed union are basically the same as those of non-union, but acting to a lesser degree. By definition, the fracture will eventually heal, though it is often difficult for clinicians to decide whether they are dealing with delayed union or non-union. In any event, if the delayed union is going to take some considerable time to heal, it is often better to revise the treatment and create a more stable fixation and speed up the repair. This will improve the animal's quality of life by reducing the prolonged convalescence.

MALUNION

Malunion includes:

- Deviations in the limb axis (angular deformities)
- Rotational limb deformities (healing of the distal fragment in a position of internal or external rotation with respect to the proximal fragment)
- Shortening of the limb (due to overriding fragments, severe angulation, comminution, bone loss, compression of the fracture).

Premature slowing or closure of the physis as a complication of fractures can produce limb deformity and shortening but this is not classified as a malunion because it is a result of arrested or asynchronous growth of the physis and not an abnormality of fracture healing.

Malunions may be considered as being either functional or non-functional (Nunamaker *et al.*, 1985). With a functional malunion, the animal has good clinical (limb) function; the deformity is often slight and only of cosmetic concern. Generally these cases can be left untreated, except in special circumstances (e.g. a show dog). A non-functional malunion implies an alteration of clinical (limb) function or the potential for such – for example, altered stresses on a joint may not produce clinical problems until several months later.

Angular deformities place abnormal stresses on adjacent joints by changing the axial alignment of a bone. This can cause poor limb function, or lead to secondary osteoarthritis due to abnormal joint loading. The direction of angulation affects joint function and adaptation; for example, lateral or medial angulation of the femur has a far more serious effect on the stifle than cranial or caudal angulation. Rotational deformity is not uncommon with femoral malunions; compensation may occur with a slight rotational deformity but extreme rotational deformity results in an awkward gait and secondary hip subluxation or patellar subluxation/luxation. Malunion may also result in limb shortening and if this is not too severe the animal can compensate by holding the joint of the affected limb at a greater angle of extension, or the joint of the contralateral limb in a greater angle of flexion, or a combination of both. In a young animal accelerated growth of other long bones in the limb can compensate for a shortened bone in the same limb.

Malunion can affect range of joint motion or alter the functional angle of the joint. The abnormal stresses placed on ligaments and joint capsule can sometimes result in periarticular fibrosis. A malunion of an articular fracture is a common cause of osteoarthritis later in life. Malunion can also result in secondary soft tissue problems such as interference with muscle and tendon function.

Causes

Fractures that are untreated because of neglect or failure of diagnosis are obvious causes of malunion (Anson, 1991). In such situations muscle pull on the bone fragments will cause rotation. Similarly, conservative treatment such as might be indicated for pathological fractures associated with nutritional secondary hyperparathyroidism can result in malunion, although this might be preferable to the complications that could occur with attempts at internal fixation.

Closed reduction and the use of casts or splints may be associated with a degree of malunion. Accurate closed reduction can be difficult either because of a very mobile fracture or because of muscle contraction. Post-manipulation radiographs are essential in checking on the adequacy of reduction. During internal fixation of a fracture the surgeon, especially if inexperienced, can sometimes create a potential malunion by inadequate or increased reduction of the fracture. Rotation and angulation of the distal fragment are the most common mistakes. It is important to have adequate aseptic access to the limb to check on the position of landmarks, joints, etc. A limb hidden by drapes can lead to this kind of complication.

Often when surgically repairing displaced non-unions, it can be difficult to identify the original cortices of the bone because of the extensive callus and remodelling that has occurred and in these cases a degree of malunion may occur after repair. An inability to maintain fracture reduction due to inadequate fixation and/or comminution may result in some degree of deformity of the bone post-operatively but with eventual healing. Bending or loosening of implants during the initial post-operative period can have a similar sequel. Premature removal of fixation before the fracture is healed, followed by weightbearing by the patient, can lead to deformity at the fracture site with eventual healing.

Diagnosis

This is often a simple task. The gross appearance of the limb, supported by radiographic examination, generally shows the problem (Figures 26.14, 26.15 and 26.16). However, proper attention should be paid to the animal's functional abilities. Any disturbance of gait should be noted. Consideration must be given to any potential problems in the future. This should include osteoarthritis due to abnormal stresses placed upon a joint, as a result of the deformity, and the effect on joint

stability and function. Varus or valgus deformities close to joints will place stresses on the joint capsule and ligaments. On the convex side of the joint there is increased tension, resulting in stretching and laxity of the supporting tissues. The converse is true on the concave side of the joint, where contractions and atrophy are observed (Hierholzer and Hax, 1985). Muscle mass and strength should be noted and the owner questioned on the animal's exercise tolerance. Limb length should be compared with the unaffected leg. Greater expectations and demands are placed on the working or hunting dog. The cosmetic appearance may be very important for the show dog. Damage to tendons/muscles or altered function of these structures should also be assessed.

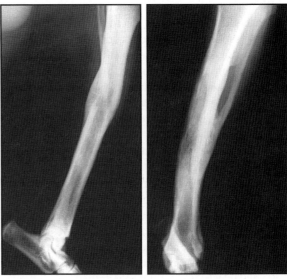

Figure 26.14: Lateral and craniocaudal radiographs of the tibia showing a malunion mid-shaft fracture. There is slight caudal and lateral displacement of the distal fragment. Limb use was good and treatment was not necessary. This is classified as a functional malunion.

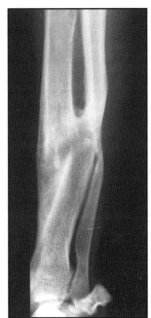

Figure 26.15: Lateral radiograph of the radius and ulna showing a lower third malunion fracture. Although a malunion, extensive remodelling of the radius and ulna is occurring to help to straighten the limb. The potential for remodelling is far greater in the young animal; the dog was 8 months of age when he first sustained the fracture. This is a functional malunion which required no treatment.

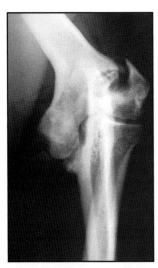

Figure 26.16: Craniocaudal radiograph of the elbow joint, showing an old malunion fracture of the lateral condyle which has recently refractured. The malunion fracture had probably predisposed this animal to the second fracture. Osteoarthritis had also developed, associated with the original malunion. The re-fracture of the lateral condyle was fixed using a lag screw but no attempt was made to correct the pre-existing malunion. The original malunion has to be classified as non-functional.

Treatment

Functional malunions generally do not require correction. Non-functional malunions generally require an osteotomy/ostectomy to correct angular and rotational deformities and to lengthen the bone (Table 26.2). In some cases compensatory surgery can be undertaken to correct complications associated with the malunion rather than correct the malunion itself – for example, correction of patellar luxation associated with a rotational malunion of the femur using a tibial tuberosity relocation. Another example would be correcting coxofemoral instability by triple pelvic osteotomy or intertrochanteric osteotomy.

Salvage procedures can be used in some instances at a later time when complications become apparent – for example, arthrodesis as a treatment of osteoarthritis

---

Transverse
This is used primarily for rotational deformities. Compression plating of the flat osteotomy surfaces provides the best stability. K-wires can be temporarily placed in the bone prior to making the osteotomy and used as markers to gauge the amount of de-rotation.

Cuneiform – closed wedge
This type of osteotomy is mainly used for axial deformities. A wedge of bone is removed from the point of maximal deformity. Compression of the osteotomy should result in a rapid healing. This technique is simple and gives good stability. Its main disadvantage is in causing bone shortening.

Cuneiform – open wedge
A transverse osteotomy is carried out and the bone straightened by creating an open wedge on the concave surface of the bone. The bony defect is filled with an autogenous cancellous bone graft and buttress (plate) fixation is applied. The primary advantage is the gain in limb length in addition to the correction of axial deformity. The disadvantages include the requirement for a bone graft, longer healing time due to the defect and potential problems with fixation stability.

Cuneiform – reversed wedge
This is used to correct angular deformities. The size of the wedge is calculated as for the closed wedge technique but is then halved. The wedge is removed with its base on the convex surface of the bone and is then reversed and inserted on the concave side of the bone. Although it is not difficult to plan this technique, it can be difficult to execute surgically. The wedge may not fit easily on the concave surface and can easily displace. The wedge has no blood supply and is incorporated more slowly into the healing osteotomy site.

Oblique
This simple technique allows correction of deformities in any of three planes (medial/lateral, cranial/caudal and rotational). The osteotomy is best supported by an external fixator. The most proximal and distal fixation pins can be inserted parallel to the respective joint surface and thereby act as markers for correction of the deformities. Bone contact may not be good at the osteotomy site, resulting in delayed healing, and thus a cancellous bone graft should be considered. The technique allows correction of all components of a deformity and some increase in bone length also, if necessary. The main disadvantage is an inherently less stable fixation because of less cortical bone contact. Exact pre-operative planning is difficult and most of the correction is done by direct 'eye-balling' by the surgeon.

Dome or crescentic
Theoretically this is a useful technique since the crescentic osteotomy acts as a ball and socket, and three-plane corrections of a deformity can be made (Sikes *et al.,* 1986; Stevens, 1988). The osteotomy line has to be accurately planned and is initially made with a series of drill holes; the osteotomy is then completed with a high speed air drill and fine burr or a small oscillating bone saw. Bone plates provide the most secure fixation. Unfortunately it is technically very difficult to achieve this osteotomy and it must be done carefully.

Step
A step osteotomy allows distraction and lengthening of a bone. An autogeneous cancellous bone graft is recommended. Lag screws can be used to secure the arms of the step but additional support in the form of a plate or external fixator is mandatory. The amount of bone length that can be created is limited and fissure fractures of the step are not uncommon.

Corticotomy/osteotomy and distraction osteogenesis
This concept has already been mentioned. Gradual distraction at the site of transection using a ring external fixator can result in significant lengthening of the bone and soft tissues. This treatment is the technique of choice for the correction of shortened bones but can also correct rotational and angular deformities.

Table 26.2: Osteotomies used in the treatment of malunions.

Aetiology

There are several hypotheses but no firm conclusions on the cause of these tumours. Proposed aetiological factors include :

· Metal implants (Bennett *et al.*, 1979; Gillespie *et al.*, 1988)
· Corrosion (Furst and Haro, 1969; Sinibaldi *et al.*, 1976; Black, 1981)
· Excessive tissue damage
· Altered cellular activity.

Fracture-associated sarcomas may result from a two-stage carcinogenic event. The first stage may be mutagenesis of the cell by binding of metal to DNA, and the actual carcinogenic event may occur during multiple mitoses resulting from excess callus formation, excess bone formation and the response to infections or instability of the implant. There are certainly other examples of sarcoma formation occurring in bone which has pre-existing disease causing altered cellular activity, e.g. Paget's disease in humans (McKenna *et al.*, 1966), nutritional hyperparathyroidism in cats (Riser *et al.*, 1968) and infarcts of bone in humans and dogs (Riser *et al.*, 1972; Mirra *et al.*, 1974).

Diagnosis

The history of a previous fracture and its treatment is very important. Typically these tumours are associated with lameness or a gradually increasing mass which is noted by the owner. The lameness may be of acute or gradual onset. Pain is an obvious feature on palpation of the bone. Occasionally there is involvement of the musculature leading to impaired muscle function and flexion with contracture. The latter may result in reduced joint motion. Loss of bodily condition may also be present.

The radiographic appearance may be mistaken for chronic infection and, as already mentioned, infection may be present as a complicating factor although there are rarely clinical signs of chronic infection such as sinus tracts. The radiographic features include extensive new bone formation, smooth borders, soft tissue mineralization, areas of bone resorption (cortical loss) and occasionally pathological fracture lines. Loosening of implants, if present, may be seen. The histological examination of a biopsy specimen can be unrewarding because of the absence of classic anaplastic cells. Thus, the most helpful parameters are the combination of history, clinical examination and radiographic appearance. Repeat radiographs at an interval of 2 to 3 weeks can help to consolidate the diagnosis.

Treatment

The treatment of these fracture-associated tumours in the dog has all the same problems as that for the spontaneous osteosarcoma. The fracture-associated tumours have the same tendency to metastasize as the spontaneous ones and with a similar time scale. Amputation can be considered and chemotherapy with cisplatin (alone, or in combination with doxorubicin) can improve survival after amputation. Because of their diaphyseal nature, limb-sparing procedures are theoretically possible but most of these tumours are large when diagnosed, with a significant soft tissue involvement, which makes limited salvage procedures technically very difficult.

Prevention

The overall incidence of fracture-associated sarcoma is very low and does not justify the routine removal of implants after fracture repair. However, in cases of complicated fracture repair, such as non-union (and even delayed union) and certainly with osteomyelitis, removal of the implant is justified and recommended.

Table 26.3: Fracture-associated sarcoma.

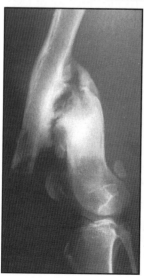

Figure 26.17: Lateral radiograph showing a malunion fracture of the femur. Although complete radiographic union had not occurred, clinical union was present and the fracture was stable. Lameness was evident but limb use was surprisingly good. Craniocaudal angulation of the femur is less of a problem than medial/ lateral angulation. Limb shortening has occurred in this case because of the overriding at the fracture site. Although this is a non-functional malunion, surgical correction was not attempted.

secondary to a non-corrected malunion. Malunited articular fractures, if causing minimal clinical problems, are sometimes better managed by arthrodesis at a later time if and when the clinical problem becomes unacceptable.

FRACTURE-ASSOCIATED SARCOMAS

Fracture-associated sarcomas occur at or close to an old healed fracture site. The fracture usually occurred five or more years previously (Stevenson, 1991). Several examples have been reported in the literature (Sinibaldi *et al.*, 1976; Madewell *et al.*, 1977; Bennett *et al.*, 1979; Van Bree *et al.*, 1980; Stevenson *et al.*, 1982; Stevenson, 1991) but the incidence of these tumours is very rare (Table 26.3).

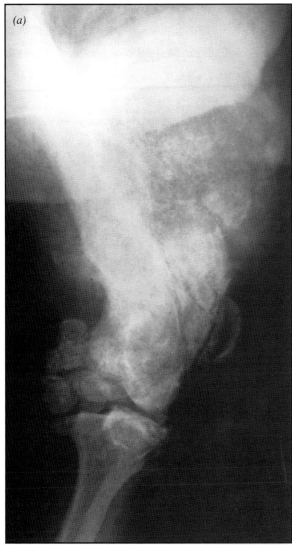

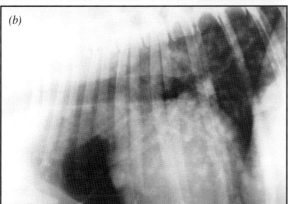

Figure 26.18: (a) Lateral radiograph of the femur showing extensive mineralized densities within the soft tissues and considerable periosteal reaction along the diaphysis. There is also loss of bone cortex and there are areas of radiolucency within the femoral shaft. This dog originally had a fracture of the femur; the fracture was plated, osteomyelitis occurred and a non-union resulted. The osteomyelitis was treated and the fracture was re-plated. Healing occurred and limb use was good, but lameness returned 5 years later, when the fracture-associated sarcoma was diagnosed. (b) The lateral thoracic radiograph of this case shows secondary tumour deposits in the lungs. Euthanasia of this patient was recommended.

Most of these sarcomas occur in the diaphysis of long bones, particularly the femur. Over 85% of fracture-associated sarcomas occur in the diaphysis of long bones (Figure 26.18a) and not the metaphysis, as with spontaneously occurring osteosarcomas. The bone most frequently involved is the femur (49%), followed by the humerus (24%), tibia (22%) and the radius (5%) (Stevenson, 1991). Occasionally sarcomas develop within 6 to 9 months of internal fixation of a metaphyseal fracture: these are probably manifestations of a pre-existing spontaneous osteosarcoma; and in some cases the original fracture may have been a pathological fracture since the tumour, even though not apparent radiographically, may have weakened the bone.

Metal implants, if present, are usually loose and bacterial contamination of the tumour is often a feature. All subtypes of osteosarcoma have been noted and metastases to lungs (Figure 26.18b), visceral organs and other bones have been reported. The original fracture usually occurs between the ages of 1 and 3 years and the lag period until tumour diagnosis averages approximately 6 years. They are most often encountered in larger breeds of dog and are also seen in the cat. Fracture-associated sarcomas are most likely to be seen where fracture complications have occurred, especially infection and non-union.

REFERENCES

Anson LW (1991) Malunions. *Veterinary Clinics of North America. Small Animal Practice* **21**, 761–780

Aro HT and Chao EYS (1993) Bone healing patterns affected by loading, fracture fragment stability, fracture type and fracture site compression. *Clinical Orthopaedics* **293**, 8–17

Bassett CAL, Mitchell SN and Gaston SR (1982) Pulsing electromagnetic field treatment in ununited fractures and failed arthrodeses. *Journal of the American Medical Association* **247**, 623–628

Bennett D, Campbell JR and Brown P (1979) Osteosarcoma associated with healed fractures. *Journal of Small Animal Practice* **20**, 13–18

Black J (1981) Chemical and foreign-body carcinogenesis. *Biochemical Performance of Materials* **1**, 128–147

Brown A and Bennett D (1989) The use of gentamicin-impregnated methly-methacrylate beads for the treatment of bacterial infective arthritis. *Veterinary Record* **123**, 625–626

Fang J, Zhu Y-Ym, Simley E *et al.* (1996) Stimulation of new bone formation by direct transfer of osteogenic plasmid genes. *Proceedings of the National Academy of Sciences, USA* **93**, 5753–5758

Frost HM (1989) The biology of fracture healing. An overview for clinicians. Part II. *Clinical Orthopaedics* **248**, 294–309

Furst A and Haro RT (1969) A survey of metal carcinogenesis. *Progress in Experimental Tumor Research* **12**, 102–133

Gillespie WI, Frampton CMA, Henderson RI *et al.* (1988) The incidence of cancer following total hip replacement. *Journal of Bone and Joint Surgery* **70**, 539–542

Hierholzer G and Hax PM (1985) Indications for corrective surgery after malunited fractures. In: *Corrective Osteotomies of the Lower Extremity After Trauma*, ed. G. Hierholzer and H. Muller, pp. 9–28. Springer-Verlag, Berlin

Ilizarov GA (1989) The tension–stress effect on the genesis and growth of tissues. *Clinical Orthopaedics* **238**, 249

Iwasaki M, Haruhiko N, Nakata K *et al.* (1995) Chondrogenic differentiation of periosteum-derived cells by transforming growth factor-β and basic fibroblast growth factor. *Journal of Bone Joint Surgery* **77-A**, 543–554

Kenwright J and Goodship AE (1989) Controlled mechanical stimulation in the treatment of tibial fractures. *Clinical Orthopaedics* **241**, 36–47

Kenwright J, Richardson JB, Cunningham JL *et al.* (1991) Axial movement and tibial fractures: a controlled randomised trial of treatment. *Journal of Bone Joint Surgery* **73-B**, 654–659

Kershaw CJ, Cunningham JL and Kenwright J (1993) Tibial external fixation, weight bearing and fracture movement. *Clinical Orthopaedics* **293**, 28–36

Kirker-Head C (1995) Recombinant bone morphogenetic proteins: novel substances for enhancing bone healing. *Veterinary Surgery* **24**, 408–419

McKenna RJ, Schwinn CP and Soong KY (1966) Sarcomata of the osteogenic series (osteosarcoma, fibrosarcoma, chondrosarcoma, parosteal osteogenic sarcoma and sarcomata arising in abnormal bone). *Journal of Bone and Joint Surgery.* **48A**, 1–26

Madewell BR, Pool RR and Leighton RL (1977) Osteogenic sarcoma at the site of a chronic nonunion fracture and internal fixation device in a dog. *Journal of the American Veterinary Medical Association* **171**, 187–189

Mirra JM, Bullough PG and Marcove RE (1974) Malignant fibrous histiocytoma and osteosarcoma in association with bone infarcts. *Journal of Bone and Joint Surgery.* **56A**, 932–940

Noordeen MHH, Lavy CBD, Shergill NS *et al.* (1995) Cyclical micromovement and fracture healing. *Journal of Bone and Joint Surgery* **77-B**, 645–648

Nunamaker DM, Rhinelander FW and Heppenstall RB (1985) Delayed union, nonunion and malunion. In: *Textbook of Small Animal Orthopaedics*, ed. CD Newton and DM Nunamaker, Lippincott, Philadelphia

Olmstead ML (1991) Complications, an overview. *Veterinary Clinics of North America, Small Animal Practice* **21**, 641–646

Reuter A and Brutscher R (1988) Die Behandlung ausgedehnter Knochendefekte am unterschenkel durch die Verschiebeostomie nach Ilizarov. *Chirurg.* **59**, 357

Riser WH, Brodey RS and Biery DN (1972). Bone infarctions associated with malignant bone tumors in dogs. *Journal of the American Veterinary Medical Association.* **16**, 411–421

Riser WH, Brodey RS and Sherer JF (1968) Osteodystrophy in mature cats, a nutritional disease. *Journal of the American Veterinary Radiological Society.* **9**, 37–45

Sharrard WJW, Sutcliffe ML, Robson MJ and MacEachern AG (1982) The treatment of fibrous non-union of fractures by pulsing electromagnetic stimulation. *Journal of Bone and Joint Surgery* **64-B**, 189–193

Sikes RI, Olds RB, Renegan W *et al.* (1986). Dome osteotomy for the correction of lone bone malunions: case reports and discussion of surgical technique. *Journal of the American Animal Hospital Association.* **22**, 221–226

Sinibaldi K, Rosen H and Liu SK (1976) Tumors associated with metallic implants in animals. *Clinical Orthopaedics* **118**, 257–266

Stevens PM (1988) Principles of osteotomy. In: *Operative Orthopaedics*, ed. MW Chapman, pp. 515–527, Lippincott, Philadelphia

Stevenson S (1991) Fracture-associated sarcomas. *Veterinary Clinics of North America. Small Animal Practice* **21**, 859–872

Stevenson S, Hohn RB, Pohler OEM *et al.* (1982) Fracture associated sarcoma in the dog. *Journal of the American Veterinary Medicine Association* **180**, 1189–1196

Sumner DR, Turner TM, Purchio AF *et al.* (1995) Enhancement of bone ingrowth by transforming growth factor-beta. *Journal of Bone and Joint Surgery* **77-A**, 1135–1147

Sumner-Smith G (1990) Osteomyelitis. In: *Canine Orthopaedics*, 2nd edn, ed. WG Whittick, pp. 571–581. Lea and Febiger, Philadelphia

Sumner-Smith G (1991) Delayed unions and non-unions. *Veterinary Clinics of North America. Small Animal Practice* **21**, 745–760

Szentimrey D, Fowler D, Johnston G and Wilkinson A (1995) Transplantation of the canine distal ulna as a free vascularised bone graft. *Veterinary Surgery* **24**, 215–225

Van Bree H, Verschooten F and Hoorens J (1980) Internal fixation of a fractured humerus in a dog and late osteosarcoma development. *Veterinary Record* **107**, 501–502

Weber BG and Cech O (1976) *Pseudoarthrosis*. Hans Huber, Bern/Stuttgart/Vienna

Index

For rapid location of specific surgical procedures, see **operative techniques**